Avoiding the Medicaid Trap

ALSO BY ARMOND D. BUDISH

Golden Opportunities:
Money-Saving Strategies from Government Programs
Everyone Over Fifty Should Know About,
with Amy Budish

Avoiding the Medicaid Trap

How to Beat the

Catastrophic Costs of

Nursing-Home Care

COMPLETELY REVISED AND UPDATED THIRD EDITION

Armond D. Budish

HENRY HOLT AND COMPANY   NEW YORK

Henry Holt and Company, Inc.
Publishers since 1866
115 West 18th Street
New York, New York 10011

Henry Holt® is a registered
trademark of Henry Holt and Company, Inc.

Published in Canada by Fitzhenry & Whiteside Ltd.,
195 Allstate Parkway, Markham, Ontario L3R 4T8.

Library of Congress Cataloging-in-Publication Data
Budish, Armond D.
    Avoiding the Medicaid trap: how to beat the catastrophic costs of
nursing-home care / Armond D. Budish—Rev. and updated 3rd ed.
p. cm.
Includes index.
1. Nursing homes—Economic aspects—United States. 2. Finance,
Personal—United States. I. Title.
RA997.B795 1995
338.4′336216′0973—dc20   94-42813
                                                      CIP

ISBN 0-8050-3426-9

First Edition—1989

Printed in the United States of America
All first editions are printed on acid-free paper.

10 9 8 7 6 5 4 3 2 1

The Durable General Power of Attorney form on page 147 is reprinted
with permission from the June 1, 1987, issue of *Family Circle* magazine.
Copyright © 1987 The Family Circle, Inc.

Publisher's Note: This publication is designed to provide accurate and authoritative information
in regard to the subject matter covered. It is sold with the understanding that the publisher and author
are not engaged in rendering legal, accounting, or other professional services. If legal advice or other
professional assistance is required, the services of a competent professional should be sought.

Contents

Acknowledgments

This new edition of *Avoiding the Medicaid Trap* would not have been possible without the help, support, and understanding of a lot of people.

First, I again would like to thank my wife Amy, who should actually be listed as a coauthor, given the number of hours she spent working on the manuscript. Amy is my partner, my inspiration, and my number-one editor.

My good friends Michael Hodes and David Pessin provided a great deal of advice and guidance to illuminate the complexities of the new Medicaid laws. I would like to give a very special thanks to their colleague Bill Gatesman, who spent many hours updating the state-by-state tables and assisting with a variety of other writing and editing challenges.

Henry Holt and Company has been my partner in presenting critical information to older people and their families for more than six years. I would like to express my sincere thanks to the family of Donald Hutter, who initiated our relationship and served as the inspiration behind this book; I miss him. After Don's passing, Bill Strachan, Alison Juram, and Greg Hamlin stepped in to make this book as successful as it has been. I hope our partnership in consumer protection will continue for years to come.

Long-term care insurance is a difficult subject to understand and explain, and no one is better than my friend Zachary Sochacky. Thanks to Zach for his great help in the preparation of the insurance chapter.

In the book are frequent references to a report prepared by Edward Neuschler for the National Governors' Association. That report contains a wealth of information, and I appreciate Mr. Neuschler's and the National Governors' Association's permission to provide portions of it to you.

Thanks also to Laurie Steiner, an attorney in my office, who helped prepare many of the forms, my law partner Michael Solomon, who allowed me the time to prepare this edition (without too much complaining), and Pam Guenther, Geri Nowak, Debbie Stacho, and Maria Stacho, who made sure the book was completed on time.

Thanks to Esther Peterson, Edith Furst, and my agent Barbara Lowenstein, whose guidance helped shape the proper approach; and David Guralnik, who encouraged me to pursue this effort.

I can't omit Arthur Hettich. Arthur had the wisdom to give me my first "big break" by accepting my articles for *Family Circle* magazine. I would also like to thank Ellen Stoianoff and Susan Ungaro, my editors at *Family Circle*, Annette Winter, my editor at *Modern Maturity*, and my editors at the Cleveland *Plain Dealer*, who have all recognized the importance of providing reader-friendly legal information.

I must thank the late congressman Claude Pepper and his staff for their enthusiastic support when this project was just getting off the ground.

Finally, thanks to my kids Ryan and Daniel, who hopefully won't have to worry about me in my old age, and to my parents, for whom I wish a long and healthy life—I love you all.

Prologue: The Most Dangerous Book in the Country

Avoiding the Medicaid Trap is the book "they" don't want you to have—the book that has been described by Medicaid officials as the most dangerous book in the country. Why? Because this book reveals how middle-class Americans and their families can hang on to a portion of their life savings when faced with long-term nursing-home care. Sounds pretty subversive, right?

Who doesn't want you to read this? First and foremost it is your elected officials, who would prefer to sweep issues of long-term care under the rug, who pretend that annual nursing-home charges of $50,000 to $90,000 are not a problem, and who by their inaction allow millions of older Americans to lose their life savings. It is the Medicaid Department bureaucrats in each state, who want to look good to their bosses (those busy elected officials who prefer reelection to legislative action) by keeping departmental expenditures low, even if it means refusing to help older Americans through the Medicaid maze. Finally, it is unscrupulous nursing-home insurance salespeople, who have tried to eliminate government assistance in order to coerce middle-class Americans into purchasing their unaffordable products.

Six years ago the first edition of *Avoiding the Medicaid Trap* was published. It was the first book to explain step-by-step how middle-class Americans could protect their homes and at least a portion of their other assets from the ravages of expensive nursing-home care by using the only program that provides any assistance in covering typical nursing-home charges: Medicaid. But as you will see in the following chapters, qualification for these benefits is difficult—you must first spend most or all of your savings. And changes mandated by the Omnibus Budget Reconciliation Act of 1993 (OBRA 1993) have made qualification tougher than ever, even threatening to take people's most precious possessions—their homes. So is all lost? Should you just give up and hand over your bank account? No!

By purchasing household items, prepaying funeral expenses, gifting assets to children, creating specialized trusts, and a host of other techniques, you can shelter at least a portion of your savings by accessing Medicaid. *Avoiding the Medicaid Trap* blew the shroud of secrecy off the Medicaid program, revealing invaluable asset protection strategies. As a result, millions of older Americans and their families learned how to preserve a measure of financial stability in the face of ever-rising health care costs.

I appreciate the kind notes of thanks so many readers have sent to me. Since their words are the most powerful endorsement, I'd like to share a few with you.

John Kerr kindly said, "I appreciate your concern regarding the ongoing problems of the elderly and especially those who are institutionalized." Alfred Pflaum thanked me for "championing causes of the elderly," noting that "our elected officials are much too busy feathering their own nests while neglecting and ignoring the needs of the middle class citizens who have elected them." And Helen Lukacs wrote, "I want to thank you for the help and information you are giving the older generation; it's more than the big guys are doing." Conrad Doedderlein: "Medicaid took everything my mother had, we got nothing. I want to make sure my children don't go through the same thing. Thank you." Dora Kwaczalo: "I want to thank you for all the good instruction I have received by reading . . . *Avoiding the Medicaid Trap*. The more I read it the more I educate myself."

Six years ago, when I originally wrote *Avoiding the Medicaid Trap*, I had two goals in mind. First, I wanted to provide middle-class individuals and families with the tools under the Medicaid program to help protect a fair portion of their savings. Second, I hoped that the result of this book would be to push the federal and state governments to change the rules, to develop a health care strategy with heart—and to make my book obsolete. Why should people have to give up all of their money, property, pride, and dignity to obtain basic health care, coverage that is provided in every Western country but ours? My hope, perhaps naive, was that our elected officials, who had been too timid to directly address the problem of long-term care on a comprehensive and fair basis, would be forced to do so as more and more citizens strained the limits of our existing system by making themselves eligible for Medicaid.

Unfortunately, our elected officials still haven't gotten the message. Their solution to the health care crisis was heartless: toughen the Medicaid rules to make it harder than ever to qualify for benefits. They even decided to try to prevent me from telling the truth about long-term care and Medicaid.

In my own state of Ohio, an executive task force appointed by the governor recommended that any attorney, financial planner, or other professional bold enough to advise the public about how they could *legally* plan to obtain Medicaid benefits would be criminally prosecuted and have their licenses yanked. Called the "Budish bill," this proposal was obviously directed squarely at me. I suppose I should have been flattered, but instead I was sickened by the widespread influence of self-serving legislators this initiative so clearly illustrated. The task force did not come up with this idea on its own. A national long-term care insurance lobbying organization that would like nothing better than to silence me (and force unsuspecting Americans into inappropriate insurance policies that they really can't afford) sent its number-one hit man to Ohio to push the Budish bill. Thankfully, enough angry voices were raised to make legislators reconsider, and the Budish bill met the timely death it deserved.

When the Ohio legislature proposed to take away protection for people's homes under Medicaid, I criticized the legislation in my syndicated newspaper column and warned people to contact their state legislators. Thousands of older Americans did just that, flooding their representatives with calls and letters about the harm that would be caused by tightening the Medicaid rules and taking people's homes.

The following is just a sampling of the outrage reflected in people's letters to their elected officials. Walter and Ruth Griffith made this plea for fairness:

> *Please do not* take away our home and any savings we may have. . . . We have always supported ourselves and our children, paid all taxes, bought our home, educated children, etc., with hard-earned money.
>
> My husband has been retired now for 8 years and I am nearly 62 years and unemployed.
>
> I also have a mother nearing 92 years of age, living in her own home. What does she have to look forward to? What do we have to look forward to?
>
> I might add my parents, as well as my husband's, went through the Depression, by the "skin of their teeth" *without* receiving any government assistance of any kind. . . .
>
> I realize people cannot expect a free ride. [B]ut there again, please take into consideration the fact that most people have been independent all their lives and have contributed to the economy. Please represent us *fairly* and *do not* take away our homes and every asset we may have.[1]

Here's what John and Jane Surdock had to say:

> Our home took 51 years of work to have it and it should be ours till we die. Dear God, help us to stay out of a nursing home and in our house.[2]

Jim Baechle didn't mince any words:

> Highway robbery! Grand larceny! A slap in the face for every decent person. . . . Will the ongoing insensitive, corrupt and greedy behavior of our so-called representatives (and those they cater to) never end? How sick, how out of touch with reality are these maggots. . . .
>
> On a personal note, my father has been seriously ill for some time. Our family has no idea what the future holds. It's been tough on all of

us, especially my mother. Don't you think there's enough sadness and stress within a family such as ours without having to worry about simply existing in the event that long-term, nursing home care would be our only option?[3]

Mrs. R. J. McCarthy asks why she should save, if savings will just go to the nursing home:

> Should I bother to hold on to my condo? I came here to cut expenses, but when I think of the possibility of losing it to a bunch of bureaucrats, I wonder if maybe I should shelve my frugality, sell my condo, rent a place and start spending. Had hoped to maybe leave at least this place to the kids. . . .
>   This is a pretty sad commentary, but many of my friends share it with me. We all pray for a sudden, *fatal* heart attack.[4]

People who work with elderly patients are particularly aware of the problems they face. Isabel Kennedy described these problems well:

> I am a home health aide and work for the elderly in their own homes. I see their needs and sometimes poverty conditions. I help them stay in their homes as long as they can but I know someday these people will need a nursing home, as I will also. It would be cruel to cut the funds for these dear people because they are too old to care for themselves.[5]

How did elected officials respond to an onslaught of heart-rending letters like these? One would think that in the face of an avalanche of opposition by common citizens, they surely would see the light and back down. But instead of compassion, they responded with passionate letters to the editors of Ohio newspapers, condemning me and my attempts to inform the public of the terrible, unfair burden their legislation would cause.

These attacks on me have not just been in Ohio. During the federal congressional hearings on OBRA 1993, which resulted in the loss of the last vestiges of protection for the homes of older and ill Americans, my work again came under attack.

In the November 30, 1992, issue of *Newsweek*, my work on behalf of older Americans was featured in an article entitled "Planning to Be Poor." The subtitle read, "With a Little Help, the Nursing Home Won't Get Your Savings—Your Kids Will." Written by Melinda Beck with Mary Hager in Washington and Karen Springen and Todd Barrett in Chicago, the article explains in detail the devastating impact of long-term care costs: "If you end up in a nursing home, your savings may be wiped out faster than you can get an attendant to answer your call button." The authors recognized that the people most at risk are "simply middle-class Americans desperate to survive." In fact, the article goes so far as to offer a legislative solution: "If the federal government had a program, like Medicare, that paid for nursing-home care for everyone, then families wouldn't have to spend their savings—or compete with the poor for scarce funds." What was the response to this well-reasoned presentation? The silence from Washington was deafening. Syndicated talk show host Rush Limbaugh consequently used his national platform to condemn me and other elder advocates.

There is some good news. Over the last six years, change has occurred. In the absence of public policy initiatives that would address the core of the problem, the public is at least becoming more attuned to the need to plan for financial security using the Medicaid program. People are coming to understand the overwhelming financial devastation that can occur, without adequate planning, when a loved one must enter a nursing home.

However, what I find unconscionable is that the government has not taken steps to help citizens. In fact, the only attention to the crisis has been focused on finding ways for Uncle Sam to preserve his assets. OBRA 1993 made it much harder for middle-class Americans to qualify for Medicaid. Several of the most wicked changes are:

- Lengthening the ineligibility period following the giving of gifts from thirty months to thirty-six months for most people, and much longer for those who don't understand the rules.
- Jeopardizing the use of one of the most beneficial tools, the standard Medicaid trust.
- Requiring states to grab the homes of Medicaid recipients as repayment for money Uncle Sam spent on nursing-home care. This is the most devastating action, threatening the most cherished possession of older Americans.

Although the president and Congress have talked

about providing basic comprehensive care for everyone, their concept of basic care does *not* include coverage of the most costly health care of all—long-term nursing-home care. Isn't it ironic that our government can find enough money to give congressmen *huge* pensions and superlative health benefits while there doesn't seem to be enough to provide basic benefits for the long-term care needs of older citizens. As long as this is our government's health reform policy, older Americans will continue to be forced to make painful choices for themselves. Those who choose to retain the right to age with dignity will ignore Uncle Sam's pleas to play the game blindly by his rules and undertake health care planning using the critical tools described in this book.

Perhaps someday soon Americans will have a stroke of good luck and Uncle Sam will have to place *his* mother in a nursing home. When that day arrives, perhaps we will see a coherent, caring health care policy that has been shaped by the legitimate needs of our citizens rather than by the self-serving interests of health industry lobbyists and campaign fund–hungry legislators. Let us hope . . .

Avoiding the Medicaid Trap

Introduction

The toughest decision you may ever have to face is to place your parent or spouse into a nursing home. No one ever wants to take that step. But there may come a time when there's just no choice—a loved one has had a stroke, develops Alzheimer's disease, or is stricken with some other severely debilitating condition and requires full-time care and attention, which you just can't provide.

If you find yourself in this situation, you would not be alone. More than a million times a year, Americans find that their options have run out and their only alternative is to obtain nursing-home care.

The decision to institutionalize a parent or spouse raises many tough questions. Are you being selfish and breaking your sacred marriage vow of commitment to a partner in sickness and in health? Are you abandoning your parent when he or she needs you most? Will it be the "kiss of death" to be moved from a familiar home environment to an impersonal facility? Will your parent or spouse receive adequate medical care? Will the staff treat him or her with kindness and respect? Although many nursing homes offer excellent services, we've all heard horror stories.

While issues like these create extreme emotional trauma, that trauma often pales in comparison with the financial shock of receiving the bill for long-term nursing care. The late Claude M. Pepper, a U.S. congressman from Florida and once a leading advocate for senior citizens' rights, recognized that "the single greatest fear of our senior citizens, and of all Americans, [is] that a long-term catastrophic illness may strike and, because of the absence of public or private coverage, they will become destitute."[1]

With nursing-home bills of $3,000 to $5,000 a month ($36,000 to $60,000 a year) or more, that fear is well-founded. More than a million Americans every year become victims of health care cost impoverishment, having been forced to give up their homes and their savings to pay the bills for long-term care.

The trauma faced by millions of older Americans and their families is succinctly summarized by Eleanor Csontos:

> Have you ever had to put your mother or father in a nursing home? I did, our mother. My brother and I cried for a couple of weeks, the trauma of going and seeing her there. Yes—she had savings and a house. The nursing home got it all in 23 months. . . . This . . . is *totally unfair*.[2]

Jack Ossofsky, past president of the National Council on Aging, describes exactly the kind of devastating impact a long-term illness can have within just a few weeks or months of entry into a nursing home:

> For an older couple of average income, a diagnosis of Alzheimer's disease spells the impoverishment of the well partner within 4 months, as the couple is forced to spend down to meet medicaid assets and income requirements for nursing home care. . . . [W]e are forcing Americans to impoverish themselves to get minimal coverage for the needs they face.[3]

1

The people who are being harmed are middle-class Americans who acted responsibly, who did their best. Even that wasn't good enough. Here's a sad story passed on to me by Alfred Pflaum about his ninety-two-year-old mother:

> This widow of forty years worked till she was seventy, at minimum wage I assure you, and was able to acquire the massive fortune through scrimping and saving of $21,000, and oh how proud she was of that achievement. She never asked for or wanted charity, never asked her son for help, and as she put it—"I will persevere." Her first nine months in a nursing home wiped out that lifetime of hard work.[4]

Listen to the story of Grace Still:

> In 1982, [my mother] was diagnosed with Alzheimer's disease. Although Dad was disabled himself, he wanted to take care of Mom. He did for several years. . . . Mom was a strain for him to handle even with an aide to help him. Every time we could provide the care ourselves in our home we did. But both my sister and I are single parents working full-time jobs.
>
> It broke our hearts but Mom became too much for all of us to handle, and we had to place her in a nursing home. The tragedy of Mom's stay in the nursing home is the cost. Most of their life savings, almost $30,000, is gone now. . . .
>
> My Dad worked hard as a machine operator for thirty years. He always took good care of Mom, my sister and me, and provided us with a good living. . . . It is heartbreaking for him to see her receiving welfare because his life savings have been wiped out, and his own health is failing. . . .
>
> It is a disgrace to our great nation that our elderly must be absolutely destitute or dying before they can receive help.[5]

After placing his wife of forty-nine years in a nursing home, Nathan Mendelsohn was faced with a similar crisis.

> Rose had a stroke in 1982. . . . For months, I cared for her myself, keeping the house, dressing and bathing her, and then carrying her downstairs for the day. But I am 77 years old and I am not as strong as I used to be. Caring for Rose at home in our two-story house got to be too much of a strain for me. . . .
>
> Medicare coverage and all other insurance coverage stopped. I began paying $2300 a month for the nursing home. In six months' time, I spent $20,700 for her nursing home care.
>
> Besides paying for the nursing home, I had to pay my rent, and had to pay for food, gas and electricity each month. . . .
>
> I have little left from the money that we gained from the sale of our home. I am 77 years old. If something should happen to me, I don't know what I would do. I do not want to be a burden to my family.[6]

Health care professionals witness the financial devastation wrought by the system, and many are deeply troubled by it. Linda O'Donnell, a registered nurse working with Alzheimer's patients, describes the tragic case of the Smiths:

> Mr. and Mrs. Smith are both 75 years old. They have been married for the past 46 years. Mr. Smith worked as an auto worker since graduating from high school. He frequently worked overtime in order to pay off his home and save for the future. . . . Mr. Smith managed to save $50,000 upon his retirement at the age of sixty-five. . . . The money Mr. Smith acquired was to be used to travel and enjoy their well-deserved retirement and also offer their children an opportunity "to get ahead."
>
> But tragedy struck. Mrs. Smith was diagnosed with Alzheimer's disease one year after Mr. Smith retired. For a short time Mr. Smith was able to care for his wife at home with the help of his children. . . .
>
> After three short years of this, they exhausted approximately $17,000. Then Mr. Smith was forced to place Mrs. Smith into a nursing home, and because of their assets she was considered private pay, with a cost of $3,000 per month. Mrs. Smith still lives at the nursing home 7 years later, as a Medicaid recipient. . . .
>
> Unfortunately, their dreams of vacations in Florida . . . are only dreams. The children remain lower middle income with little hope of a break. . . . Mr. Smith's trips are only as far as the nursing home to visit his wife.[7]

[W]ith the blink of an eye, long term care places many middle income families into poverty.

Nursing-home patients and their families are often stripped of everything—their homes, their savings, their dreams for a future. Spouses of nursing-home patients may be left destitute and even forced onto the welfare rolls. When that happens, what incentive is left for nursing-home patients, whether married or unmarried, to try to get better and return home—to homes they no longer own and daily living expenses they can no longer afford? This is a cruel joke.

The prospects of losing an entire life's savings drives some older Americans to think the unthinkable, as revealed by the following letters:

Eleanor Melzak:

> I am a seventy-four year old widow who made a few astute investments—investments to see me through my golden years—and now if I need nursing home care, these investments will be taken from my children.
>
> I still work, and if I feel myself getting closer to a nursing home, I'll take my life![8]

Linda Ellis:

> The suicide rate in the ill elderly will most assuredly rise. They will have little options left—death or bankruptcy—a wife or husband "left behind" in a home that could possibly be lost to pay nursing home costs. Not a bright prospect for anyone, would you say?[9]

H. E. Gallagher stated:

> Perhaps the only solution . . . is to have everyone over seventy years of age commit suicide. There is a bit of that as it is.[10]

These notes are written not by "crazy people" but by ordinary citizens who have been pushed to the edge by an uncaring system.

One of the few members of Congress who understands the problems facing the elderly is Congressman Robert A. Borski of Pennsylvania, who asks, "Why should our citizens bankrupt themselves, become dependent on the state and be robbed of their dignity and self-esteem because they suffer from 'uncovered' or chronic illnesses?" Why indeed! Borski goes on: "What is most disheartening is that . . . the financial devastation is unnecessary."[11]

In fact, the financial devastation *is* unnecessary. You don't have to sit by idly waiting while a financial nightmare becomes reality. The tips in this book can save you and your family *thousands of dollars*. By planning ahead, or assisting your parents or spouse to plan ahead, you can help maintain a loved one's dignity and preserve family savings from being completely consumed by nursing-home costs.

Successful planning means having to address facts that we usually don't feel comfortable discussing—illness, incompetency, death. If you have older parents, they, like most of us, probably want to believe that by not talking about such depressing issues, they'll always be independent. Nobody likes to think he or she will be struck down by a catastrophic illness or injury that requires long-term care. And when you consider that of all persons entering nursing homes, over 80 percent are not married at the time, you can see why children had better sit up and listen too, because they are likely to be the ones who must assist a parent with preparing a suitable Medicaid plan and making the complex arrangements for a nursing-home admission.

If planning can be so helpful, why don't we hear more about ways that older Americans can protect their assets? Why doesn't the government *promote* planning?

The answer is simple: it would cost Uncle Sam a lot of money. And government officials are unwilling or unable to confront head-on the issues of long-term care, to come up with a rational program providing basic care for middle-class Americans.

In fact, government bureaucrats will even go out of their way to prevent you from finding out how to protect yourself and your family. In a lengthy letter to the editor of the Cleveland *Plain Dealer*, Paul Offner, then Medicaid director for the state of Ohio, responded to an article I had written promoting Medicaid planning, stating:

> Unfortunately, there are numerous lawyers like Budish running around, and there are more people following his advice. The result, eventually, will be that legislatures will have to find some way to penalize this willful divestiture of assets to become Medicaid-eligible. I hope your readers will turn their backs on those who would turn us all into an army of cynics playing

the loopholes and seeking the unethical short-cuts in life.

Offner went on to say that Medicaid planning is "reprehensible" and that those who partake in it are "selfish."

If trying to help your parents or spouse avoid losing their life savings is selfish, so be it. But it's certainly not reprehensible. What *is* reprehensible is that so many politicians and Medicaid bureaucrats have shut their eyes to this colossal problem and are allowing families to be devastated by nursing-home costs.

Not every governmental official believes that it is wrong to try to help one's parents or spouse protect their life savings. The late Congressman Claude Pepper, former chairman of the Subcommittee on Health and Long-Term Care, Select Committee on Aging, expressed his "enthusiastic support" for this book and its goal of helping older Americans protect their savings and avoid impoverishment.

> The advice in this book is crucial to older Americans, to help them protect their savings and avoid impoverishment. I am enthusiastic in supporting this publication which presents important information not to my knowledge found anywhere else.

Unfortunately, there was only one Claude Pepper—and no one has stepped in to even try to fill his shoes. Few politicians are willing to stand up for older Americans.

Is it immoral, as Medicaid bureaucrats and politicians suggest, to consider ways to avoid poverty? Absolutely not! Do you believe *they* are lying awake at night worrying about how you are going to pay the bills?

Let's debunk two myths right now. First, while Medicaid is critical for the financial security of middle-class Americans, wealthy Americans are not cashing in on Medicaid. As a result of this book, my other writings, my frequent television and radio appearances, and my legal practice, I speak daily with older Americans and their families; I can vouch for the fact that it is *not* the wealthy who are transferring assets or taking other steps to get Medicaid benefits. Raymond J. Hanley and Joshua M. Weiner, a senior research analyst and a senior fellow at Brookings Institution in Washington, D.C., confirm my view in a syndicated newspaper article published in 1992, call-

ing asset transfers by older people "a non-problem."[12] It doesn't even make sense for rich people to give away their wealth or put it into specialized trusts to qualify for Medicaid—they'd lose more in estate and capital gains taxes than they would gain in Medicaid benefits.

Second, few if any people are out to save every penny and to place the entire burden of nursing-home care onto the government. Most people recognize their ethical obligation to pay a fair share; but people, quite properly, do not feel it is right to have to spend every last penny on catastrophic nursing-home charges. Retirees Walter and Ruth Griffith exemplified this sentiment when they wrote to their governor:

> We realize people on Medicaid cannot expect a free ride. But then again . . . [the law should not] take away our homes and every asset we may have.[13]

Charles Morelli expresses the same view:

> I am a retired high school administrator. My wife and I live comfortably on my pension, but we live within our income. We, too, have some savings. However, [with a catastrophic illness] we could be devastated in a short time.
>
> This does not mean we don't want to carry our load. However, . . . if something should happen to one of us that requires long-term health care, please, leave the other one with some dignity and the ability to survive.[14]

Most middle-class Americans pay large amounts of their income into the "system" over the years, to support the vast array of government programs, with little expectation of any direct return. Then, the one time these individuals do ask for some support, when facing financial devastation due to a serious illness, they are criticized for being "selfish" and "immoral."

Sue Hildebrand says it better than I ever could:

> The middle class receives the shaft from everywhere, whether it's bearing the brunt of paying income tax or our inability to obtain financial aid for our college students. . . . Denying Medicaid benefits to elderly people who have worked hard and contributed to others all their adult lives is a pitiful way to balance a budget.[15]

Mrs. Mildred Stith says:

> As a law abiding citizen, taxpayer and senior citizen who expects fair treatment (no handouts), I think it's reprehensible that those of us who have given the most in our productive years, and continue to give, now are faced with the possibility of the most being taken away from us.[16]

And Shirley Hazle raises the right questions when she asks,

> Some bureaucrats think it is ethical for our senior citizens to pay for entitlement programs throughout their lifetime in taxation and to pay more for their nursing home care to help with the cost of caring for Medicaid beneficiaries, but then these same bureaucrats think it is unethical for these citizens to transfer any assets to benefit their own heirs. Is this just?[17]

The answer to Shirley's question should be clear: it is not just to force older Americans into poverty, and it is not immoral to try to protect a portion of one's life savings.

Isn't it far more immoral that our government forces its citizens into poverty to obtain nursing-home coverage? The goal of sound public policy should be to prevent this sort of financial devastation. As stated by noted attorneys Michael Gilfix and Peter J. Strauss in their article "New Age Estate Planning: The Emergence of Elder Law," "Reasonable asset preservation has been at the top of the national legislative agenda for years; it is not the creature of a creative, scurrilous lawyer trying to find that illicit edge for his or her client."[18]

In fact, for years Americans have been allowed to take advantage of tax protections and deductions to preserve their assets from taxes—with our politicians' blessings. What is the ethical difference between Americans using tax deductions to protect assets from Uncle Sam and the middle class using gifts or trusts to protect some assets from a nursing home? Why criticize the elderly? As Gilfix and Strauss so aptly state:

> Planning to preserve a portion of one's estate when facing long-term care is conceptually tantamount to arranging one's personal finances to take maximum advantage of tax protections and

deductions. In both circumstances the attorney advises the client about opportunities presented by law and regulations to minimize the loss of assets. Tax planning and tax advice are and have been "mainstream" for decades. Asset preservation planning in the face of long-term care is not yet mainstream, but is rapidly emerging.[19]

So it's not Medicaid planning that's immoral, it's our government policies. These policies force our elderly to leave everything—money, property, pride, and dignity—at the door of the nursing home as they enter.

Other Western countries have adopted far more humane systems than what we have in the United States. For example, the Canadian government guarantees its citizens long-term nursing-home care without requiring residents to impoverish themselves and their families.

"Today the United States of America and South Africa are the only industrial nations in the world that don't have a comprehensive health care program for the people. Is that the kind of company this great America wants to be in with respect to this particularly critical matter?"[20]

The American Association of Retired Persons (AARP), the leading voice for the interests of older Americans, has recognized the critical role of the Medicaid program for middle-class Americans, at least until comprehensive coverage is otherwise provided. As AARP stated in its testimony to Congress on OBRA 1993,

> AARP is concerned about proposed efforts to further "tighten" rules governing estate planning and the transfer of assets in the absence of a comprehensive long-term care program which addresses the needs of people of all ages and incomes. Without such a program, middle income families would continue to be vulnerable because they would not readily qualify for Medicaid; could not afford to pay for care out-of-pocket; could not afford meaningful private insurance protection; and would not have the resources necessary to prepare for their financial future. Thus, in the absence of a comprehensive social insurance program, average Americans needing long-term care would continue to face the likelihood of having their life savings wiped out.

A variety of proposals to fund long-term care for middle-income Americans have been introduced. Many senior citizen advocate groups have urged funding by taxes—maybe "sin taxes" on alcohol and tobacco—to spread the burden of cost from families with members in nursing homes to the general population. Others have suggested developing a system in which private insurance would cover the first year or two and the government would then step in to pay nursing-home expenses after that. Yet others have suggested funding basic care through the terrible "T" word—raising income taxes. Another feasible option would be the creation of a Medicare Part C to provide basic coverage of long-term care, at home, in the community, and in nursing homes, by charging a premium similar to the funding mechanism of Medicare Part B.

We will all be better off when our government officials address the real issue of making affordable, quality health care available to all Americans. The Federal Affairs Health Team of the AARP, in response to the passage of OBRA 1993, stated, "The Association continues to believe that the solution to the budget deficit is not deep cuts in Medicare and Medicaid. The record of the last decade clearly shows that real, long-term deficit reduction will require confronting the critical condition of our health care system through comprehensive health care reform."[21] Until that day arrives, the Medicaid program will be the primary government program available to help older Americans and their families meet long-term care costs.

Older Americans need to plan ahead. Esther Peterson, a consumer movement pioneer and longtime advocate for the elderly, who herself is in her eighties, hits the nail on the head:

We've done very poor planning. When you get up into your older years, you don't want to be a burden. You want to be independent and want to protect whatever resources you have. We have been so slow in waking up to this.[22]

One of my clients, Emma Kmet, admitted the same thing, saying, "I feel I should have started this [planning] sooner, to be aware of what's all available. It makes you feel more secure as to what you can do."

It's easy to delay, to put off thinking about catastrophic illness. But delays can be costly. As stated by another of my clients, Joseph Weinberg, "procrastination is the thief of time." In this case, procrastination will prove to be the thief of your pocketbook as well.

It's time to wake up and start planning. Perhaps someday we will see the adoption of a humane government policy on nursing-home financing, and then every older American will be able to get whatever care is best for him or her without being financially, as well as emotionally, devastated. But until then, the financial burden rests with the family.

The tips in this book are intended primarily to benefit middle-income Americans. As Senator John Heinz of Pennsylvania once stated, "The greatest threat to the financial security of middle-income Americans is the cost of long-term medical care."[23] Those persons with very little income and assets probably are adequately protected by existing laws; the Medicaid rules were designed specifically to help the poor. The wealthy can and should pay their fair share. But if you are one of the great majority of Americans falling in between, this book can save you and your family thousands of dollars.

1 | What, Me Worry About Nursing-Home Costs?

If you think a nursing home is not in your future, take a look at these horrifying statistics: Persons aged sixty-five to sixty-nine years face almost a one-in-two risk of entering a nursing home.[1] In a report entitled "The Risk of Nursing-Home Use," doctors Christopher Murtaugh, Peter Kemper, and Brenda Spillman determined that seven in ten couples turning sixty-five can expect that at least one of the two will require nursing-home care. And if you and your spouse are lucky enough to have four living parents, there is a 90 percent chance that at least one of them will wind up in a nursing home.[2] As you can see, you don't need a crystal ball to predict what's in store for many of us.

Surprised by such a high risk? You shouldn't be. As Esther Peterson points out, there are many paths that lead to the door of a nursing home:

> Most people think of catastrophic illness as a massive heart attack, a bone-crushing auto accident, or cancer. But the biggest catastrophe of all may well be the crippling, chronic conditions—such as senility, Alzheimer's disease, severe arthritis, osteoporosis, or the long-term effects of a stroke.[3]

Don't expect the health care picture to get any brighter, because America is rapidly graying—our older population is the fastest-growing segment in the country. Right now well over thirty million Americans are sixty-five and older, and seven million require long-term care. Government statistics show the number of people over age eighty—those most in need of long-term care—to be over six million now and doubling by the year 2010. There are now 2.5 million elderly in nursing homes. In thirty years, double that number will wind up institutionalized. Within the next fifty years, more than one in five citizens, about sixty million strong, will be elderly, and more than nineteen million of them will need long-term care.[4]

A poll conducted for the AARP and the Villers Foundation determined that long-term care and its costs already touch many of us. Sixty percent of respondents in the poll had some personal experience, through family or friends, with long-term care. More than half of the respondents expected that within the next five years, someone in their own families would require long-term care.

Former congresswoman Mary Rose Oakar of Ohio highlighted these issues in congressional hearings:

> All of us can recite at least one incidence when a loved one or close friend has needed extended assistance at no fault of their own. Perhaps it is one of our parents, perhaps one of our children or a neighbor. It is normally a situation of great misfortune where the health of the individual is suddenly swept away to expose the fact that our lives are precarious and in need of constant care. How many of us now have a parent or a close friend facing not only the frustrations of poor health but also financial ruin due to an extended illness or injury? Almost everyone can relate at least one occurrence of such a

tragedy. This is not the problem of an isolated few.[5]

Of course, this probably comes as no great surprise. In all likelihood, you too know someone whose life has been traumatized by the financial strains brought on by illness and long-term care.

The High Costs of Nursing-Home Care

The costs of nursing-home care are soaring and are already far beyond the means of most of us. The average cost of nursing-home care is about $3,000 a month, or $36,000 a year. And that's if you're lucky. In many metropolitan areas, like New York City, nursing-homes charge as much as $50,000 to $85,000 annually. And even if nursing homes around you are charging "only" $36,000 a year, don't breathe a sigh of relief yet; the costs go up each year at a pace far outstripping inflation.

The average nursing-home stay is more than two years; many elderly citizens will spend far more time there. Consider Alzheimer's disease, which has struck more than 7 percent of the nation's elderly over age sixty-five. Although victims must often be placed in a nursing home, Alzheimer's disease does not necessarily reduce a person's life expectancy. A patient with Alzheimer's lives an average of eight years after the symptoms first appear, with much of that time often spent in a nursing home.

Long-term illnesses like Alzheimer's disease are emotionally devastating for the victim's family. With care costs of at least $3,000 a month, these illnesses can also be financially devastating.

How Nursing-Home Costs Devastate a Family

Here's how it all adds up:

High nursing-home costs + Lengthy stays = Disaster for your family

Anyone who has had a family member or friend enter a nursing home knows only too well the accuracy of this formula. California congressman Edward R. Roybal, chairman of the House Select Committee on Aging, put this formula into words:

Millions of elderly and non-elderly Americans are at great personal financial risk of being impoverished by high and sustained long term care costs. With over 200 million Americans underinsured against long term care costs . . . *a host of personal catastrophes are in the making.*[6]

How long will your family be able to hold out? How long will it take to dissipate the nest egg your parents or spouse worked so hard to build during their lifetimes? The sad answer is: not long.

By using table 1.1, you can estimate how long your (as an older person) or your parent's financial resources would last. For example, if your mother is living alone, has an income of between $6,000 and $10,000, and has average assets for that income range, the nursing home would get everything after she spent just thirty-two weeks in the facility. If she were fortunate enough to recover so that she could leave the nursing home and return to the community after that time, she would be facing life on the welfare rolls! The figures in table 1.1 explain why elderly Americans and their families fear not only the health impact of a long-term illness but also the financial devastation that often follows.

If facts and figures leave you cold, let a few people tell you, in their own words, about what it means when a catastrophic health problem necessitates full-time care. For instance, Mrs. Bellamy:

I'm writing to tell you about my husband. My son had to put him in a nursing home today. He has had two strokes. I've waited on him, and me sick. See I live by a pacemaker and can hardly walk because of arthritis. The doctors said I could no longer care for him because I couldn't lift him or give a bath or give him IV's. So he had to go to a nursing home.

We are both 74 years old and I feel God has been good to us both. He worked until he was 70 years and paid into Social Security ever since 1937. He sure wasn't lazy.

Now, all of our life savings are gone. Henry and I together got $831 in Social Security. Today the nursing home will take [most of his income] . . . which sure will be rough going, even with the sickness I have.[7]

TABLE 1.1

Average Number of Weeks to Poverty for Unmarried Older Americans in Nursing Homes

AVERAGE ASSETS AND ANNUAL INCOME	AVERAGE NUMBER OF WEEKS TO POVERTY	
	If Age 65	*If Age 75*
$4,860–6,075	8	9
$6,075–9,720	32	36
$9,720–15,000	97	110

SOURCE: Adapted from "Long Term Care and Personal Impoverishment: Seven in Ten Elderly Living Alone Are at Risk," a report presented by the Chairman of the House Select Committee on Aging, One Hundredth Congress, First Session, Comm. Pub. No. 100-631 (October 1987), p. 15.

TABLE 1.2

Risk of Impoverishment for Unmarried Americans in Nursing Homes

NUMBER OF WEEKS IN NURSING HOME	PERCENTAGE OF SINGLE ELDERLY WHO BECOME IMPOVERISHED	
	Based on Income and Assets	*Based on Income Alone*
13	48%	69%
26	58	84
39	63	91
52	67	94

SOURCE: Adapted from "Long Term Care and Personal Impoverishment: Seven in Ten Elderly Living Alone Are at Risk," a report presented by the Chairman of the House Select Committee on Aging, One Hundredth Congress, First Session, Comm. Pub. No. 100-631 (October 1987), p. 9.

And Samuel L. Baily:

> My mother died of Huntington's Disease [a hereditary terminal brain disorder that results in the gradual loss of control over both the body and the mind]. . . . I am at risk for HD and I have a wife and three children whom I love and for whom I wish to provide as best I can. We are not wealthy, but we do have some savings and a house. I believe I should pay my fair share, but I do not believe I should be forced to strip my family of these assets if I should get HD. My options at present are to divorce my wife or to commit suicide, neither of which I intend to do.[8]

These are not unique cases. The ruination brought upon the elderly and their families by unbearable nursing-home costs is widespread, touching virtually every American in all walks of life.

The late representative Claude Pepper, in a hearing before his House Select Committee on Aging, Subcommittee on Health and Long-Term Care, recognized that these stories "could be matched in every city in America and in every part of this nation. People have suffered similarly to these people. . . . Every one of them lost their homes. Every one of them lost their savings. And every one of them suffered terribly in America."

The House Select Committee on Aging produced a report entitled "Long Term Care and Personal Impoverishment: Seven in Ten Elderly Living Alone Are at Risk."[9] The findings of that report were astounding: after about thirteen weeks in a nursing home, nearly one-half of the elderly living alone had used up their financial resources; within one year of entering a nursing home, two-thirds of older Americans living alone had lost everything (see table 1.2). (While tables 1.1 and 1.2 address unmarried individuals, the financial impact of one spouse's nursing-home stay on a married couple's resources is almost as damaging.)

As Tables 1.1 and 1.2 clearly demonstrate, it's just a matter of time—and not much time at that—until a loved one is forced into poverty after entering a nursing home. The way to change that picture is to plan ahead and follow the steps described in the next chapters.

2 | Who Pays the Bill?

Perhaps you never worried about nursing-home costs because you always assumed that someone else—maybe Medicare, maybe private insurance—would pick up the tab. Surprise! You and your family had better start to worry, because chances are that no person, no government program, and no insurance coverage will step in and help you shoulder the financial burden of a nursing-home stay.

As Congressman Borski recognized,

> If you have the misfortune of getting a long-term catastrophic illness in the United States of America, no one will help you. Not the United States Government and Medicare, not Medigap insurance policies and no one until you have exhausted all of your financial resources, until they ask you to become virtually penniless, until you lose your home, until you lose all of your money, and unfortunately until you lose all of your pride.[1]

Nursing homes are a big business. When a loved one enters a nursing home, someone has to pay the bill. But who that someone will be is often misunderstood. People often expect that one or more of the following resources will take care of the payments:

- Medicare
- Private insurance
- Veterans Administration benefits
- Medicaid
- Personal assets and savings

Relying solely on the last option can be ruinous. It doesn't take a trained mathematician to figure out what will happen to your savings if you have to foot the entire bill.

The reality is that only one of these sources—Medicaid—is of much help, leaving most older Americans at risk of losing everything to a nursing home.

Medicare

Medicare is widely available, covering more than thirty million Americans. It is federal health insurance for all persons over age sixty-five who are entitled to monthly Social Security or railroad retirement benefits. Even persons under sixty-five are eligible if they have received Social Security disability benefits for two years. Medicare offers protection for sick people, and since people who enter nursing homes tend to be very sick, then one would think that Medicare must cover these long-term care costs.

Let's explode a dangerous myth right now: *neither Medicare nor private insurance will pay for nursing-home costs*. It can't be said any more clearly. Do not count on Medicare to pay for a nursing home.

Of all those persons receiving Medicare benefits, only one-tenth of 1 percent of them are covered for nursing-home care. Yet people assume otherwise: an AARP survey indicates that 80 percent of Medicare beneficiaries believed that they were adequately protected from the high costs of long-term care by

Medicare and their private policies.[2] In fact, Medicare pays less than 2 percent of the nation's long-term nursing care bill. Why does Medicare pay so little? Because Medicare coverage is extremely limited. It provides coverage of home health and skilled nursing care in only a very few situations—typically when a person is suffering an acute illness and needs rehabilitation or therapy to recover. There is no Medicare coverage for custodial care.

At most, Medicare will pay for the first twenty days of nursing-home costs and up to eighty additional days after you pay $89.50 a day (these are 1995 figures). Any stay longer than one hundred days and your family is on its own. Since statistics show that an older person is likely to remain in a nursing home for an average of two years, Medicare is not going to solve the cost problem.

It's tough to qualify for even this limited one hundred–day coverage. Medicare will pay nursing-home costs only when:

- The care a person receives is "medically necessary," which means skilled care, not intermediate or custodial care.
- The nursing-home care is preceded by three days in a hospital, and the illness or condition treated in the hospital is the same for which the person will be treated at the nursing home.
- The nursing home is a Medicare-approved skilled nursing facility with a registered nurse available seven days a week, twenty-four hours a day.
- The patient is assigned to a bed that is Medicare-certified for reimbursement.
- As a practical matter, only a nursing home can provide the level of skilled care required.

These conditions are rarely satisfied. "Skilled care" generally includes medical or therapeutic services that can be performed only by or under the supervision of nurses, physical therapists, or other medically trained professionals. For example, if a doctor or nurse observes a patient's condition, develops a plan of treatment or care, prescribes medications, inserts a catheter, administers injections, applies surgical dressings, treats skin problems, or provides physical or speech therapy, the care should qualify as skilled.

Skilled care is very different from custodial care, which is much more typically required for long periods. "Custodial care" includes the services that help people dress, bathe, eat, take medication, and carry on other normal living activities. Individuals with no special medical training can do the job. If a loved one is stricken with Alzheimer's disease, Parkinson's disease, senility, or a stroke, he or she may need custodial care, not skilled care, for a long time. Medicare will not cover these costs.

Besides entering a nursing home to obtain needed skilled services, other options are available that address the diverse long-term care needs of older people, options that may or may not be covered by Medicare. They include:

- *Home health care.* Just as the name implies, this type of health care is provided in the client's home. Services can range from skilled nursing care, speech, and physical and occupational therapy to homemaker or companion services. Even minor home repairs and yard work may be included.

  Medicare provides extremely limited coverage, and only when: the need is certified by a doctor; the care includes part-time or full-time skilled nursing care, physical therapy, or speech therapy; the patient is homebound; and the agency providing the home care is Medicare-certified. Otherwise your parent or spouse is on his or her own.

- *Hospice care.* Created to address the special needs of the terminally ill, hospice care is designed to ease patient suffering, not to cure or rehabilitate. Services can be provided at home or in a hospice facility. Either way the costs are high, but Medicare will pay a substantial portion.

- *Adult day care.* Through adult day care, non-medical care is offered to people at home, or at a center when just companionship or minimal assistance is needed during the day. Costs generally are not covered by Medicare or Medicaid.

- *Respite care.* With respite care, very short term health or custodial care is provided at home or in a nursing home in order to give family members who normally care for the individual a rest. The patient will probably have to pay most or all of these costs.

- *Meals on Wheels.* This service provides hot meals at a client's home. Although costs are not covered by Medicare or Medicaid, fees for these services are sometimes met under other federal or state governmental programs.

What's the bottom line? Forget Medicare as your one-stop answer to payment for long-term care needs. If you (or a loved one) can qualify for Medicare at all, and chances of that are slim, at most you will get some help toward your bills for one hundred days. If you initially qualify for Medicare by meeting all of the requirements, don't assume that you're on easy street; if the level of care you require becomes downgraded to custodial services, you will lose your Medicare coverage—even if the hundred-day period hasn't yet expired. On average Medicare covers less than two weeks of a person's nursing-home stay. After one hundred days you will be on your own no matter what.

Private Insurance

Private insurance is even less helpful than Medicare, covering only about 1 percent of all nursing-home costs. Again, many older Americans have been sadly misled into believing that their so-called Medigap, Medifil, MedSupp, or MediCal supplemental insurance policies will pay for any necessary long-term care. Here is a typical story, by Jack J. Lomas:

My aunt . . . is confined to a nursing home, stripped of all her worldly earnings. . . .

My aunt worked from the time she was fourteen, for over fifty years, in a textile mill, toiling long hours for very little money. In the process, she lost her hearing and her health. She has cataracts, colitis and a chronic heart condition, in addition to arthritis in her legs and spine and other chronic health problems. The country she worked so hard to support in her youth and vigor has turned its back on her during her time of need.

She purchased Blue Cross–65 Special and a supplemental insurance policy from AARP to pick up what Medicare did not pay. She thought she was well taken care of. But when she went into the nursing home, her life savings, almost $13,000, were eaten up in just six months. Medicare, Blue Cross–65 Special and AARP will not cover the expenses because the care she needs is called custodial. Because she suffers from chronic illness, none of the insurers will pay for her medical care to keep her comfortable.[3]

Congressman Borski stated at a congressional hearing:

Older Americans unknowingly pay exorbitant prices for policies which do not provide relief from the high medical costs associated with chronic illnesses. . . . Clearly, the private insurers are not picking up the tab for extended nursing care.[4]

The late Congressman Pepper shared that view:

Senior citizens buy hope in the form of one or more insurance policies, not realizing that there is no public or private insurance policy, or combination of such policies, that will protect them when a catastrophic illness strikes and provide them with the comprehensive coverage they desperately want.[5]

Many folks *believe* they are protected, yet very few people in the entire country actually have policies that cover long-term nursing-home care.

Is it sheer coincidence that so many of our nation's elderly have mistakenly concluded that their supplemental private Medigap insurance policies cover long-term care? Stanley J. Brody, professor of health care systems at the Wharton School of the University of Pennsylvania and director of the Research and Training Center for Rehabilitation of Elderly Disabled Individuals, thinks not: "Media marketing methods by private insurers . . . lull elderly consumers into believing they are covered for long-term care." In other words, many in the Medigap insurance industry have intentionally set out to deceive older Americans in order to make a buck.

In fact, many insurers haven't been satisfied to sell one policy to a misinformed consumer; some have been known to use scare tactics and high-pressure techniques to sell several overlapping policies to a single person.

As Esther Peterson warns, "High-power salesmen have talked people into thinking they need things. I talked to one woman who had seven policies. Only one of them was worth anything." One woman from Arkansas was duped into buying twenty-eight Medigap policies, none of which paid her a single penny toward her nursing-home charges.

Gail Shearer, manager in charge of policy analysis for Consumers Union (publisher of the magazine *Consumer Reports*), also had few kind words for private long-term insurance providers. Acording to Shearer, private policies are marketed to the elderly "often through deceptive marketing techniques," and as a result of confusion, "older Americans waste $3 billion annually on private health insurance."[6]

The good news is that states and the insurance industry itself have been tightening up on these unfair marketing ploys. And the standardization of Medicare supplement insurance policies mandated by the federal government has put the brakes on the overenthusiasm of salespeople. Consumers can easily comparison shop to verify what a policy actually includes, and salespeople will be penalized for any misrepresentations.

Today about one hundred private insurers offer long-term care coverage. These insurance policies, which are not the same as Medicare supplement policies, have evolved quite a bit in the last six years, and they continue to change and improve on a daily basis. Many policies now offer extremely useful protection. While pitfalls still exist, a wise consumer can select a policy that will provide financial security and peace of mind. Now for the bad news: the policies are very expensive, with premiums far exceeding the budgets of most older Americans.

The pros and cons of long-term care insurance are discussed in chapter 16. Suffice it to say for now that private insurance probably isn't the answer, certainly not the complete answer, when people must face the nursing-home cost dilemma.

Veterans Administration Benefits

If an older person is a veteran, he or she may be entitled to limited nursing-home coverage. VA benefits are available only if (1) the patient was in a VA hospital and is being discharged directly into a nursing home, or (2) the patient's need for a nursing home stems from a service-connected disability, which is defined as an injury or disease incurred or aggravated in the line of duty.

Even if you or a loved one should qualify, Uncle Sam generally won't give you VA benefits for any

more than six months unless you are suffering from a service-related disability.

Medicaid

Medicaid *will* cover long-term care in a nursing home; in fact, about 40 percent of our nation's nursing-home costs are paid by Uncle Sam and the states through the Medicaid program. Medicaid has become the largest payer—by far—for long-term care.

But there's a trap, and it's a huge one. To qualify for Medicaid, a person must either be poor or become poor. A typical example of what happens when you are unlucky enough to fall into the Medicaid trap was poignantly described by one adult child during testimony before a congressional committee:

> Pop had to be put in a nursing home at a cost to my mother of about $2,400 per month, and neither Medicare nor Medicaid could help because my parents had a nest egg. The law is without pity. Had my father lived for just 2 more years in a nursing home, my mother would have had to spend the rest of her life in poverty, but God called Pop to his eternal rest in 1 year, rather than 2. My mother and I can never forget the terrible feeling of relief we had when Pop died. We can only live with it in shame. We loved him.[7]

Medicaid bureaucrats like to say that lower- and middle-income Americans must "spend down" their resources before Medicaid coverage begins. That's a nice euphemism—"spend down." In plain English it means that a person must turn over his or her life savings to the nursing home before Medicaid will pay a cent.

The House Select Committee on Aging accurately describes the picture:

> Medicaid coverage comes with a heavy price for persons needing long term care as well as their spouses. . . . [T]he bottom line is that elderly persons must essentially impoverish themselves, and probably their spouses, before they are protected by Medicaid.[8]

Put simply, if your parents are not poor before one of them enters a nursing home, with nursing-home costs as high as they are, they will be before long. According to the U.S. Department of Health and Human Services, about one-half of the people receiving Medicaid coverage for nursing-home costs had too much money or property to qualify when they first entered but became impoverished, and so qualified for Medicaid, after entering the home.

How many people are losing their life savings because they were unlucky and became ill enough to require nursing-home care? The figures represent a terrible human tragedy and national embarrassment. Upward of one million people each and every year qualify for Medicaid assistance by first exhausting their own resources.

Yes, Medicaid will help pay nursing-home costs, but often the price is personal degradation and financial ruin.

Personal Assets and Savings

If you (or your parents) do pay for the nursing home, you will pay until the money runs out. About one-half of all long-term care is paid by elderly Americans and their families. A spouse has a legal obligation to pay medical costs—including nursing-home bills—for an ill spouse unless he or she qualifies for Medicaid. Children and their family members do *not* have any legal obligation to pay.

Most older citizens have annual incomes of less than $13,000. When you compare this figure with average annual nursing-home costs of $36,000, you can see that older Americans have a real problem.

If a person starts early in life, can he or she save enough to avoid impoverishment? That would be the ideal solution. Unfortunately, it's not very realistic. Let's say that starting at age forty, your father put $1,000 each year into an interest-bearing account. Sound good to you? Well, it's not good enough. Twenty-five years later, he wouldn't have saved enough to pay for even one year in a nursing home!

As you can see, a family's life savings is at serious risk when a loved one enters a nursing home. Uncle Sam and insurance carriers have not created an equitable and affordable safety net to protect the average American. This means that you will have to develop your own plan of action, unless you don't mind playing the dangerous game of nursing-home Russian roulette.

3 | How Much Can an Older Person Keep from the Nursing Home?

For most older people, the general rule is very simple: just about everything you have (your income and life savings) must go to the nursing home to pay expenses. Only when your assets run out will Medicaid step in. As shown in the preceding chapter, the practical application of this rule is a formula for financial ruin for older Americans and their families.

The Medicaid eligibility rules have always been difficult for people to meet. But in August 1993, Congress passed OBRA 1993, which made the rules even tougher.

Why were these changes made? Our elected officials were frustrated because desperate middle-class Americans were working within the rules of the system to obtain Medicaid benefits for nursing-home expenses without first going completely broke. The financial impact of OBRA 1993 on middle-class Americans is devastating. Now it is more essential than ever for older Americans and their families to understand the new Medicaid rules so that they can take the legally correct steps to protect a portion of their life savings.

This book will not burden you with all of the details of the Medicaid qualification rules as they now stand. But it is important to understand some of them, in order to formulate your protection plan.

To qualify for Medicaid, a person entering a nursing home must:

1. Be at least sixty-five, blind, or disabled (as defined by the state).
2. Establish residency in the state which would provide Medicaid benefits.

3. Need the type of care provided in a nursing home (most states have preadmission screening programs).
4. Meet the income limitation test.
5. Meet the assets limitation test.

When a person meets these criteria, Medicaid generally will cover long-term nursing-home care.

The first requirements are pretty straightforward—to obtain Medicaid, a person must be sixty-five, blind, or disabled. Most people would not consider a nursing home until their disability was so great that they had no other option. Residency generally poses no problem either. A person is considered a resident in a state in which he or she intends to stay indefinitely. States cannot establish residency waiting periods—a person can move from one state to another, move right into a nursing home, and immediately obtain Medicaid benefits.

In the third condition above, the "type of care" requirement should not pose a problem. People generally don't go into nursing homes by choice; they enter because they need the care and have no other choice. The last two requirements, the Medicaid income and assets limitation tests, are tricky; they are described below. Since different rules apply to married and nonmarried people (widows, widowers, divorced, or never married), we'll look at each group separately.

Nonmarried Individuals

INCOME LIMITATION TEST

Eligibility Standards

For purposes of the Medicaid eligibility rules, "income" is defined broadly. Both earned income (cash or in-kind payments for work) and unearned income generally are included. Social Security, pensions, worker's compensation, unemployment, alimony, rents, interest, dividends, annuities, gifts, and even regular contributions of food and shelter are all considered unearned income. Only a few types of things you receive are not counted as income for Medicaid purposes; these include medical insurance reimbursements, food stamps, insurance proceeds, loan proceeds, and reparation payments to Holocaust survivors.

In most states and in the District of Columbia, there is no limit on the amount of income you may have in order to qualify for Medicaid. In these states, listed in table 3.1, you meet the eligibility standards whether your income is $20 a month or $2,000 a month. Most of your income goes to pay the nursing home and the remaining charges are covered by Medicaid. Income eligibility is easy in these states.

If you don't live in one of these no-income-limit states, you may face unbearable hardships. In the income cap states listed in table 3.2, you can meet the eligibility standards only if your income is below the limits set by law.

Let's say you live in Florida, which sets a monthly income limit of $1,374. As long as your income is below that figure, you pass the income test. If your income is $1,000 a month, most of that would be paid to the nursing home and Medicaid would pay the rest of the bill.

But if your monthly income is $1,375, just a dollar over the limit, you'd be in big trouble. Your income exceeds the cap, so you can't get Medicaid. Sadly, this leaves some people with too much income for Medicaid but not enough to pay the nursing home.

Example 1

Your mother has spent all of her savings on medical costs. She gets $700 a month in Social Security and $800 a month in pension benefits. Unfortunately, the state says that no one with income of over $1,374 a month can get Medicaid.

Nursing homes in her area run $4,000 a month. She can't afford to pay the cost herself and you don't have the funds to make up the difference. What happens? She may have to get used to sleeping on a park bench, because the nursing home doesn't have to keep a nonpaying resident who can't qualify for Medicaid.

TABLE 3.1

States with No Limit on Income for Older Individuals Seeking Medicaid Coverage for Nursing-Home Costs

California	New Hampshire
Connecticut	New York
District of Columbia	North Carolina
Georgia	North Dakota
Hawaii	Ohio
Illinois	Oregon
Indiana	Pennsylvania
Kansas	Rhode Island
Kentucky	South Carolina
Maine	Tennessee
Maryland	Utah
Massachusetts	Vermont
Michigan	Virginia
Minnesota	Washington
Missouri	West Virginia
Montana	Wisconsin
Nebraska	

SOURCE: Edward Neuschler, *Medicaid Eligibility for the Elderly in Need of Long Term Care* (Washington, D.C.: National Governors' Association Center for Policy Research, 1987), updated for 1995 by Hodes, Ulman, Pessin and Katz, P.A., an elder law and estate planning firm in Towson, Md. (hereafter "National Governors' Association Report").

TABLE 3.2

States with a Monthly Income Limit of $1,374 or Less for Older Americans Seeking Medicaid Coverage for Nursing-Home Bills

Alabama	Louisiana
Alaska	Mississippi
Arizona	Nevada
Arkansas	New Jersey
Colorado	New Mexico
Delaware	Oklahoma
Florida	South Dakota
Idaho	Texas
Iowa	Wyoming

SOURCE: National Governors' Association Report.

The severe income limits set by the states listed in table 3.2 create terrible problems for older Americans. Thankfully, there are planning solutions to this dilemma—see chapter 14.

How Much Income Can an Older Person Keep?

Say your widowed or divorced mother is eligible under the income limitation test. In that event, almost all of her income must go to the nursing home. Only if her income (and assets) isn't enough to pay the whole bill will Medicaid step in.

Only a small amount of her income does not have to go to the nursing home. In particular, she will be able to protect:

- A monthly allowance ranging from $30 to $75, depending on the state, for personal, nonmedical needs, such as clothing, toiletries, books, and magazines. Don't spend it all in one place! The specific amounts allowed are listed in table 3.3.

- In most states, credit toward the nursing-home bill for any funds spent for health insurance premiums, including Medicare premiums, and other medical expenses not covered by Medicaid, such as glasses, dentures, hearing aids, and over-the-counter drugs. Federal law actually requires *all* states to provide this credit, but not all of them do.

- In just about half of the states, an allowance to help maintain a home in anticipation of returning within three to six months after entering a nursing home. As table 3.4 shows, in most states about $200 to $400 a month can be kept, with figures ranging from $75 to over $800 a month. Generally this home maintenance allowance is available only for unmarried individuals and only upon a physician's statement that the patient should be able to return to the home within six months; if the nursing-home stay exceeds six months, this allowance normally cuts off after that time.

Here's an example of how these rules work:

Example 2

Your mother lives in New York and enters Sunny Hills nursing home. The doctor assures her that she'll be able to return home within a few months. Her monthly income is $1,000. She may keep:

$ 50	personal-needs allowance (from table 3.3)	
65	medical insurance premium	
534	home maintenance allowance (from table 3.4)	
$649	total monthly allowance	

The nursing home would get the rest of her income, $351 a month.

To qualify for Medicaid, a person must pass the income limitation test. In no-income-limit states that generally means that one's income must be less than the nursing-home costs; in states that set an upper limit for income, a person's income must fall below the limit as well. Once you qualify, you will be able to keep only a small portion of your income (see the list on this page). The rest will go to pay the bills.

ASSETS LIMITATION TEST

As if it weren't bad enough that most of your income will go to a nursing home, the assets limitation test that also must be met is even worse. Under this test, almost all of your assets must be turned over to the nursing home before Medicaid will pay any nursing-home charges. If you're not poor going into the nursing home, it won't take long to get there.

For purposes of the Medicaid assets limitation test, assets include almost all money and property. Most states define assets as "cash or liquid assets or any real or personal property that an individual (or spouse, if any) owns and could convert to cash." Assets include cash, savings and checking accounts, CDs, stocks, bonds, mutual fund shares, promissory notes, cars, and real estate. Even assets that carry a penalty (for example, loss of interest, such as early liquidation of a CD, or payment of tax, such as withdrawal of an IRA) will be included as part of your assets. The bottom line when it comes to valuing your bottom line for the Medicaid assets limitation test is that just about any resource having a cash value will be defined as an asset and will count against you, pushing you toward (and often over) Medicaid's asset limitation ceiling.

NOTE: Many retirement plans give participants a one-time right, at retirement or upon reaching

TABLE 3.3

Personal-Needs Allowance Protected Out of Individual Income

STATE	AMOUNT	STATE	AMOUNT
Alabama	$30	Montana	$40
Alaska	75	Nebraska	40
Arizona	66.10	Nevada	35
Arkansas	30	New Hampshire	40
California	35	New Jersey	35
Colorado	34	New Mexico	30
Connecticut	40	New York	50
Delaware	36	North Carolina	30
District of Columbia	70	North Dakota	45
Florida	35	Ohio	30
Georgia	30	Oklahoma	30
Hawaii	30	Oregon	30
Idaho	30	Pennsylvania	30
Illinois	30	Rhode Island	40
Indiana	30	South Carolina	30
Iowa	30	South Dakota	30
Kansas	30	Tennessee	30
Kentucky	40	Texas	30
Louisiana	38	Utah	30
Maine	40	Vermont	40
Maryland	40	Virginia	30
Massachusetts	65	Washington	36.62
Michigan	30	West Virginia	30
Minnesota	45; varies	Wisconsin	40
Mississippi	44	Wyoming	30
Missouri	30		

SOURCE: National Governors' Association Report.

a fixed age, to elect to receive either a lump sum or a monthly annuity. When it comes to Medicaid planning, this decision could cost you money. Here's why: Prior to making this election, the funds in a pension would likely be counted by Medicaid as an available asset only if the funds can be obtained without having to leave the job. However, once a person elects taking a lump sum, watch out—the funds are no longer protected and will usually be considered an available asset that can be counted against Medicaid eligibility. On the other hand, a person who opts for monthly annuity payments (and who cannot change back to a lump sum payment) will not be considered as having assets available, although the monthly payments received will count as income. A few states have taken the position that once a person has begun taking regular monthly pay-

ments from an IRA or other retirement fund, the principal will not be considered an available asset, even if the Medicaid applicant or spouse could reach and obtain the principal.

Now, I don't want to overstate the case. An older person will be allowed to keep some of his or her assets, up to a maximum total value of about $2,000 (plus certain exempt assets, as described on pages 19–20), depending on his or her state of residence. What a comfort to know that for a lifetime of hard work and "doing without," your parent will get to keep a grand sum of about $2,000. Table 3.5 lists the amount of assets each state allows a single person to protect from a nursing home.

In addition to about $2,000, a few specific items, called exempt assets, are excluded from the maxi-

TABLE 3.4

States Providing a Home Maintenance Allowance

STATE	AMOUNT[a]	FLAT OR MAXIMUM[b] AMOUNT	MAXIMUM NUMBER OF MONTHS AVAILABLE
Alaska	$808	Flat	6
California	$192	Flat	6
Colorado	$208	Maximum	6
Connecticut	$460	Maximum	6
Delaware	$ 75	Flat	None
District of Columbia	$418	Maximum	None
Idaho	$212	Flat	6
Illinois	Varies	Maximum	3
Iowa	$446	Maximum	6
Maryland	$342	Flat	6
Massachusetts	Varies	Maximum	6
Montana	$425	Flat	6
New Hampshire	$243	Flat	3
New Jersey	$150	Maximum	6
New York	$534	Flat	6; subject to extension
North Carolina	$242	Flat	6
North Dakota	$369	Flat	6
Oregon	Varies	None	None
Pennsylvania	$478.40	Flat	6
Rhode Island	$558.33	Flat	6
South Carolina	$446	Flat	6
Utah	$361	Flat	6
Vermont	$376	Flat	6
Virginia	Varies	Flat	6
Washington	$180	Flat	6
West Virginia	$175	Flat	None
Wisconsin	Varies	None	6

[a] "Varies" indicates that a home maintenance allowance is provided but that the amounts vary according to a state formula.
[b] "Flat" indicates that the amount in column two is the home maintenance allowance in all cases; "maximum" indicates that the amount in column two is the most that will be permitted under a formula adopted by the state.

SOURCE: National Governors' Association Report.

mum asset allotments listed in table 3.5. These exempt assets are items you can keep "off the top," meaning that they are Medicaid-neutral and won't be counted against you when Uncle Sam is taking stock of your assets to determine whether you pass or fail his asset limitation test. Although these exempt assets vary from state to state, they most commonly include:

- A person's home. This is protected as long as a spouse or a dependent relative is living there. Even without an occupant the home may still be protected—most states will allow the house to remain protected as long as its owner *intends* to return there; in some states the house will remain protected for a limited time. Table 3.6 shows the rules adopted in each state for protecting a home.
- Household goods and other personal items, up to a total (equity) value of $2,000.
- One wedding ring and one engagement ring, regardless of value.
- One car (or other vehicle) with a current market value of up to $4,500. There is no limit on value if the car is necessary to get to work or to receive medical care, or if the car

TABLE 3.5

Amount of Assets a Person Can Protect from a Nursing Home

STATE	AMOUNT	STATE	AMOUNT
Alabama	$2,000	Montana	$2,000
Alaska	2,000	Nebraska	4,000
Arizona	2,000	Nevada	2,000
Arkansas	2,000	New Hampshire	2,500
California	2,000	New Jersey	2,000
Colorado	2,000	New Mexico	2,000
Connecticut	1,600	New York	3,200
Delaware	2,000	North Carolina	1,500[a]
District of Columbia	2,600	North Dakota	3,000
Florida	2,000	Ohio	1,500
Georgia	2,000	Oklahoma	2,000
Hawaii	2,000	Oregon	2,000
Idaho	2,000	Pennsylvania	2,400
Illinois	2,000	Rhode Island	4,000
Indiana	1,500	South Carolina	2,000
Iowa	2,000	South Dakota	2,000
Kansas	2,000	Tennessee	2,000
Kentucky	2,000	Texas	2,000
Louisiana	2,000	Utah	2,000
Maine	2,000	Vermont	2,000
Maryland	2,500	Virginia	2,000
Massachusetts	2,000	Washington	2,000
Michigan	2,000	West Virginia	2,000
Minnesota	3,000	Wisconsin	2,000
Mississippi	2,000	Wyoming	2,000
Missouri	999.99		

[a]Soon to be increased to $2,000.

SOURCE: National Governors' Association Report.

has been adapted for a handicapped person.
- All property used in an income-producing trade or business. This includes cash accounts of the business. For example, if your mother has a small business in her house making handwoven rugs, the looms are exempt, as is the computer she uses to keep her books.
- Up to $6,000 equity in nonbusiness property (personal and real estate) if essential to the person's support. To be considered necessary for support, the property should either produce income or produce goods or services necessary for one's daily activities (such as land to grow food for one's own use). Income-producing property should produce net annual income of at least 6 percent of the amount of protected equity (for example,

$360 or more income with equity of $6,000).
- Cash surrender value of all life insurance if the total face value of all life insurance on any one person doesn't exceed $1,500.
- Burial plots for the person and his or her immediate family.
- Up to $1,500 per person for burial costs if kept separate from other resources. Some states allow you to enter into an irrevocable contract and prepay your burial expenses. Often such burial contracts can exceed the $1,500 a person limit.

Most states have adopted the asset protection rules (other than for a home) described above. Table 3.7 lists the most significant variations adopted by the remaining states.

The assets limitation test can and usually does

TABLE 3.6

Rules for Protecting a Person's Home from a Nursing Home

STATE	YOU MUST INTEND TO RETURN[a]	A DOCTOR MUST CERTIFY LIKELIHOOD OF RETURNING	TIME LIMIT ON PROTECTION
Alabama	Yes; subject to lien[b]	No	No
Alaska	Yes	Yes	No
Arizona	Yes	Yes	6 mos.
Arkansas	Yes	No	No
California	Yes	No	No
Colorado	Yes	No	No
Connecticut	Yes; subject to lien[b]	Yes	9 mos.
Delaware	Yes	Yes	6 mos.
District of Columbia	Yes	Yes	6 mos.
Florida	Yes	No	No
Georgia	Yes	No	No
Hawaii	Yes	No	No
Idaho	Yes	Yes	6 mos.
Illinois	Yes; subject to lien[b]	Yes	No
Indiana	Yes	Yes	No
Iowa	Yes	No	No
Kansas	Yes	No	No
Kentucky[c]	No	No	No
Louisiana	Yes	No	No
Maine	Yes	No	No

(continued on next page)

have a devastating impact on nursing-home residents and their families. It requires individuals to spend virtually their entire life savings on nursing-home care before Medicaid helps. Planning is essential for those who believe there should be another option.

Married Individuals

The Medicaid laws are only a little more generous for married couples. Lawmakers threw a few crumbs to a nursing-home resident's spouse-at-home—but certainly not enough to make a meal out of—while the meat and potatoes still go to the nursing home.

INCOME LIMITATION TEST

Eligibility Standards

In general, the eligibility standards for someone who is married are the same as for an unmarried individual—if one's income is below the amounts set forth in tables 3.1 and 3.2, one should pass the income eligibility test.

But let's say your husband is entering a nursing home. How much of his and your total joint income will be considered his and how much will be considered yours? How is income to be divided between spouses?

Just about every state has answered these questions by assuming that, barring unusual circumstances, income belongs to the spouse whose name is on the check. (In a flash of bureaucratic brilliance, this policy was called the "name-on-the-check" rule.) Money paid to your husband from his pension or Social Security is considered to be his; income paid to you is considered to be yours—even if the two of you use the incomes jointly. Income designated for both of you is split evenly.

In community property states—Arizona, California, Idaho, Louisiana, Nevada, New Mexico, Texas, and Washington—the rule might be slightly different. You and your spouse may each be considered to own one-half of any income, regardless of whose name is on the check. A bright spot of compassion actually exists: states that apply community property

TABLE 3.6 *(continued)*

Rules for Protecting a Person's Home from a Nursing Home

STATE	YOU MUST INTEND TO RETURN[a]	A DOCTOR MUST CERTIFY LIKELIHOOD OF RETURNING	TIME LIMIT ON PROTECTION
Maryland	Yes; subject to lien[b]	No	No
Massachusetts	Yes	Yes	No
Michigan[c]	No	No	No
Minnesota	Yes	Yes	6 mos.
Mississippi	Yes	No	No
Missouri[c]	No	No	No
Montana	Yes	Yes	No
Nebraska	Yes	Yes	6 mos.
Nevada	Yes	No	No
New Hampshire	Yes	No	No
New Jersey	Yes	Yes	6 mos.
New Mexico	Yes	Yes	No
New York	Yes	No	No
North Carolina	Yes	Yes	6 mos.
North Dakota	Yes	Yes	6 mos.
Ohio[c]	No	No	6 mos.
Oklahoma	Yes	Yes	12 mos.
Oregon	Yes	Yes	6 mos.
Pennsylvania	Yes	No	No
Rhode Island	Yes; subject to lien[b]	No	No
South Carolina	Yes	No	No
South Dakota	Yes	Yes	No
Tennessee	Yes	No	No
Texas	Yes	No	No
Utah	Yes	No	No
Vermont	Yes	No	No
Virginia	Yes	Yes	6 mos.
Washington	Yes	No	No
West Virginia	Yes	No	No
Wisconsin	Yes	Preferable	No
Wyoming	Yes	No	No

NOTE: This table assumes that the nursing-home resident has no spouse or dependent relative at home. If he or she does, the house is protected when it comes to Medicaid eligibility.

[a]Intent is entirely subjective and does not have to be supported by medical evidence of ability to remain home. The statement by a nursing-home resident that he or she intends to return home must usually be made in writing.

[b]States have been permitted to adopt lien laws, allowing them to place liens on the homes of nursing-home residents receiving Medicaid. However, a lien may not be placed on a home if: the nursing-home resident's spouse or dependent children are living there, or if a sibling who has an ownership interest in the home has been living there for at least a year. A nursing-home resident can probably block the imposition of a lien just by stating in writing his or her intent to return home. To date only five states have adopted lien laws, but it is likely that many more states will soon follow suit.

[c]Kentucky, Michigan, Missouri, and Ohio protect the home without regard to a person's intent or ability to return.

SOURCE: National Governors' Association Report.

rules instead of the name-on-the-check rule generally will do so only when it benefits the spouse-at-home, and the name-on-the-check rule is applied when it works to the financial advantage of the spouse-at-home.

As with unmarried individuals, the income test for eligibility is usually easy to pass. As long as you don't live in an income cap state (see tables 3.1 and 3.2), you'll qualify for Medicaid if your income is less than what the nursing home charges. If you live in an in-

Assets Excluded from Medicaid Asset Eligibility Limits (Other than the Home)

STATE	HOUSEHOLD GOODS	RINGS[a]	CAR	INCOME-PRODUCING PROPERTY	LIFE INSURANCE	BURIAL PLOTS	BURIAL COSTS
Alabama	Excluded	1 set excluded	Excluded	Excluded up to $6,000 if property produces 6% return on excluded equity	Excluded if face value is below $2,500	Excluded	Excluded
Alaska	Excluded up to $2,000	1 set excluded	Excluded up to $4,500		Excluded if face value is below $1,500	Excluded	Excluded up to $1,500
Arizona	Excluded	Excluded	Excluded up to $4,500 for single person, unlimited for married couple	Excluded up to $6,000 if property produces 6% return on excluded equity	Excluded if face value is below $1,500	Excluded	Excluded up to $1,500
Arkansas	Excluded up to $2,000	1 set excluded	Excluded up to $4,500 if used for medical purposes	Excluded up to $6,000 if property produces 6% return on excluded equity	Excluded if face value is below $1,500	Excluded	Excluded
California	Excluded	1 set excluded	Excluded	Excluded if for business use	Excluded if face value is below $1,500	Excluded	Excluded up to $1,500; unlimited if in irrevocable contract
Colorado	Excluded	1 set excluded	Excluded up to $4,500 or if used for medical purposes	Excluded up to $6,000 if property produces 6% return on excluded equity	Excluded if face value below $1,500	Excluded	Excluded up to $1,500 if in revocable contract, unlimited if in irrevocable contract

TABLE 3.7 (continued)

Assets Excluded from Medicaid Asset Eligibility Limits (Other than the Home)

STATE	HOUSEHOLD GOODS	RINGS[a]	CAR	INCOME-PRODUCING PROPERTY	LIFE INSURANCE	BURIAL PLOTS	BURIAL COSTS
Connecticut	Excluded	1 set excluded	Excluded up to $4,500 or if used for medical purposes	Not excluded	Face value for nonterm and nongroup is excluded up to $1,500	1 excluded	Excluded up to $4,800 if in irrevocable contract or up to $1,200 if in revocable contract contract, reduced, by face value of life insurance policy
Delaware	Excluded	1 set excluded	1 vehicle excluded	Excluded on a case-by-case basis	Excluded up to $1,500	Excluded up to $1,500	Excluded up to $5,000 if in burial trust
District of Columbia	Excluded	1 set excluded	1 vehicle excluded	Excluded as asset but counted as income	Excluded if value does not push resources over $2,600	Excluded	Excluded up to $1,500
Florida	Excluded up to $2,000	1 set excluded	1 vehicle excluded	Excluded	Excluded up to $2,500	Excluded	Excluded up to $1,500
Georgia	Excluded	Excluded	Excluded	Excluded	Whole life insurance up to $5,000 face value per policy	As many as needed for family excluded	No limit if prepaid, $5,000 limit if designated from other resource
Hawaii	Excluded	1 set excluded	Excluded up to $4,500 of value	Not excluded	State cash value not excluded	1 per person excluded	Excluded up to $1,500
Idaho	Excluded up to $2,000	1 set excluded	Excluded if used for medical purposes	Not excluded	Excluded up to $1,500	Excluded	Excluded up to $1,500
Illinois	Excluded up to $2,000	1 set excluded	Excluded up to $4,500 or if used for medical purposes	Not excluded	Excluded up to $1,500 cash value	Excluded	Excluded up to $1,500

State							
Indiana	Excluded	1 set excluded	1 vehicle excluded if used for medical purposes	Not excluded	Excluded up to $1,400	Excluded	Excluded
Iowa	Excluded up to $2,000	1 set excluded	1 vehicle excluded up to $4,500 or if used for medical purposes	Excluded up to $6,000 if property produces 6% return on excluded equity	Excluded up to $1,500	1 per person excluded	Excluded from $4,000 to $6,000; itemized listing needed if above $4,000
Kansas	Excluded	1 set excluded	1 vehicle excluded	Not excluded	Excluded up to $2,000	Excluded	Excluded up to $3,000, $1,500 in irrevocable trust and $1,500 in revocable trust
Kentucky	Excluded	Excluded	1 vehicle excluded if used for medical purposes	Excluded up to $6,000 if property produces 6% return on excluded equity	Excluded up to $1,500	Excluded	Excluded
Louisiana	Will not exclude items of unusual value	Depends on value	Excluded if used for medical purposes	Not excluded	Cash value not excluded unless receiving a disability payment, and then only the payment income is counted	1 plot excluded	1 prepaid funeral excluded up to $1,500
Maine	Excluded	Excluded	Excluded		Excluded up to $1,500	Excluded	Excluded
Maryland	Excluded	1 set excluded	Excluded up to $4,500 in equity value; entire value excluded if necessary for employment or medical purposes or if modified for handicapped person	Excluded up to $6,000 if property produces 6% return on excluded equity	Excluded up to $1,500	Excluded	Excluded up to $5,000 if in irrevocable trust

TABLE 3.7 (continued)

Assets Excluded from Medicaid Asset Eligibility Limits (Other than the Home)

STATE	HOUSEHOLD GOODS	RINGS[a]	CAR	INCOME-PRODUCING PROPERTY	LIFE INSURANCE	BURIAL PLOTS	BURIAL COSTS
Massachusetts	Excluded	Excluded	Excluded up to $4,500	Not excluded	Excluded up to $1,500	Excluded	No limit on pre-paid burial fund if in irrevocable trust; up to $1,500 in separate burial fund also allowed
Minnesota	Excluded	1 set excluded	1 vehicle excluded				
Mississippi	Excluded	Excluded	1 vehicle excluded	Excluded up to $6,000 if property produces 6% return on excluded equity	Depends on face value	Excluded for immediate family	Excluded if in irrevocable contract, regardless of value
Missouri	Excluded	1 set excluded	1 vehicle excluded	Possible exclusion, but very stringent standards	See burial costs	Excluded	Excluded up to $1,500 for pre-paid burial costs; any remainder can be applied toward life insurance
Montana	Excluded	1 set excluded	1 vehicle excluded	Not excluded	Excluded up to $1,500	Excluded	Excluded
Nebraska	Excluded	1 set excluded	1 vehicle excluded up to $4,500 maximum value or if used for medical purposes		Excluded up to $1,500	Excluded	Excluded up to $1,500
Nevada	Excluded	1 set excluded	Excluded	Not excluded	Excluded up to $1,500 under complex formula	Excluded	Excluded up to $1,500 unless there is excluded life insurance; if in irrevocable contract, more may be excluded

State							
New Hampshire	Excluded	1 set excluded	1 vehicle excluded				Excluded if in irrevocable contract
New Jersey	Excluded up to $2,000	1 set excluded	Excluded up to $4,500 or if used for medical purposes	Excluded up to $6,000, if property produces 6% return on excluded equity	Excluded up to $1,500 face value	Excluded	Burial funds excluded up to $1,500 if in revocable contract, unlimited if in irrevocable contract
New York	Excluded	1 set excluded	Excluded		Insurance policy with cash value up to $1,500, with beneficiary being nursing home or estate, or excluded unless there is an excluded burial trust	Excluded	Burial trust up to $1,500 excluded unless there is an excluded insurance policy
North Carolina	Excluded	1 set excluded	Excluded up to $4,500 or if used for medical purposes	Excluded up to $6,000 if property produces 6% return on excluded equity	Excluded up to $1,500 face value	Excluded for immediate family	Excluded up to $1,500, fully excluded if in irrevocable trust
North Dakota	Excluded	1 set excluded	1 vehicle excluded		Excluded up to $1,500	Excluded	Excluded up to $3,000 if in burial fund with contract
Ohio	Excluded unless of unusual value	1 set excluded	Excluded if used for medical or employment purposes	Excluded if equity is less than $6,000	Excluded up to $1,500	1 per family member excluded	Excluded only if in irrevocable agreement
Oklahoma	Excluded	1 set excluded	1 vehicle excluded	Excluded up to $6,000 if property produces 6% return on excluded equity	Excluded up to $1,500	Excluded	Excluded up to $6,000 if in irrevocable contract

TABLE 3.7 (continued)

Assets Excluded from Medicaid Asset Eligibility Limits (Other than the Home)

State	Household Goods	Rings[a]	Car	Income-Producing Property	Life Insurance	Burial Plots	Burial Costs
Oregon	Excluded	1 set excluded	Excluded up to $4,500 or if used for medical purposes	Excluded up to $6,000 if property produces 6% return on excluded equity	Excluded up to $1,500 face value	Excluded	Excluded up to $1,500
Pennsylvania	Excluded	1 set excluded	1 vehicle excluded	Excluded up to $6,000 if property produces 6% return on excluded equity	Excluded up to $1,500 face value	Excluded	Irrevocable prepaid contract excluded
Rhode Island	Excluded	1 set excluded	1 vehicle excluded		Excluded up to $1,500	1 excluded	Excluded up to $1,500
South Carolina	Excluded	1 set excluded	Excluded	Excluded up to $6,000 if property produces 6% return on excluded equity	Excluded up to $1,500 face value	Excluded for immediate family except for grandchildren	Excluded up to $1,500; unlimited exclusion after 30 days if in irrevocable contract
South Dakota	Excluded unless of unusual value	1 set excluded	Excluded up to $4,500 or if used for medical purposes	Excluded up to $6,000 if property produces 6% return on excluded equity	Excluded up to $1,500	Excluded	Excluded up to $1,500
Tennessee	Excluded	1 set excluded	1 vehicle excluded up to $4,500	Excluded up to $6,000 if property produces 6% return on excluded equity	Cash surrender value is counted unless designated as a burial policy, and then up to $1,500	Excluded	Excluded up to $1,500; excluded entirely if in irrevocable trust if reasonable
Texas	Excluded	1 set excluded	Excluded up to $4,500 or if used for medical purposes	Excluded up to $6,000 if property produces 6% return on excluded equity	Excluded up to $1,500 face value	Excluded	Excluded up to $1,500 unless there is excluded life insurance; excluded entirely if in irrevocable contract

State							
Utah	Excluded	1 set excluded	Excluded up to $6,000 if property produces 6% return on excluded equity	1 vehicle excluded	Excluded up to $1,500	Excluded	Excluded up to $1,500; excluded entirely if in irrevocable trust
Virginia	Excluded	1 set excluded	Excluded up to $6,000 if property produces 6% return on excluded equity	1 vehicle excluded	Excluded up to $1,500 face value	Excluded	Up to $2,500 can be excluded
West Virginia	Excluded un-less of unusual value	1 set excluded	Excluded up to $6,000 if property produces 6% return on excluded equity; counted as income if connected to homestead	1 vehicle excluded	Cash surrender value is countable	Excluded	Excluded if in irrevocable trust

[a]One set refers to one wedding and one engagement ring.

SOURCE: National Governors' Association Report.

come cap state, you'll qualify if your income is less than the cap.

If you live in an income cap state that is also a community property state (Arizona, Idaho, Louisiana, Nevada, New Mexico, and Texas), you may even get a break. Let's say your spouse's income is $2,000 a month and yours is $400 a month. His income under the name-on-the-check rule would be over the income cap, but you are entitled to half of the total income under community property rules. Half of $2,400 is $1,200, leaving your spouse with only $1,200, which is below the income cap. This rationale has been successfully applied in Arizona and New Mexico, but it is not yet clear whether other community property states will agree with this interpretation.

How Much Can a Nursing-Home Spouse Keep?

Once you have determined that your nursing-home spouse is eligible for Medicaid under the income test, put aside your calculations and start again to find out exactly how much of his or her income can be kept. These rules are much different from the eligibility rules.

Again, use the name-on-the-check rule to allocate income between you and your spouse. If income is paid in your spouse's name it will be considered his or hers; income paid in your name is considered yours. Income paid jointly to both of you is considered to be shared equally. If others, such as children or business partners, are named on the income payment, the income is considered as a pro rata payment to each named person (for instance, for three people it would be a one-third division). Payments received from a trust are considered in the same way as income from any other source, unless the trust says otherwise. This will be important when it comes to planning for a nursing-home spouse.

In years past, this method of income allocation often left a spouse-at-home with no income. Example 3 presents a typical example of "the way we were."

Example 3

Your father worked his entire life, building up his pension and Social Security. While your father was working outside the home, your mother took care of the unpaid chores, raising the children and maintaining the house. She earned praise but no pension. On your father's retirement, your folks were able to live reasonably well on his stream of income. That happy picture changed when your father entered the nursing home, because the fruits of his labors flowed straight into the nursing home's coffers. Your mother was left with no alternative but welfare.

Statistics show that women have suffered unfairly under this allocation system. Because women typically live longer and earn less, the wife-at-home has been the one who most often has become destitute. In an attempt to deal with this problem, the law now provides a basic living allowance to support the spouse-at-home.

Spouse-at-Home Basic Living Allowance

The amount of the basic living allowance provided by Congress for the spouse-at-home is determined by a complicated formula. This should come as no surprise when you consider that it was created by the same Congress that brings you the tax code. To calculate the amount a nursing-home spouse can protect for his or her spouse-at-home:

1. Take 150 percent of one-twelfth of the official poverty line income for a family of two. At this writing, that should be $1,230 a month.
2. Subtract any income otherwise available to the spouse-at-home (income paid in his or her name plus one-half of joint income) from the amount in number 1.
3. For the principal residence of the spouse-at-home, add monthly rent or mortgage payments (including principal and interest); real estate tax; homeowner's or renter's insurance costs; the state utility allowance or, if your state doesn't have one, actual average utility payments; and, for a condominium or cooperative, required maintenance charges (minus any included utility costs).
4. Take 30 percent of the amount in number 1 above; today that is $369.
5. Calculate the amount by which the figure in number 3 exceeds the figure in number 4.
6. Take your figures from numbers 2 and 5 and add them together.

The amount in number 6 gives you the basic living allowance that a nursing-home spouse can protect from his or her income for the spouse-at-home. (Note that the official poverty line income is adjusted periodically and is effective July 1 of each year. Contact your local Medicaid or human services office for updates each summer.)

Here are two examples of how this formula works:

Example 4

The income of your father, who is in a nursing home, is $2,000 a month, and the income of your mother, who remains at home, is $200 a month. Your mother has rental and utility costs of $600 a month.

1. 150 percent of one-twelfth of the poverty line is $1,230 a month.
2. Subtract $200 (your mother's income) from the amount in number 1, and you get $1,030.
3. The residence costs for your mother are $600 a month.
4. 30 percent of the amount in number 1 is $369.
5. Number 3 exceeds number 4 by $231 ($600 minus $369).
6. Numbers 2 and 5 together total $1,261 ($1,030 plus $231). So of your father's income of $2,000 a month, $1,261 would go to your mother (in addition to her $200) and $739 (less other adjustments, discussed next) would go to the nursing home.

Example 5

Your father's income is $3,000 a month, and the income of your mother, who remains at home, is $400 a month. Your mother pays mortgage, utility, and insurance costs of $800 a month.

1. 150 percent of one-twelfth of the poverty line is $1,230.
2. Subtracting your mother's $400 income from the amount in number 1, you get $830.
3. Your mother pays residence costs of $800.
4. 30 percent of number 1 is $369.
5. Number 3 exceeds number 4 by $431.
6. Numbers 2 and 5 together total $1,261. So of your father's income of $3,000 a month, $1,261 would go to your mother (in addition to her $400) and $1,739 would wind up paid to the nursing home.

Still, Congress wanted to make sure that a spouse-at-home didn't get too much money, so it put an $1,870.50 a month cap (this is the 1995 amount; it increases slightly each year) on the basic living allowance for a spouse-at-home. (Note that states may just decide to allow all spouses-at-home a flat amount between $1,230 and $1,870.50 as the basic living allowance, without regard to the complicated formula. More than twenty states, including California, Georgia, Illinois, New Hampshire, New York, South Carolina, and Wisconsin, have set the allowance at the highest amount, $1,870.50.)

Following is a worksheet to help you calculate the basic living allowance.

SPOUSE-AT-HOME BASIC LIVING ALLOWANCE WORKSHEET

Monthly Amount

1. 150 percent of one-twelfth of poverty line (through July 1, 1995): _____ $1,230
2. (a) Income of spouse-at-home: _____
   (b) Number 1 minus number 2: _____
3. (a) Monthly rent or mortgage payments (principal and interest): _____
   (b) Real estate taxes per month: _____
   (c) Homeowner's or renter's insurance per month: _____
   (d) Average utility costs per month: _____
   (e) Condominium or cooperative maintenance charges (minus included utility costs) per month: _____
   (f) Numbers 3(a)–(e) added together: _____
4. 30 percent of amount in number 1: _____ 369.00
5. Number 3(f) minus number 4: _____
6. Number 2(b) plus number 5 is the basic living allowance: _____

By allowing a nursing-home spouse to give his or her spouse-at-home this basic living allowance, Congress has helped ensure that the spouse-at-home won't be left without any income, although as examples 4 and 5 show, most of a nursing-home spouse's income is still likely to go to pay for long-term nursing care.

However, the basic living allowance will not help a spouse-at-home much, if at all, if his or her income is near or above the minimum allowance set by the state ($1,230 a month unless set higher). Looking at example 4, if your mother's monthly income was $1,200, only $261 of your father's income could be paid to his spouse.

There are two important exceptions to the basic living allowance rules discussed above. First, a spouse-at-home may ask a court to order a nursing-home spouse to pay a monthly amount above the basic living allowance. If successful, a court order takes precedence. At this time, very few state courts (with New York as the principal exception) have issued support orders increasing the allowance to the spouse-at-home. And support orders are not a panacea anyway—even if a spouse-at-home can use a support order to preserve more income, the spouse would have to hire a lawyer and go to court to get the order, a process that can be costly and time-consuming (and thus difficult for the spouse of a nursing-home candidate or resident to manage).

Second, if the basic living allowance does not allow the spouse-at-home enough income, a higher amount may be permitted by the state Medicaid office after what is called a "fair hearing." However, exceptions are made only in *very rare circumstances* when it can be shown that the spouse-at-home will suffer *significant* financial duress unless more income is allowed.

So far we've been talking about using the nursing-home spouse's income to supplement that of the spouse-at-home. But what if the income of the nursing-home spouse is not sufficient to bring up the income of the spouse-at-home to the basic living allowance? In that case the spouse-at-home should be permitted to keep additional assets that would produce more income.

As discussed below, the law severely limits the amount of assets a couple may keep when one spouse enters a nursing home. That amount should be increased if necessary to provide the spouse-at-home the required minimum income.

Let's go back to example 5. Your mother is supposed to get $1,661 a month ($1,261 from your father and $400 of her own) to live on. But she has only

$400 a month of her own income, mostly from the $74,820 of assets she is allowed to keep after spending down her life savings under the assets limitation test discussed below. If your father's income was only $800, that would not be enough to provide your mother with her full allowance. The law says that your mother should be permitted to keep more assets than would otherwise be allowed, as much as necessary to generate sufficient income (via interest and dividends) to bring her up to the basic living allowance amount. In this case it might take more than $100,000 to produce the extra $461 a month in interest needed for your mother. Your mother would have to petition the state Medicaid office to allow her to keep additional assets.

Personal-Needs Allowance

Not only can a person protect the basic living allowance from the nursing home, but he or she can also keep about $30 a month (depending on the state—see table 3.3) for personal needs, such as toiletries, books, and magazines.

Unreimbursed Medical Expenses

A nursing-home resident may also hang on to enough income to pay medical expenses that are not reimbursed by Medicaid or some other third party.

Family Allowance

A spouse is not the only person who is entitled to some of the nursing-home resident's income. Certain family members can get one-third of the difference between $1,230 and their own income. For example, a dependent child with income of $330 a month should be entitled to $300 a month (one-third of $900) from the nursing-home parent.

To be entitled to income from the nursing-home resident, you must:

- Be a minor or dependent child, dependent parent, or dependent sibling of the nursing-home resident or the nursing-home resident's spouse; and
- Reside with the nursing-home resident's spouse.

Family members come after the spouse. They collect only if there is income remaining after the spouse's basic living allowance.

ASSETS LIMITATION TEST

As explained earlier, a single person (widow, widower, divorced, or never married) is permitted to keep only about $2,000 of an entire life's savings. Married couples get to keep more, but the law is still very harsh.

In general, a nursing-home resident and his or her spouse can keep a total of $74,820 or one-half of their combined life savings, whichever is *less*. At a minimum, every couple is entitled to shelter $14,964. Here's how this works:

1. Take the total value of all of the couple's assets on the day one spouse enters a nursing home (or a hospital, if earlier, and there is no return home). Count assets in the names of the nursing-home spouse, the spouse-at-home, and both spouses jointly. If either spouse has a partial interest in an asset with someone other than the spouse, add the value of that partial interest as well.

2. Now cut the total in half. If the result is less than $14,964, then $14,964 can be sheltered. If the amount is more than $74,820, then $74,820 can be protected. And if the amount falls in between, then that's what can be kept.

Here are three examples:

Example 6

Your father, who is entering a nursing home, has assets in his name, including CDs and bank accounts, totaling $50,000. Your mother, who is still at home, has assets in her name of $80,000, and they have jointly held assets of $40,000. Total value of all assets is $170,000. One-half would be $85,000. Since that is more than $74,820, your mother could keep the maximum of $74,820, your father would get to keep about $2,000 (the amount listed in table 3.5), and the nursing home would get the rest—$93,180—before Medicaid would provide any help.

Example 7

Your assets at the time you enter a nursing home total $15,000 and the assets of your spouse, who is remaining at home, come to $5,000, for a $20,000 total. Since one-half is less than the $14,964 minimum, your spouse keeps $14,964, you protect $2,000, and the nursing home gets $3,036.

Example 8

Your father, who is in a nursing home, has assets of $45,000 and your mother, at home, has assets of $35,000, for total combined assets of $80,000. One-half is $40,000—so your mother gets $40,000, your father gets $2,000, and the nursing home will get $38,000.

A growing number of states, including California, Florida, Georgia, Illinois, New York, North Dakota, Vermont, Washington, and Wisconsin, will allow you to keep $74,820 without going through this rigamarole of figuring your total worth and cutting it in half.

The protected assets (up to $74,820) should promptly be moved into the name of the healthy spouse. Otherwise they may lose their protection.

Example 9

Your mother, your sister, "and/or" you are all named on your mother's bank account. Any one of you can write checks and withdraw funds. Your mother's money created the account and her Social Security number is listed. In this case the entire amount in the account will be counted as hers when Medicaid tallies up her assets for the assets limitation test.

If the account has *your* name listed first, is in your Social Security number, and was created by your funds, the account should be considered yours, even if your mother (the Medicaid applicant) is also named on the account with you "or" her. If your mother was named only for convenience purposes and there was no intent to actually give her an ownership interest, the law of most states would say that the account should be considered yours.

PROTECTED ASSETS

Even before a married couple calculates their assets, they can exclude the assets listed on pages 19–20 and in table 3.7. In fact, the exempt assets are even better for married couples than they are for singles; they can protect their home, household goods and furnishings, personal effects, and a car, *without limita-*

tion on their value. These items are protected *off the top*. For example, if a couple owns a house worth $100,000 and has other combined assets of $80,000 (as in example 8), their home plus $42,000 of the remaining assets will be sheltered. As will be discussed in chapter 7, wise use of the legal exemptions for certain assets can be an important nest egg planning tool.

RECORD KEEPING

If a couple is paying full fare for nursing-home costs because they are not yet poor enough to qualify for Medicaid, they will want to be great record keepers. They must be able to show the Medicaid office the value of their assets *at the time the spouse was first institutionalized*. Otherwise they could end up paying more to the nursing home than is legally required.

Let's look back at example 8. At the time your father first entered the nursing home, your parents were "too rich" and he was not eligible for Medicaid. Not until your parents spent $38,000 on care (or used some of the planning tools described in upcoming chapters) would he qualify. At the time he applies for Medicaid, after your parents' assets are down to $42,000, Medicaid will want some proof that the assets were originally $80,000. If your parents can show assets of only $70,000 at the time your father was institutionalized, then they may be required to spend another $5,000 on the nursing home (using one-half of $70,000 instead of one-half of $80,000) before Medicaid will pay anything.

IMPACT OF THE LAW ON MARRIED COUPLES

The law allows married couples to keep more of their life savings than it does single people; keeping $74,820 is surely better than keeping only about $2,000, right? Not necessarily! Even with the more generous allotment, many couples wind up being wiped out by nursing-home costs anyway.

If your parents have barely been making ends meet on their income from CDs, stocks, and bonds, how will they live on half or less? Income generated by, say, $200,000 buys a lot more groceries than does the income from $74,820.

Yet when one spouse enters a nursing home, the daily living expenses for the spouse remaining at home often are hardly reduced. Whether it's one or two living under one roof, certain basic expenses won't go away—the rent or mortgage payments, real estate taxes, and utilities all stay home too. Car-related costs often go up, owing to driving to and from the nursing home.

So if you were barely getting by on investment income of $10,000 a year and that income gets cut to $3,500 a year, you've got big problems. You'll wind up dipping into principal each year to make up the difference, until your life savings are gone. For married couples, like singles, the Medicaid law might leave you with a roof over your head but unable to afford the costs of repairing the leaks.

When the spouse in the nursing home dies, the financial picture for the surviving spouse won't get any better—and in many cases things get worse. The income and asset limitations together can have a devastating impact on older Americans. To illustrate, let's look at example 10, which combines examples 4 and 6.

Example 10

Your father and mother were doing quite well; they had combined assets of $170,000 and a combined monthly income of $2,200—the result of careful planning.

Then your father becomes ill and enters a nursing home. He won't qualify for Medicaid until your parents' assets have been spent down to $74,820 (the maximum amount that can be kept and still be Medicaid-eligible).

After your father qualifies for Medicaid, your mother would continue to receive her monthly income of $200 and a basic living allowance of $1,261 from your father.

Then your father dies, eliminating a substantial portion of his income and the basic living allowance for your mother. Your mother is left with assets of $74,820 and a monthly income of $500 (perhaps she gets a slightly increased Social Security check, but she loses your father's pension).

In a situation like example 10, you can guess what would happen to your mother. The effect could be catastrophic—unless they take steps to protect themselves.

Joint Assets

Questions of how to divide jointly held assets under the Medicaid laws used to arise, but the OBRA 1993 rules have set the record straight. The value of assets owned by a Medicaid applicant (whether married or unmarried) "and" another person or persons, where every person must sign off to sell, withdraw, or transfer the asset, should be calculated pro rata (for example, if property is owned by Bob and Joe, each owns half). But the value of assets owned by a Medicaid applicant "or" others, where any *one* owner can sell, withdraw, or transfer the asset, typically will be counted as an asset owned entirely by the Medicaid applicant. This rule doesn't make much difference when it comes to assets owned by husband and wife, because all of the couple's assets are considered for Medicaid. But this rule can have a big impact when it comes to assets owned by a Medicaid applicant (or spouse) and children or others.

Example 11

Your father added you to his house deed years ago, and the two of you own the house jointly with rights of survivorship. Since the deed is in the names of your father "and" you and both signatures are needed to sell or transfer the property, it will be considered one-half his and one-half yours for Medicaid purposes.

CHAPTER 3 SUMMARY CHECKLIST

How Much Can an Older Person Keep from the Nursing Home?

As a general rule, older people's income and assets will go to pay nursing-home bills—Medicaid won't pay until their assets have dwindled.

An *unmarried* nursing-home resident generally can protect only a limited amount of income and assets and still qualify for Medicaid:

Income

✔ Personal-needs allowance of $30 to $75 a month.

✔ Monies spent for health insurance and other medical expenses not covered by Medicaid.

✔ Home maintenance allowance of about $200 to $400 a month.

Assets

✔ About $2,000.

✔ Home, regardless of value, but often only for a limited time.

✔ Limited amount of household goods and other personal items, up to $2,000 in value.

✔ One car, up to $4,500 in value; no limit on value if used to get to work or medical appointments.

✔ One wedding ring and one engagement ring.

✔ Property in an income-producing trade or business.

✔ Up to $6,000 equity in nonbusiness property essential for support (for example, farm equipment to grow your own food).

✔ Life insurance with a cash surrender value of $1,500.

✔ Burial plot.

✔ Funeral costs of up to $1,500 per person or an irrevocable burial contract.

If a nursing-home resident is married, the couple generally can protect income and assets as follows:

Income

✔ Basic living allowance for the spouse-at-home, from $1,230 to $1,870.50 a month, based on a complicated formula.

✔ Personal-needs allowance for the nursing-home spouse of about $30 a month.

✔ Unreimbursed medical expenses (must be documented).

Combined Assets

- ✔ Half of the couple's combined assets or $74,820, whichever is less.

- ✔ Home (regardless of value).

- ✔ Household goods (regardless of value).

- ✔ Personal effects (regardless of value).

- ✔ Car (regardless of value).

- ✔ Property in an income-producing trade or business.

- ✔ Up to $6,000 equity in nonbusiness property essential for support.

- ✔ Life insurance with a cash surrender value of $1,500.

- ✔ Burial plot.

- ✔ Burial costs of up to $1,500 per person or an irrevocable burial contract.

4 | Why Can't Older People Protect Their Nest Eggs Just by Giving Them Away?

By now the thought may have occurred to you: Why don't people simply get rid of their assets right before entering a nursing home? Maybe give them away to their kids? Then the parent in the nursing home could tell the Medicaid bureaucrats that he or she has no assets, and Medicaid would pick up the nursing-home tab. If the parent recovered enough to return home, the children would return the assets. If the parent is married, maybe both spouses could give away their assets to their children, who would use those assets to care for the healthy parent; that arrangement would benefit the healthy parent and, eventually, the children.

Unfortunately, Uncle Sam won't let a person give away his or her life savings and then immediately qualify for Medicaid coverage. Transfers of property for less than fair market value made right before a person enters a nursing home generally are not considered valid transfers for Medicaid purposes.

For purposes of the transfer-ineligibility rules, transfers include any voluntary gift or transfer of an asset for less than its fair market value. Involuntary transfers, such as those resulting from a divorce or foreclosure, do not disqualify a Medicaid applicant no matter when the transfers occurred.

Ineligibility Penalty

Almost any gift or transfer of assets (money or property) by a Medicaid applicant or spouse will make the applicant ineligible for Medicaid for a period of time. Under either the old rules or the new, the ac-

tual length of the ineligibility period will depend on the amount of the transfer. Each state sets an average cost of nursing-home care, usually ranging from $3,000 to $4,000 a month. (Some states, like New York, also set different amounts based on region.) For example, the current rate in Texas is just over $2,000 a month; in Michigan it is $2,500 a month; in California it is just over $2,900 a month; in Maryland and Ohio it is $3,000 a month; in Pennsylvania it is just over $3,500 a month; and in New York City it is over $5,500 a month. These amounts change annu-

> **OBRA 1993, signed into law August 10, 1993, made big changes in the rules and penalties for gifts and transfers of assets. People who gave away assets to others—usually family members—on or before August 10, 1993, would be ineligible for Medicaid coverage in a nursing home for as much as thirty months (two and a half years) from the date of the gifts.** *Gifts made on or before August 10, 1993, still fall under the old rules.* **Under the new law, people who transfer assets *after* August 10, 1993, could be required to wait much longer. The rules are far more complicated, but the impact of the new law will be that most people who transfer assets will have to wait up to thirty-six months before becoming eligible for Medicaid benefits. Not playing by the new rules of the game could make you ineligible for Medicaid for as long as you live.**

ally, so check with your local Medicaid office for current rates.

NOTE: If the rate selected by your state seems ridiculously low and totally unrealistic, you may be able to challenge the amount. Not surprisingly, this is complicated and would require a lawyer's assistance.

To figure the ineligibility period, divide the value of the gift by the average cost of nursing-home care set by your state. In most states the ineligibility period will begin with the month of the first transfer of assets. For example, if a gift was made in May, May will count as the first month of the penalty period. However, under OBRA 1993, states are permitted to delay the ineligibility period one month; this means that a gift made in May would trigger an ineligibility countdown period beginning in June, giving the state a one-month money-saving bonus.

Example 12

Your state fixes the average cost of nursing-home care at $3,000 a month. The ineligibility period is one month for every $3,000 given away. A transfer of $3,000 makes your parent ineligible for one month, the month in which the transfer takes place. A $30,000 gift triggers a ten-month penalty ($30,000 divided by $3,000 a month); a $60,000 transfer brings a twenty-month penalty.

For gifts or transfers made on or before August 10, 1993, the maximum ineligibility period is thirty months. So a gift of $300,000, which might have triggered a penalty period of one hundred months ($300,000 divided by $3,000, assuming a $3,000 monthly average care cost), would be capped at thirty months. Under the new rules, the potential ineligibility period can be *unlimited* without proper planning. A gift of $150,000 causes a fifty-month ineligibility assuming $3,000 monthly average cost of care ($150,000 divided by $3,000 a month); a gift of $300,000 creates a one-hundred-month penalty!

Here are three examples of how the penalty works using both the old rules and the new rules:

Example 13

Six months before your father enters a nursing home, he gives $18,000 to you and his other children. Average nursing-home costs in his state are $3,000 a month. Under either the new

or the old Medicaid law, he would be ineligible for Medicaid for six months ($18,000 divided by $3,000 a month) as a result of the transfer.

Example 14

On January 10, 1993, your mother entered a nursing home and transferred cash and a house worth a total value of $150,000 to your brother. The average nursing-home costs in your mother's state were $3,000 a month. Taking the $150,000 value and dividing by $3,000 a month leaves fifty months of ineligibility. However, because the transfer occurred before August 10, 1993, the effective date of OBRA 1993, your mother would wait only thirty months—the maximum delay allowed under the old rules. She would become eligible for Medicaid on July 1, 1995 (thirty months later).

Example 15

On January 1, 1994, your father entered a nursing home and transferred his house and cash to your sister. The value totaled $150,000 and the average nursing-home costs in his state were $3,000 a month. Taking the $150,000 value and dividing by $3,000 a month results in an ineligibility penalty of fifty months. Remember, under the new rules there is no cap on the amount of time you can be penalized for asset transfers.

Look-Back Period

The potentially unlimited ineligibility period created by OBRA 1993 would devastate the life savings of many middle-class Americans, if that is all the law did. But there is a saving grace included in the law: a thirty-six-month "look-back" period for most gifts or transfers (six months longer than under the old law).

This means that the state can "look back" only thirty-six months to see if any gifts or transfers were made by the Medicaid recipient or his or her spouse. If no gifts or transfers were made within those thirty-six-months, then there is no ineligibility period.

If you're already on Medicaid when you enter a nursing home, the look-back period starts the day you enter the facility. If you're already in a nursing home when you apply for Medicaid, the look-back period begins the day you apply. If you made no gifts within the prior thirty-six months, you won't be penalized—no matter how much you may have given away more than thirty-six months earlier. (The new law also gives states the option of extending this look-back period to Medicaid applicants who are not in or going into nursing homes.)

Does all of this sound complicated? It is, but several examples should help clarify how the look back works.

Example 16

On December 31, 1993, your mother transferred the family home, worth $150,000, to you and your brother. Assuming the average cost of nursing-home care in your state is $3,000 a month, her ineligibility period for Medicaid benefits would last fifty months from the date of the gift. But thanks to the look-back rule, she may not have to wait that long.

If she waits to apply for Medicaid until three years have passed from the date of the gift (January 1, 1997), she should then qualify for benefits. Why? Medicaid can only look at those thirty-six months; the bureaucrats will ask for and look through financial records (including monthly bank and brokerage statements, and settlement sheets and deeds for any real estate transactions) for January 1, 1994, through December 31, 1996, to see if any gifts were made. Since no gifts were made within the last three years, your mom would be in the clear.

Example 17

Let's take the same facts as in example 16. But instead of waiting the full three years, your mother jumps the gun and applies for Medicaid too early—on December 1, 1996. Medicaid would look back at financial records for three years, find the gifts, and rule her ineligible for the full fifty months. She would not be eligible for Medicaid until February 1, 1998 (fifty months from December 1994).

In other words, even though the ineligibility period can be unlimited, wise timing of the Medicaid application can limit the ineligibility period to three years. But the new rules create a terrible trap for the careless or uninformed.

Let's look back at example 17. Your mother applied too early and was ruled ineligible for fifty months. Can she wait a couple of months, until the three-year look-back period has passed, and reapply

for coverage? Or is she stuck with the full fifty-month ineligibility period without the right to reapply? Nothing in the law seems to prohibit a person from reapplying, but the law is not crystal clear (do you want to be the test case?). You'll be better off watching your calendar and not applying until the time is right.

Keep in mind that the look-back and ineligibility periods apply only to gifts or transfers made by a Medicaid recipient or his or her spouse. Both spouses can still spend money on personal purchases and routine living expenses, such as clothes, debts, home repairs, or vacations, without worrying about triggering any penalty for transfers.

What if more than one gift or transfer is made? If a transfer is made, triggering an ineligibility period, and then another gift is made while the first ineligibility period is still running, do the periods run concurrently or consecutively?

Let's say you transfer $30,000 on January 1, 1995, triggering a ten-month period of ineligibility (with an average care cost of $3,000 a month). Your ineligibility for Medicaid will last through October 31, 1995. Then on June 10, 1995, you make another gift, this time of $15,000, triggering a five-month period of ineligibility. Does the new, five-month penalty run concurrently, during the months of June, July, Au-

---

WARNING

Some experts believe that the OBRA 1993 rules create a sixty-month (five-year) look-back period for transfers into certain irrevocable trusts; the federal Health Care Financing Administration is taking this position. Others disagree, believing that the law requires only a thirty-six-month look-back period for transfers into irrevocable trusts. Watch out—the language is ambiguous enough to raise questions that may have to be resolved by the legislature or courts. The law also seems to create a sixty-month look-back period for transfers from a revocable trust established by a Medicaid applicant or spouse to others (not to themselves). Again, the law is not clear on this. Don't be too "trusting" of any expert who advises you not to worry because the law is perfectly clear!

gust, September, and October 1995, so you'd still qualify for Medicaid on November 1? Or is the new, five-month ineligibility period tacked on to the first penalty period, resulting in a fifteen-month penalty?

Prior to OBRA 1993, most states allowed the ineligibility periods to run concurrently, giving Medicaid applicants a nice break. OBRA 1993 changed the rule: all transfers or gifts within the look-back period are now added together, and the ineligibility period runs from the date of the earliest transfer or gift within the look-back period. The two examples that follow illustrate the impact the new rule can have on your eligibility.

Example 18

On January 1, 1995, you give your son $30,000. On June 10, 1995, you make another gift of $15,000. November 15, 1995, you enter a nursing home and apply for Medicaid.

During the prior three years, you made two gifts totaling $45,000. This $45,000 transfer creates a fifteen-month period of ineligibility (assuming a $3,000 monthly average cost of care), which begins to run with the January transfer. You won't qualify until April 1, 1996.

Example 19

On May 10, 1994, you gave your daughter your savings bonds, worth $150,000. Then on October 17, 1996, you give her another $30,000. In August 1997 you enter a nursing home and apply for Medicaid.

The three-year look-back period dates back to August 1994, three years prior to your Medicaid application. The only transfer within that period was $30,000 on October 17, 1996; the earlier gift is no longer considered because it was made more than three years earlier. The October 17, 1996, gift created a ten-month period of ineligibility (assuming a $3,000 monthly average cost of care), running from October 1996 through July 1997. As of August 1, 1997, you qualify for Medicaid.

Permissible Transfers

Certain transfers, regardless of the date on which they were made, will not affect an individual's eligi-

bility for Medicaid. A Medicaid applicant will not be ineligible if:

- The person (or spouse, if applicable) transfers a home, whether before or after entering a nursing home, to any of the following:

  1. His or her spouse.
  2. Any child who is under twenty-one, blind, or permanently and totally disabled.
  3. A brother or sister who already has some ownership interest in the house and who was residing in the home for at least one year immediately before the person was admitted to a hospital or nursing home.
  4. Any child who was residing in the house for at least two years immediately before the parent's admission to a hospital or nursing home and who provided care for the parent that allowed him or her to stay at home rather than in an institution.

- The person transfers any other assets:

  1. To his or her spouse.
  2. To any child who is under twenty-one, blind, or permanently and totally disabled, or to a trust solely for the child's benefit.
  3. To a trust solely for the benefit of a disabled individual under sixty-five years old.

- The person can prove to the state Medicaid bureaucrats that:

  1. He or she intended to dispose of the assets for their market value.
  2. He or she transferred the assets solely for some purpose other than to qualify for Medicaid assistance.
  3. All assets transferred have been returned to the transferor.

- The person can show that denial of Medicaid eligibility would cause an undue hardship.

When it comes to planning, these exceptions to the transfer-ineligibility rules can be very important. The three examples that follow illustrate why.

Example 20

The day after your father enters a nursing home, he transfers the family home to his wife's name. The transfer does not make him ineligible for Medicaid because spouses can pass any assets between themselves with no penalty. When his wife dies, the home passes under her will or trust to her children, and your father remains eligible for Medicaid. Had he not transferred the home, he would have lost his Medicaid eligibility because the home would have been his again and no longer would have qualified as an exempt asset (see chapter 10).

Example 21

You have been living with and caring for your mother for three years. Without your help, institutionalization would have been necessary. But you haven't been well lately yourself and can no longer manage to take care of her. So, reluctantly, you admit her to a nursing home. If your mother transfers the house into your name, the transfer will protect the house from the nursing home and she will still be eligible for Medicaid.

Example 22

A few months ago your mother gave you $30,000 to pay for your child's education. She was in good health at the time. Shortly after, she suffered a stroke and entered a nursing home. Will the gift keep her from getting Medicaid coverage? Not necessarily.

The government will presume the worst, that she made the gift to qualify for Medicaid. But the presumption is arguable. If you can show that the gift was simply made to help pay for her grandchild's education, not for Medicaid qualification, she shouldn't be penalized. Your substantiating evidence might be proof that your mother had also paid for her other grandchildren's educations and that she was in good health at the time of the gift (not contemplating imminent institutionalization).

NOTE: Under the language of the Medicaid laws, the exception to the transfer-ineligibility rules for assets transferred solely for some purpose other than

to qualify for Medicaid assistance conceivably could allow a person to transfer his or her house, household goods, and other exempt assets (see pages 19–20) to any other person at any time. Since possession of an exempt asset does not affect a person's Medicaid eligibility, it could be argued that any such transfer would necessarily be for some purpose other than Medicaid qualification. This interpretation of the law would be helpful because you or your loved ones could freely transfer a house or exempt assets, which would then continue to be protected even if the items subsequently lost their exempt status. (Let's say, for example, that your parents own a car worth $10,000 when your dad enters a nursing home. At that time it is exempt. But if your mother dies, a portion of the car's value is no longer exempt. Your father might lose the car unless your parents had previously transferred it).

While this argument is reasonable and has been accepted by some states, others have expressly rejected it. I would not recommend taking this approach without first consulting a lawyer.

Transfers of Joint Assets

Assets held jointly with others have been dealt with specially under OBRA 1993. As discussed earlier (see page 35), an asset owned by a Medicaid applicant "and" another person should be considered one-half the applicant's for Medicaid purposes; an asset owned by a Medicaid applicant "or" another person, where either one could draw out funds, is considered entirely the applicant's.

When a co-owner (not the Medicaid applicant) of a joint asset pulls out some or all of the funds or removes the name of the Medicaid applicant, is that a gift or transfer by the applicant, triggering an ineligibility period? Before OBRA 1993, some states said yes, others said no. I regularly (and successfully) argued that withdrawal of an asset by a co-owner was not a gift or a transfer by the Medicaid applicant. But OBRA 1993 says that when any person takes any action to reduce or eliminate the applicant's ownership or control of a joint account, then that will be considered a transfer by the applicant. In other words, withdrawals (by anyone) from a joint account now trigger an ineligibility period.

Example 23

Your mother and you own some stock, in her name "and" your name. The stock is worth $50,000. The two of you sell the stock and the entire $50,000 is put into your name. Your mother has made a gift to you of $25,000, which triggers an ineligibility period.

Example 24

Your mother and you are named on her bank account, with $50,000 in her name "and/or" your name. Either one of you can make withdrawals from the account. You go to the bank, withdraw the $50,000, and put it in your name alone. Since your mother had rights to the entire $50,000 before the withdrawal (see page 35), the withdrawal will be considered an asset transfer, triggering an ineligibility period based on the transfer of $50,000.

Transfers by a Spouse After Medicaid Qualification

After your spouse qualifies for Medicaid, if you then give or transfer any assets, will that trigger a loss of benefits by creating an ineligibility period for your spouse? The answer is not clear under OBRA 1993.

On the one hand, OBRA 1993 broadly says that any transfers made by a Medicaid applicant or spouse within the time of the look-back period will create an ineligibility period. Under this broad statement, transfers by a spouse after a Medicaid applicant begins to receive Medicaid coverage might create an ineligibility period and cause the Medicaid recipient to lose benefits until the period expires. On the other hand, this view is inconsistent with other parts of the Medicaid laws. For example, the law says that after a Medicaid applicant obtains coverage, assets in the name of a spouse-at-home are protected.

Example 25

You and your spouse spend down your assets to $74,820 (the maximum allowed before Medicaid qualification can begin); your spouse goes on Medicaid. The $74,820 is transferred into your name. Those assets are protected. If they grow over the years due to wise investment, the increased amount should still be protected.

Two years later you inherit $50,000 from your sister. That inheritance is also protected and does not cause your spouse to lose benefits.

If you then transfer $50,000 to your children, the transfer should not cause your spouse to lose his Medicaid benefits. After all, you are clearly not making the transfer to qualify for coverage, since your spouse is already covered and your assets are protected.

I believe that transfers of assets by the spouse-at-home *after* the nursing-home spouse goes on Medicaid should not create an ineligibility period. But this is another ambiguity in the law that may require clarification by the court or legislature. Please note that the federal government (Health Care Financing Administration) seems to agree with my position.

Perhaps the thought crossed your mind: Why can't I cheat a little by "forgetting" to tell the Medicaid bureaucrats about a few of the assets that were given away just before going into a nursing home? After all, my assets are a drop in the bucket compared with the whole federal Medicaid budget; Uncle Sam will never miss the contribution.

Forget it! Medicaid bureaucrats will go back through an applicant's financial history—tax returns, bank statements, brokerage account statements, and so forth—to check out statements on the application. They will often examine records for the previous three to five years.

For example, your father's federal income tax return for 1993 may show interest income of $5,000. The IRS will conclude that to generate that income, he must have had somewhere in the neighborhood of $100,000 of income-generating assets. If those assets don't appear on his Medicaid application, the Medicaid bureaucrats will get suspicious and start asking a lot of tough questions. If Medicaid determines that your father lied on his application, kiss Medicaid funding good-bye. In fact, he may not have to worry about Medicaid at all if he lies on his application, because he may become entitled to free room and board—in jail! While there are lots of strategies available to protect your life savings, lying is definitely not one I would recommend.

CHAPTER 4 SUMMARY CHECKLIST

Why Can't Older People Protect Their Nest Eggs Just by Giving Them Away?

✔ Gifts or transfers of assets can be made to protect them from nursing-home costs.

✔ Most gifts or transfers trigger an ineligibility period for Medicaid benefits.

✔ To figure the ineligibility period, divide the value of the gift by the average cost of care set by the state.

✔ The maximum ineligibility period for gifts or transfers made on or before August 10, 1993, is thirty months; there is no cap on the ineligibility period for gifts or transfers after that date.

✔ The state can "look back" only thirty-six months for most gifts or transfers; transfers into irrevocable trusts may cause a sixty-month look-back period. In general, gifts or transfers made more than thirty-six months (sixty months if into an irrevocable trust) before your Medicaid application will *not* cause you to become ineligible for Medicaid benefits.

✔ Certain asset transfers do not disqualify a person from Medicaid no matter when he or she applies:

• A person (or spouse) can transfer his or her home, before or after entering a nursing home, to any of the following:

1. His or her spouse.
2. Any child who is under twenty-one, blind, or permanently and totally disabled.
3. A sibling who already has some ownership interest in the house and who was residing in the house for at least one year immediately before the person was admitted to a hospital or nursing home.
4. Any child who was residing in the house for at least two years immediately before the parent's admission to a nursing home or hospital and who provided care for the parent that allowed him or her to stay at home rather than in an institution.

• A person can transfer any other assets:

1. To his or her spouse.
2. To any child who is under twenty-one, blind, or permanently and totally disabled, or to a trust solely for the child's benefit.
3. To a trust solely for the benefit of a disabled individual under sixty-five years old.

• A person can transfer any assets that he or she intended to dispose of for market value.
• A person can transfer any assets solely for a purpose other than to qualify for Medicaid.
• A person can transfer any assets and still qualify for Medicaid if denying Medicaid would cause him or her an undue hardship.

5 | Estate Recoveries: The State Giveth and the State Taketh Away

The most devastating aspect of the new Medicaid law may be estate recoveries. Why? Because the special protection for the foundation of most families' estates—the family home—has been undermined.

As discussed earlier, Medicaid laws have provided and continue to provide special protection for the family residence. If one spouse enters a nursing home, he or she may qualify for Medicaid and the other spouse may keep the family residence for as long as that person continues to live there. For married couples, the house is exempt from the normal rules that require them to spend down their assets before becoming eligible for Medicaid benefits (see pages 19–20 and 33–34). Many states even allow unmarried nursing-home residents to keep their homes after spending other nonexempt assets (see pages 19–20 and table 3.6).

Under the old law, the house usually passed free and clear to the heirs at the owner's death. This simple transfer may be gone. Under the new OBRA 1993 law, your spouse can still keep the home when you qualify for Medicaid coverage. The critical difference is that now, when you both die, the state can force the sale of the house to recover the total cost of Medicaid benefits it paid for your nursing-home care. Your heirs could easily lose what was to be theirs.

The state will send in its band of bill collectors to grab the house and sell it, then use the money from the proceeds to pay itself back for the Medicaid benefits previously paid. The state may even put a lien on the house while you are still alive as a condition to receiving Medicaid! A lien makes it impossible to sell the property without the state's knowledge or ability to collect. Prior to OBRA 1993, a few states had estate recovery procedures; now all states are required to adopt similar programs.

In other words, unless you take steps to protect it, kiss the house good-bye.

Recoveries Against Estates and Liens

The state can go after assets from only two sources:

1. Assets held in the name (estate) of the Medicaid recipient when he or she dies (and the spouse dies, if applicable).
2. Assets against which a lien has been placed by the state.

ASSETS HELD AT DEATH

When a Medicaid recipient dies, he or she probably won't have much left, other than a home, household goods, other exempt assets, and up to $74,820 at the most. It is these assets that the state may grab when the Medicaid recipient (and spouse) dies.

The state can grab any assets in the deceased's name alone that would pass to heirs under a will at death. These are called probate assets.

What about assets that would avoid probate, such as bank accounts held jointly and survivorship with children or a home held in a standard revocable living trust? Can these assets be intercepted by the state too?

OBRA 1993 gives states the option to grab assets that would avoid probate. At this writing, few states have decided whether to exercise this option. If your state decides not to grab probate-avoiding assets, then a wise move would be to immediately transfer any assets remaining in the Medicaid recipient's name into holdings that avoid probate, such as a living trust.

NOTE: OBRA 1993 says that states may opt to go after a life estate, a planning tool that enables you to transfer ownership of your home or other real estate while still giving you the right to live there during your life (see pages 77 and 78). To allow the state to grab a life estate at death makes no sense, since a life estate ends when you die; at your demise, the property is given away and is no longer yours. So there should be nothing left for the state to grab at your death.

ALSO NOTE: California, Connecticut, Indiana, and New York adopted plans that allow individuals who purchased private long-term care insurance to shelter a portion of their assets from the state. Assets sheltered under these plans cannot be grabbed by the state. Under OBRA 1993, no other states may create similar programs.

If the Medicaid recipient dies leaving a surviving spouse or a child who is under age twenty-one, blind, or permanently and totally disabled, the state cannot grab any assets until that individual is deceased. In addition, the state must adopt procedures to waive estate recoveries that would cause an undue hardship to beneficiaries. What constitutes "undue hardship" will depend on your individual circumstances, but you'd better be prepared to prove your point if you intend to make such a claim.

LIMIT TO ASSETS OF MEDICAID RECIPIENT

The most significant limit on the state's power to grab the house and other assets is that the state can only go after assets in the Medicaid recipient's name at death, *not assets in the spouse's name*. The law prohibits the state from grabbing the spouse's assets. As you will see in chapter 6, this creates a wonderful planning opportunity—the house and any other assets should promptly be moved to the name of the spouse-at-home.

Unfortunately, it appears that at least a few states intend to violate the law and ignore this limitation by going after either spouse's assets. If this happens to you, contact a good elder law attorney for help.

LIENS

As mentioned earlier, the state may place a lien on the home of a Medicaid recipient while he or she is still alive. But this cannot be done while the spouse-at-home is living or while either of the following people reside in the home:

- A child who is under twenty-one, blind, or permanently and totally disabled.
- A sibling who has an equity interest in the home and who resided in the home for at least one year before the Medicaid recipient became institutionalized.

In addition, a lien cannot be put on a home without a hearing, where the state is required to prove that the Medicaid recipient is not likely to return home. This procedure prevents the state from automatically putting liens on all Medicaid applicants' homes as a precondition for receiving benefits.

If a lien does get put on your home, it must be removed when the institutionalized individual returns home. In other words, bringing an institutionalized person home may be a good way to remove a lien.

If a lien gets put on the home and the family wishes to sell the house, the state cannot take the proceeds while the spouse-at-home is still alive or any one of the following individuals resides in the home:

- A child who is under twenty-one, blind, or permanently and totally disabled.
- A sibling who has an equity interest in the home and who has lived there for at least one year before the Medicaid recipient became institutionalized.
- A child of the Medicaid recipient who lived in the home at least two years before the individual was institutionalized and who provided care that allowed the individual to stay at home for that time.

CHAPTER 5 SUMMARY CHECKLIST

Estate Recoveries: The State Giveth and the State Taketh Away

The most devastating impact of OBRA 1993 is the requirement that states adopt estate recoveries. Estate recoveries mean that many Medicaid recipients will lose their prize possession—the family home.

✔ If your state decides not to grab assets that avoid probate, move any assets remaining in the Medicaid recipient's name into a revocable living trust or other probate-avoidance holdings.

✔ The state can grab only assets in the name of the Medicaid recipient, not those of a spouse. Don't let the state violate the law without a fight.

✔ The state cannot put a lien on a Medicaid recipient's home if:

• The spouse-at-home is alive; or
• A child who is under twenty-one, blind, or permanently and totally disabled is living in the home; or
• A sibling who has an equity interest in the home and who resided in the home for at least one year before the Medicaid recipient became institutionalized is still living there.

✔ Before placing a lien on a Medicaid recipient's home, the state must prove that he or she is not likely to return home.

6

How Can You and Your Family Avoid the Medicaid Trap?

By this point you may be feeling pretty depressed—and for good reason. It's become clear that hard work and a savings plan don't count for much. Financial ruin due to nursing-home costs is just a catastrophic illness away.

Although the heartbreaking scenario described below happened to a gentleman from Maine, it could just as easily have been your neighbor, relative, or best friend:

> Here I sit, the loneliest man that ever lived. I have admitted my wife of 55 years to a nursing home. She has Alzheimer's and I am caught between a rock and a hard place. I can no longer provide the round-the-clock care she requires, and I will soon be unable to pay the costs of care she now gets, which have exhausted our $160,000 in savings.[1]

The politicians have made it as tough as possible to qualify for Medicaid. A person can't protect his or her assets just by transferring them when he or she is about to enter a nursing home. But without a crystal ball, who can predict whether an individual will go into a nursing home in thirty-six months or more?

So is there any practical way to juggle assets to qualify for Medicaid—before losing everything? The answer is yes. By adopting a Medicaid strategy that fits their needs, older Americans can avoid the Medicaid trap and keep their savings from flowing endlessly into a nursing home.

The options listed below will be discussed in sub-

sequent chapters. But don't jump ahead. Your very first step in planning starts right here—you need to analyze your current financial picture.

- Move money into exempt assets.
- Transfer assets directly to children tax-free.
- Pay children for their help.
- Juggle assets between spouses.
- Transfer a home while retaining a life estate.
- Change wills and titles to property, and create a revocable living trust.
- Write a durable power of attorney.
- Set up a Medicaid trust.
- Create a family asset protection trust.
- Put the home into a house preservation trust.
- Get a divorce.
- Purchase a long-term care insurance policy.

Analyze Your Current Financial Status

In order to choose the best strategies for protecting savings from a nursing home, you must first be aware of what resources you have and where they are located.

It's amazing—I can't tell you how many times clients come in to my office with no real idea about their assets. They may tell me they've got $100,000 in their estate, only to find out that the total is actually much higher once we sort out the papers they've brought in shopping bags and shoe boxes. The following worksheet is intended to assist in gathering

MEDICAID PLANNING WORKSHEET

Part A:
Assets

(Give market values where appropriate.) Assets	Your Name Alone	Spouse's Name Alone	Joint Names (Indicate who is named and how asset is titled—"or" and "and")
Residence	$ _____	$ _____	$ _____
Other Real Estate	_____	_____	_____
Cash and Equivalents Checking account(s)	_____ _____	_____ _____	_____ _____
Savings account(s)	_____ _____	_____ _____	_____ _____
CDs and money market account(s)	_____ _____ _____	_____ _____ _____	_____ _____ _____
Marketable Securities Stocks	_____ _____	_____ _____	_____ _____
Taxable bonds	_____ _____	_____ _____	_____ _____
Tax-exempt bonds	_____ _____	_____ _____	_____ _____
Mutual funds	_____ _____	_____ _____	_____ _____
Life Insurance (from part B)	_____	_____	_____
Business Interests (from part C)	_____	_____	_____

Retirement Plans
  Pension/Profit Sharing
  IRAs
	_____
	_____
		_____
		_____
			_____
			_____

Personal Property	_____	_____	_____
Other	_____	_____	_____
TOTAL ASSETS	$ _____	$ _____	_____
Expectancies *(i.e., inheritances)*	_____	_____	_____
TOTAL ASSETS AND EXPECTANCIES	$ _____	$ _____	$ _____

Part B:
Life Insurance

Company	Type	Face Value	Present Cash Value	Insured	Owner	Beneficiary
_____	_____	$_____	$_____	_____	_____	_____
_____	_____	$_____	$_____	_____	_____	_____
_____	_____	$_____	$_____	_____	_____	_____
_____	_____	$_____	$_____	_____	_____	_____
_____	_____	$_____	$_____	_____	_____	_____

TOTAL CASH VALUE OF LIFE INSURANCE

You: $ _____   Your spouse: $ _____

(Include these amounts on Life Insurance line in part A.)

Part C:
Business Interests*

Name of Business _____

Percentage of Interest Owned by
You: _____ %   Your spouse: _____ %   Jointly: _____ %

Percentage Owned by Children
Name _____   _____%
Name _____   _____%
Name _____   _____%

Tax Basis of Business (if you know) $ _____

Book Value of Business (if you know) $ _____

YOUR ESTIMATE OF PRESENT VALUE OF BUSINESS
You: _____ %   Your spouse: _____%   Jointly: _____ %

(Include these amounts on Business Interests line in Part A.)

*This information might be found in a corporate record book, a partnership K-1 form, or possibly on a tax return.

Part D:
Appreciated Assets*

Assets	Purchase Price	Improvements (To real estate)	Current Market Value
Stock	$ _____	$ _____	$ _____
	_____	_____	_____
	_____	_____	_____
	_____	_____	_____
Real Estate *(including home)*	_____	_____	_____
	_____	_____	_____
	_____	_____	_____
Partnerships	_____	_____	_____
	_____	_____	_____
	_____	_____	_____
Other	_____	_____	_____
	_____	_____	_____
	_____	_____	_____

*This may overlap with amounts listed in Part A.

Part E:
Income

Type of Income	Your Monthly Income	Spouse's Monthly Income	Total Monthly Income
Net Salary or Wages *("take-home pay")*	$ _____	$ _____	$ _____
Social Security Benefits	_____	_____	_____
Retirement Benefits	_____	_____	_____
Interest	_____	_____	_____
Dividends	_____	_____	_____
Other	_____	_____	_____
TOTAL INCOME	$ _____	$ _____	$ _____

Part F:
Liabilities

(Give outstanding balances.) Liabilities	Your Name	Spouse's Name	Joint Names
Residence			
Primary Mortgage	$ _____	$ _____	$ _____
Second Mortgage	_____	_____	_____
Other Real Estate Mortgages	_____	_____	_____
Personal Loans	_____	_____	_____
Income Taxes	_____	_____	_____
Other Debts	_____	_____	_____
TOTAL LIABILITIES	$ _____	$ _____	$ _____

Part G:
Net Worth

	Your Name	Spouse's Name	Joint Names
Total Assets (from part A)	$ _____	$ _____	$ _____
minus			
Total Liabilities (from part F)	_____	_____	_____
NET WORTH (Assets minus liabilities)	$ _____	$ _____	$ _____

Part H:
Gifts

Gifts made in excess of $500 to an individual other than your spouse within the last three years:

Recipient _____	Date _____	Amount $ _____
Recipient _____	Date _____	Amount $ _____
Recipient _____	Date _____	Amount $ _____
Recipient _____	Date _____	Amount $ _____

the financial information necessary to design and implement your asset protection plan.

This worksheet is divided into eight sections: Assets, Life Insurance, Business Interests, Appreciated Interests, Income, Liabilities, Net Worth, and Gifts.

After completing the Medicaid Planning Worksheet, you will be ready to consider the options available for protecting your nest egg.

If you can't fill in all of the information, don't worry—and don't give up! Just do the best you can, because whatever you can supply will be helpful.

Taking this worksheet with you when meeting with an experienced elder law attorney not only will save you time and money, it will also enable the lawyer to give you the most comprehensive and personalized advice.

You now have an understanding of the critical problems facing older Americans, you understand the basics of the Medicaid laws, and you've organized your assets. Ready to move on to the "good stuff"? Let's see how you can protect your savings.

7 | Move Money Into
Exempt Assets and Pay Debts

Probably the easiest and often one of the best planning techniques available is moving savings into exempt, or protected, assets. As discussed in chapter 3, certain assets, by law, are removed from Medicaid's reach. By putting money into these exempt assets, an elderly person or couple can preserve their savings.

"Shelter" Money in the Home

For most people, the home is their largest asset. It is automatically protected as long as a spouse is living there (see pages 19–20 and 33–34). For a married couple, this makes the family home a wonderful shelter for money and other assets that would otherwise have to be spent on nursing-home costs. Even for unmarried people who intend to remain home (see pages 19–20 and table 3.6), putting money into the residence can protect those funds. (Keep in mind that the new estate recovery laws may require you to take some additional steps to protect the home.)

When I say that putting money into the home can protect it, I am *not* telling you to pull your funds out of the bank, put them into a shoe box, and hide them in the basement—*don't do that!* What I am saying is that you can pay off the mortgage, replace your thirty-year-old roof, waterproof the basement, fix the garage, buy a new water heater, furnace, or air-conditioning, repair the driveway, lower cabinets and add ramps for easier handicapped living or put on an addition. The benefits of paying off a mortgage and making home improvements and repairs are both immediate and long-term: you get to enjoy an improved environment, your home's resale value is enhanced, and, best of all, your assets are now protected from the nursing home's grasp.

MAKE HOME IMPROVEMENTS AND REPAIRS

Putting money into home improvements and repairs can serve to protect a hard-earned nest egg. As long as the improvements add value to the home or make life easier for a spouse remaining there, this strategy may be a perfect way to keep at least some of a family's savings from flying out the window.

Example 26

Your mother is doing pretty well, but your father is not and must enter a nursing home. On the date he enters, they have $100,000 total assets plus a house. They must first spend $48,000 (roughly one-half of the liquid assets) before he can get Medicaid to cover his nursing-home bills; your mother will be able to keep only $50,000 (one-half of the total assets) plus the residence (your father also gets $2,000).

To lose $48,000 would hurt and might leave your mother in a precarious financial position. This is especially true because the home now needs a lot of work. As your father's illness worsened over the years, they were afraid to spend money on the house. If your mother is left with only $50,000 after paying for the nursing home, she may not have enough to keep the house in good repair. Is there any way for them to protect more of their savings? The answer is yes.

They redo the kitchen, replace the leaking roof, and add aluminum siding. The furnace is twenty-five years old, so they buy a new one. To reduce winter heating bills, they add insulation and replace the windows. Since your mother is having trouble climbing the stairs, they add a bedroom and bathroom to the first floor. Total cost: $48,000.

The next day, your mother goes to Medicaid and applies for benefits. Since they've spent $48,000, your father qualifies immediately. They haven't really lost anything, because they've added value to the home and made it more livable for your mother; they've also cut the likely need for major home repairs. No gifts or transfers to any third person were made, so there's no waiting or ineligibility period. By this one simple technique, they've protected $48,000 that otherwise would have been consumed by nursing-home charges.

In example 26, your parents had $100,000 of unprotected assets on the date of your father's institutionalization. That's the "snapshot" date—the time that is used to measure your parents' total assets (even though they don't apply for Medicaid until later).

Since the total was $100,000, your mother is allowed to keep half, $50,000 (the funds don't have to be moved into your mother's name before making the Medicaid application, although they should be moved into her name promptly after applying for Medicaid), and your father gets $2,000. The rest, $48,000, must somehow "disappear." Most people spend it all on the nursing home. But as example 26 shows, the $48,000 can be protected by moving the funds into exempt assets.

For more on the timing of using this planning tool, see page 58.

Of course, money in a home isn't as liquid as money in stocks or bank accounts. But it is still reachable if needed. For example, combining this strategy with a reverse mortgage might be a perfect way to shelter assets while increasing income as well. A reverse mortgage provides the homeowner with a monthly income; the mortgage grows as the payments are made. But the mortgage generally does not have to be repaid until the homeowner dies. Detailed information on reverse mortgages and their

benefits is provided in *Golden Opportunities: Money Saving Strategies from Government Programs Everyone Should Know About* (Henry Holt, 1994), by Amy and Armond Budish.

PAY OFF A MORTGAGE

If your parents still have a mortgage on the home, they can pay it off. As example 27 shows, this too can provide a wonderful shelter.

Example 27

Your husband soon will be going into a nursing home. Together you have $50,000 and a house. If you do nothing, you'll have to spend down $25,000 before Medicaid will cover any of his costs.

There is $25,000 left on your home mortgage. When Medicaid figures your and your husband's assets, they don't subtract unpaid liabilities. Pay off the mortgage, though, and the next day you will qualify for Medicaid. The $25,000 that you have to spend does not have to go to a nursing home—paying the mortgage is just fine!

Of course, you can mix and match—you might use some funds to pay a mortgage and other funds to make home repairs or improvements. The money is being protected one way or the other.

What if you don't have a mortgage? Many older Americans own their homes free and clear. Can this strategy still be used? The answer is yes—you may take a mortgage and then pay it off, as shown by example 28.

Example 28

Take the same facts as in example 27, except that you and your husband own the house free and clear. Can you still protect some portion of your $50,000 nest egg?

The week before he enters a nursing home, you take out a $50,000 mortgage loan on your home. If you can take the loan from your kids or other relatives, you can avoid paying any points or fees. You now have a $50,000 mortgage and another $50,000 cash.

When your husband enters a nursing home, Medicaid takes a "snapshot" of your assets. On that day you have combined assets of $100,000 (not $50,000, thanks to the recent loan) plus the house. Medicaid won't subtract your debts (for example, the mortgage) from your cash assets.

Now you've got to spend $50,000 before he qualifies for Medicaid (one-half of the $100,000). You take $50,000 from your cash and pay off the mortages. Voilà—your husband qualifies for Medicaid and you get to keep the entire $50,000 that you originally had!

Note that this strategy of taking and then turning around and paying a mortgage is an aggressive planning technique. While it has been used effectively in some states, there is no guarantee that it will work for you. Talk to a lawyer with expertise in elder law before trying this on your own.

BUY A HOME

If your parents don't own a house or condominium, they could buy one. The same principle applies—take assets that could be reached by the nursing home and make them unreachable by sheltering them in a home. Again, since buying a home is *not* a gift or transfer of assets to a third person, there is no ineligibility period. This strategy can be used the day an individual is about to enter a nursing home.

There's no limit on the value of a house that can be bought. Whether the house is worth $50,000 or $250,000 makes no difference; if it is protected under the rules described earlier (see pages 19–20 and 33–34), purchasing a home can shelter some or all of a family's savings.

Example 29

Your parents are renting an apartment. They have combined assets of $200,000 when your father becomes ill. After he enters a nursing home, your mother will be allowed to keep only $74,820.

She takes $130,000 and buys a condominium in a retirement community. Since she now has less than $74,820, the next day, she can get Medicaid coverage for the nursing-home charges. Your father has Medicaid benefits, your mother has a safe, friendly place to live, and the condominium is protected.

If your parents already own a home, they may purchase a more expensive one, as shown in example 30.

Example 30

Your parents own a home worth $75,000. They have combined additional savings of $200,000. As in example 29, your mother would be allowed to keep only $74,820.

Your parents sell their home, netting $70,000. Your mother then adds $130,000 from their savings and buys a $200,000 home complete with special adaptations for seniors. Presto, change-o—your father qualifies for Medicaid.

For some people, moving assets into the purchase of a home can be an effective way to protect part or all of a life's savings. But, of course, not everybody wants to buy a house. If your parents are in an apartment, the reason might be that they didn't want the headaches of home ownership. In that case, buying a house to protect assets from nursing-home charges may not be practical for them.

In addition, buying a home or making home improvements can be a problem for someone preoccupied with caring for a loved one. A caregiver is likely to be emotionally and physically exhausted and may not have the energy or will to cope with buying a house or making improvements. Buying a home or hiring home repair contractors creates its own stress, perhaps requiring dealing with a bank, real estate agent, or attorney. In the right circumstances, buying a home or making home repairs or improvements can provide a nice shelter for both assets and owner, but no one strategy works for everyone.

Purchase Household Goods, Personal Items, or a Car

All states allow a nursing-home resident to protect some household goods and personal items, such as furniture and clothing. If the person is married, household goods, a car, and personal effects are protected *without regard to their value.*

This exemption offers an excellent way to protect assets. Is it time to buy a new refrigerator? Is the stove on its last legs? Instead of "making do," this may be the time to buy replacements.

Example 31

Your father has just been admitted to a nursing home, and it looks like he'll be there for the rest of his life. Together your parents have $50,000, so they must spend down $23,000 (half of the total less the $2,000 your father is allotted) before Medicaid will step in to help.

Your mother plans to visit her husband every day. The drive is fifteen miles round-trip, and her eight-year-old car is starting to need major repairs.

She takes $15,000 and buys a new car. Now she has a new, safer car to drive and only $8,000 will have to be spent on the nursing home before Medicaid coverage begins.

Be careful when using this strategy. State bureaucrats usually will not challenge you if you purchase basics like a car, furniture, or clothing. But if your taste becomes too exotic, you could be asking for trouble.

Example 32

Same facts as in example 31, except that instead of buing a new car, your mother buys a $15,000 Oriental rug. She claims that it's a household good and should be exempt. But the state may argue that it's really an investment, not a household good, and so still counts against you. Do you really want to do battle with the state? Probably not.

Protect Property Essential to Support

As discussed on pages 19–20 and in table 3.7), income-producing property used in connection with a trade or business is completely exempt; nonbusiness property that produces goods or services and is essential to a person's support is exempt up to $6,000 in value.

As example 33 shows, this protection can be a critical one.

Example 33

Your mother runs a bookkeeping service from her home. In connection with the business, she maintains a computer, software programs, and a van for house calls. When your father goes into a nursing home, your mother should be permitted to keep her business property so that she can maintain her income.

Some planners have even argued that managing a portfolio of stocks and bonds is a business, and so the stocks and bonds should be protected under this exemption. However, the Medicaid bureaucrats and courts have not yet agreed.

For farm owners, the land and equipment may all be exempt as income-producing property. Farmland that abuts the home is covered by the protection for a home in most states anyway.

When it comes to planning, the same principle applies here as it did above: if the person has a small, productive family business, he or she should consider protecting assets by upgrading equipment and making other necessary improvements.

Buy Family Burial Plots and Prepay Funeral Costs

After spending their life savings on long-term nursing-home care, some older Americans have been left without enough money for a proper burial. The nursing-home resident can avoid this sad conclusion by prepaying for burial plots and funeral costs.

Everyone dies sometime—that's a fact of life. Why not pay for your funeral and your final resting place out of funds that would otherwise go to your temporary residence, the nursing home? These costs are not cheap; by prepaying for funerals and burial plots, a couple can easily shelter $10,000 or more.

Of course, don't go overboard burying money in cemetery plots. Unlike a house or household goods, funerals are not assets that can be passed on to heirs.

Pay Off Debts

I've already explained how paying off a mortgage can help shelter assets that would have to go to a nursing home. That technique is beneficial because when calculating the amount of your assets, Medicaid will not subtract your unpaid debts from the total. For the same reason, paying off credit cards, car loans, and other debts can also be a wise move.

Example 34

Your parents have savings of $50,000. When your father goes into a nursing home, your mother gets to keep $25,000 (half of the $50,000), your father keeps $2,000, and $23,000 must be spent. If they pay all $23,000 to the nursing home, your father will qualify for Medicaid, but they will still owe debts of $10,000. When your mother pays those off, she'll be left with only $17,000 to live on.

There's a better way. If they pay off the $7,000 car loan and the $3,000 credit card debt, they will have only $10,000 left to pay to the nursing home, and your mom will be debt-free.

If you know that a parent will be going into a nursing home, hold off paying debts until *after* institutionalization. Do what you have to do—tell creditors that the check's in the mail if you have to in order to buy time. Then, once your parent has entered a nursing home, you can pay off the balance. Compare example 35 with example 34.

Example 35

Take the same facts as in example 34: $50,000 of assets and $10,000 of debts. If your parents pay the debts *before* your father enters the nursing home, they'll have combined assets of $40,000 on the date of institutionalization. Your mother and father will be allowed to keep only $22,000 (half of the $40,000 plus your father's $2,000). In example 34, when your parents' debts were paid *after* your father was institutionalized, your parents were able to keep $27,000—$5,000 more!

Prepay Upcoming Costs

To further reduce your assets for Medicaid qualification, you may prepay some upcoming costs.

Example 36

You and your husband had $50,000 when your husband entered a nursing home. He will not be able to qualify for Medicaid until your savings has been spent down to $27,000.

After moving some of the funds into exempt assets and spending some on your husband's care, the total is down to $28,500—just a little too high. Is there anything else you can do?

Consider spending some money on up-coming costs. For example, you might prepay this year's homeowner's insurance, real estate taxes, utilities, and condo maintenance fee. Don't go overboard, or the Medicaid bureaucrats may say your prepayment is an asset. But these kinds of payments should be allowed if within reason.

As you can see, paying bills and moving assets to Medicaid-proof exemptions can pay off. That's exactly how Beverly Newton and Ludvik Roch were able to shelter part of their life savings.

Beverly Newton:

My husband was diagnosed in 1989 as possible Alzheimer's, and he was doing rather well until Easter when he got violent. He was taken to the hospital and he was there just over a week, and then we had to put him in a nursing home, where he is today. He could be in a nursing home for another 10, 20 years. That's one horror of this disease, you can't plan, you don't know how long it's going to last or what condition they are going to be in or when certain levels are going to appear. It's very difficult.

We also had to spend down. We're in the process of doing that and we plan to make home improvements . . . rather than lose our money completely.[1]

Ludvik Roch:

According to the regulations, half of our savings was my wife's, so I had to spend that half. Some of it went to the nursing home. I bought an automobile, put on a new bathroom if by chance my wife would ever come home. On a colonial I had two baths but I needed one for her on the first floor, so I'm putting that in now. And I paid for a couple of funerals, so I've got that taken care of.[2]

Take a look at the following examples to see how shifting assets into exemptions can provide useful protection.

Example 37

At the time your father enters a nursing home, he and your mother have combined assets of $200,000, excluding the value of their house. Your mother is allowed only the $74,820 maximum; your father is allowed $2,000; the rest ($123,180) must be spent down or somehow protected.

Your father immediately transfers the home into your mother's name. The house has an $80,000 mortgage, which they pay off. Your mother buys a few things for the house and makes some necessary repairs, for a $15,000 total cost. Finally, she buys burial plots and prepays funeral costs for your father and herself, for a total of $13,000.

Instead of spending $123,180 entirely on nursing-home care, your parents have sheltered most of it. They moved $108,000 into exemptions, your mother gets to keep $74,820, and your father keeps $2,000. The nursing home now gets only about $15,000 of your parents' funds before Medicaid will step in. By taking these steps, your parents were able *legally* to protect $108,000 that would otherwise have disappeared, cut their monthly expenses (by eliminating the mortgage payments), and benefit from home improvements.

Example 38

At the time your father enters a nursing home, he and your mother have $30,000 and a home. Your mother would have to spend $13,000 before Medicaid would cover his bills.

Instead of pouring the $13,000 down the nursing-home drain, your mother purchases exempt assets. She spends $7,000 to prepay for funerals for her and your father. The stove, refrigerator, washer, and dryer are twenty years old, so she spends $2,500 to replace them. She needs a newer car, so she trades in her car and spends another $3,000 for that. Finally, neither your mother nor your father has bought clothes in years, so $500 goes for a few new items.

Now that they've spent down, your father immediately qualifies for Medicaid. Rather than going to the nursing home, their $13,000 has been used to make your parents' lives a little more comfortable.

Example 39

Your mother, a widow, has just entered a nursing home. She has $10,000 in the bank—well

over the $2,000 Medicaid limit. If she does nothing, $8,000 of her $10,000 will be spent on the nursing home in no time flat.

Her first step is to prepay for her funeral—that is $4,000. She doesn't drive, so getting a car doesn't make much sense for her. But you would like to visit her and have no easy way to get to the nursing home so she might want to spend $4,500 to get a car that you could use. And what do you know? Your mother now qualifies for Medicaid!

Watch the Timing

The timing for changing unprotected assets into protected assets is critical, especially for married couples. Although you may be anxious to take steps to protect your nest egg, it generally pays to wait until one spouse has entered the nursing home.

Let's go back to example 37. After your father entered a nursing home, your parents had combined assets of $200,000. Your mother then moved $108,000 into exemptions (paid off a mortgage, made home repairs, and prepaid funerals). The nursing home would receive only about $15,000; the remaining $185,000 is protected ($108,000 spent on exemptions and the $76,820 your parents are allowed by law to keep).

But if your mother had acted too quickly, she would have lost a great deal of benefit. Let's say she moved the $108,000 into exemptions *before* your father was institutionalized. On the date of his entry into a nursing home, they would have $92,000 of unprotected assets. Your mother would get to keep $46,000 (one-half of the total), your father could keep $2,000, and the nursing home would take $44,000. In other words, by acting too fast, your parents would have unnecessarily spent an extra $29,000 on the nursing home.

Why it is better to wait if you are going to move money into exemptions? Because the snapshot of assets is taken on the date of continuous institutionalization—usually the date of entry into the nursing home. Debts paid and exempt items purchased before institutionalization are paid by the Medicaid applicant and the spouse; after institutionalization, the government helps pick up the tab.

CHAPTER 7 SUMMARY CHECKLIST

Move Money Into Exempt Assets and Pay Debts

Shelter Money in the Home

✔ Make home improvements and repairs.

✔ Pay off a mortgage.

✔ Buy a home.

Purchase Household Goods, Personal Items, or a Car

Protect Property Essential to Support

Buy Family Burial Plots and Prepay Funeral Costs

Pay Off Debts

Prepay Upcoming Costs

Make Asset Protection Payments After *a Spouse Is Institutionalized*

8 Give Your Money Away

You can't have much in the way of assets if you want Uncle Sam to help pay the nursing-home tab through Medicaid. How about giving away your life savings rather than spending it on nursing-home bills? The law says that's OK.

But as explained earlier, a person cannot give away assets and immediately qualify for Medicaid. You can't write a check to your children, pull your pockets inside out, walk into the Medicaid office, and expect coverage. Almost every gift or transfer of assets triggers a waiting period for Medicaid benefits. While it's perfectly legal to give away your savings, you will have to wait until the ineligibility period runs out before coverage will kick in (see chapter 4 for details on how the ineligibility period works).

Although you may have to wait as long as three years, making a gift or transfer can still be an extremely valuable strategy. Most middle-class Americans, whether single or married, can benefit by giving away assets, as example 40 demonstrates.

Example 40

Your father has $150,000 and his income (Social Security, interest, and dividends) is $20,000 a year. If he goes into a nursing home and fails to use our planning tools, he'll spend all but about $2,000 before Medicaid will pay a penny.

If he gives away the assets, he won't be eligible to receive Medicaid benefits for three years from the date of the gift. But after that three years has passed, Medicaid will cover his costs.

Even if he has done no advance planning and is about to enter a nursing home, giving away assets may be very wise. Let's say he gives his children the $150,000 on the day he enters a nursing home. The home costs $40,000 a year—$20,000 more than his income.

The first year the children will use the interest and dividends, as well as his Social Security, to pay the nursing home. The children also will have to supplement the income with $20,000 of principal from his transferred assets. The second year the same thing is done: his income and about $25,000 of principal (probably slightly more than the year before, owing to increased prices and reduced income) is used to pay the nursing-home costs. And for the third year, the same procedure is followed. At the end of three years, the $150,000 pot has been cut to about $80,000.

But here's the great benefit: after the three years have passed, the remaining $80,000 is protected and Medicaid will start to pay your father's bills. Although not ideal, just remember that without the transfer your father's assets would continue to dwindle to nothing.

How Much Should Be Gifted?

Once they've decided to give away assets, many people go all the way, giving away their entire savings. That can be a major mistake.

A person who transfers everything becomes completely dependent on others, and that's never a good situation. If you have handed over the bank accounts and property to your children and then need money later, you'd better pray that they'll take care of you. And if a child dies or becomes divorced, your money may end up in the hands of an in-law. I don't think I have to tell any in-law jokes here—if your money passes to in-laws, your financial security could be in serious jeopardy. I'll talk more later about the risks of gifting and how you might minimize those risks. But certainly one good way to reduce or eliminate your dependence on others is to keep at least part of your savings.

Making gifts of part, but not all, of your nest egg can be wise for another reason, too. Since the length of the ineligibility period for Medicaid benefits, triggered by gifts or transfers, depends on the amount gifted, you may be able to save more money by gifting only part of your savings rather than giving it all away. Compare examples 41 and 42.

Example 41

You have CDs totaling $110,000 that make up your entire estate. It looks like you'll be entering a nursing home soon, and your Social Security and pension benefits of $1,000 a month won't come near to covering the $4,000 monthly charges.

If you give your kids the entire $110,000 and the average cost of nursing home care set by the state is $3,000 a month, you'll have to wait thirty-six months for Medicaid benefits. Over that time, your children will have to spend just about the entire amount of your CDs to cover the costs: they'll have to spend $3,000 a month from your principal to supplement your $1,000-a-month Social Security and pension income. At the end of thirty-six months, when you can get Medicaid, your life savings are gone.

Example 42

Let's take the same facts as in example 41, except this time you give your children only $54,000, and you keep $56,000.

The $54,000 gift triggers an eighteen-month period of ineligibility, not a thirty-six month waiting period (see pages 37–38). To pay the $4,000 monthly nursing-home bill, you'll again need $3,000 a month from your remaining CDs to supplement your $1,000 monthly income. Over eighteen months, your $56,000 will be spent, but when the eighteen-month ineligibility period expires, you qualify for Medicaid. And the $54,000 transferred to your children is protected.

Can Parents Require Children to Use Gifted Assets for Them?

If you could just require your children to use gifted funds for your benefit and to return them as you need them, much of the risk of making gifts would disappear. So why not condition gifts on your children, signing an agreement to return funds to you on your request?

The answer is simple: parents *cannot* put strings on gifts. If they do, they haven't really made gifts, and they won't qualify for Medicaid.

Parents' gifts to their children just to beat Medicaid, with the understanding that the assets are really to be used for the parents' benefit, could be considered a life-care contract, which would constitute an asset of the parents with a value that could disqualify them from receiving Medicaid. And in rare circumstances, the transfer of assets to children with such an "understanding" could be considered Medicaid fraud and/or tax fraud, exposing the parents to possible criminal penalties.

For all of these reasons, parents should be careful when considering whether to use gifts to children or others as a technique to keep their savings from the nursing home.

Look-Back Gifting

Remember I told you (pages 38–39) that the state will look at all gifts or transfers within the three-year look-back period, add them up, and then calculate the ineligibility period from the date of the first transfer? This may actually work to your advantage.

Example 43

On February 3, 1994, your mother made a $10,000 gift to the kids. Then in April 1995 she enters a nursing home, and she makes a $26,000 gift. She applies for Medicaid immediately. Can she qualify? Doesn't the $26,000 gift she just made render her ineligible for Medicaid?

According to OBRA 1993, the $26,000 and $10,000 gifts within the look-back period should be added together, and the ineligibility period begins to run *from the date of the earliest gift*, February 1994. At a $3,000-a-month average cost of care, the penalty period would be twelve months ($36,000 divided by $3,000 a month)—February 1994 through January 1995. Your mother should qualify for Medicaid benefits in April 1995, even though she just gave a large gift.

The making of look-back gifts can be a useful planning tool. To take full advantage of this opportunity, older Americans may wish to make small gifts to family members every few months. Then if a nursing-home stay is ever required, a large gift may be made at the last minute, without causing a loss of Medicaid benefits, because the ineligibility period will run starting from the date of the earliest gift within the three-year look-back period.

Example 44

Your dad makes a $2,000 gift to you once every three months ($8,000 a year), and he continues this practice for several years. He then enters a nursing home in March 1997. At that time he makes a $77,000 transfer to you—the rest of his funds—and applies for Medicaid in April 1997. Looking back three years from the Medicaid application, to April 1994, we find that your father made a total of $22,000 in gifts to you over the years. Adding the $77,000 gift in March 1997, he made total gifts within the look-back period of $99,000. Since the first gift within the look-back period was in May 1994, the ineligibility period of 33 months ($99,000 divided by the average cost of care of $3,000 a month) has ended, and your dad can get Medicaid, even though his last gift was very large.

If your parent hasn't been making look-back gifts regularly and is now entering a nursing home, check his past gift-giving record carefully. If you can find a gift within the last thirty-six months, say for a wedding or holiday, that gift may be used as a look-back gift to allow your parent to make a large gift now without jeopardizing his or her Medicaid eligibility.

NOTE: The federal Health Care Financing Administration, which has realized how beneficial look-back gifting can be, is now saying that this technique cannot be used, and states may adopt HCFA's position. However, the language of OBRA 1993 supports look-back gifting. While this planning tool should be viable, consult with an elder law attorney before using this strategy.

Make Gifts That Trigger No Ineligibility Period

Not every gift or transfer triggers an ineligibility period. As explained on page 40, certain transfers can be made with *no* penalty. If any of these transfers are available to you, they can provide valuable protection. Take a look at examples 45, 46, and 47.

Example 45

You are a widow, and your hard-earned nest egg totals $100,000. You recognize that your deteriorating health may cause you to need long-term care soon, and you'd like to make sure your legally blind daughter benefits from your savings.

If you give the money to your daughter, will you be prevented from getting Medicaid benefits for three years? Since your daughter is legally blind, the answer is no. There is no penalty for transferring any assets to a child who is blind or permanently and totally disabled.

Example 46

Your home is by far your largest asset. Your son has been living with you and taking care of you for the last several years. When you go into a nursing home, will he be forced out so that the house can be sold to pay the nursing-home bills? No.

The house can be transferred to your son with no penalty, since he has lived with you and cared for you for more than two years. Once your other assets are spent down to the required limits, you'll be eligible for Medicaid, and the home will be protected. Once transferred to your son, he may choose to continue to live in the house himself, rent it out, or sell it.

Example 47

You and your sister have been living in your home for years. You are now entering a nursing home, and you are afraid your sister will be put on the street if you lose the house.

If you simply transfer the entire house to your sister, you'll trigger a long waiting period. For example, if the home is worth $90,000 and the average cost of care in your state is $3,000 a month, the ineligibility period will be thirty months.

But let's say instead you sell your sister a one-tenth interest for $9,000 (one-tenth of the $90,000 value). Then you give her the rest of the home. There will be *no* ineligibility period, since you now come under the special rule for transfers to a sibling with an equity interest in the home. The law does not specify any time period that the sibling must have held an equity interest prior to the transfer; the only time period in the law is that the sibling must have lived in the home for at least a year before the Medicaid applicant was institutionalized.

Some experts argue that it should be possible to transfer any exempt assets other than a house to *anyone*, at *any time*, without penalty. Since gifts that are not made to qualify for Medicaid are not penalized, and since transferring exempt assets will not qualify a person for Medicaid (the assets are already exempt), the argument goes that transfers of exempt assets should not trigger any penalty. Consult with an experienced lawyer to determine how your state handles this argument.

Why worry about transferring exempt assets? After all, since they're exempt, they won't be included as assets for Medicaid purposes. But they may not always be exempt, as example 48 demonstrates.

Example 48

Your mother is in a nursing home. She has paintings and jewelry worth $15,000. While your father is alive, all of that is exempt. But should he die, only $2,000 would remain exempt and the rest would have to be sold to pay your mother's nursing-home costs.

Had your mother transferred her assets to you while they were exempt, before your father died, they would have been protected even

after he passed away. Then if she recovered enough to return home, you could return the assets.

Pay Children for Their Help

So far I've been talking about making gifts or transfers to children or others while receiving nothing in return. As you now know, when you do this you trigger a Medicaid ineligibility period.

If you transfer assets but receive something of fair value in return, then you have not triggered any penalty period. Paying children for help, or paying room and board while living with them, fall into this category.

Let's say that you have been helping your widowed mother with a variety of chores—driving her to the store, doing her banking, preparing meals. Maybe you have even moved into her house to provide full-time care. She could transfer assets without worrying about the transfer-ineligibility rules by paying you for services rendered.

This can be a very helpful technique if used carefully—Medicaid personnel are likely to scrutinize payments to children. Only reasonable payments can be made—for instance, a parent can't pay a child $2,000 each time the child drives him or her to the store and expect Medicaid to overlook it. But if full-time care provided at home costs $40,000 a year in your area, a child providing the same services could be fairly compensated that same amount.

Of course, most children helping their parents do so without any expectation of payment. And that's as it should be. But if a parent will be going into a nursing home, consider using a portion of assets to pay a reasonable amount for services rendered.

The Medicaid bureaucrats may presume that payments to children are really gifts (and thus should trigger an ineligibility period). To bolster your argument that the children should be allowed payments for actual services, treat the arrangements—in advance, if possible—as if it were truly an employer-employee relationship.

Put the agreement between parent and child in writing, with as much detail as possible. For example, state that the child agrees to prepare three meals per day, bathe the parent every other day, administer medications as needed, and do light housekeeping. In exchange, the parent agrees to pay a fixed amount of money per week. Both parent and child should sign the contract.

To set the price, get an independent estimate for services. One way to do this is to write a list of everything the child will be doing and submit it to an independent business that provides home care. Get a written estimate from the company and use it to fix a reasonable price for the child's services. Keep the independent estimate in your records in case the Medicaid officials ever challenge the basis for the fee.

A written contract made *in advance* of providing services is best. What if you've been helping a parent without any written agreement—can you collect "back pay"? The answer may be yes, but usually only if you convince the state Medicaid bureaucrats that you and your parent had an unwritten agreement or understanding that you would be compensated for your services. Proving your claim probably will not be easy. Statements from you, your parent, and anyone else who knew of the arrangement will help. Proof that you gave up other employment or other opportunities for employment to help your parent may also indicate that you expected compensation.

If the parent is living with the child, the parent may also pay room and board. After all, why should the child have to absorb the costs for food and shelter from his or her own pocketbook?

Again, fix a reasonable fee—don't be greedy. Call a real estate agent and get a written estimate for a fair rental fee for a room in a house under similar arrangements. Keep receipts for food in case the folks at Medicaid want proof. And put the terms in writing, signed by you and your spouse.

Be Aware of the Tax Laws

When we talk about making gifts or transfers to qualify for Medicaid coverage, we also need to discuss how the tax laws come into play. Three types of federal taxes may be involved: (1) gift or transfer tax, (2) capital gains tax, and (3) income tax. If you are careful, none of these should pose a problem.

GIFT OR TRANSFER TAXES

I probably get more questions about gift taxes than anything else. The most common question: "If I give

away more than $10,000, won't I have to pay tax?" The answer is no, unless the total estate of the gift giver is worth more than $600,000.

People generally have heard about two laws. First, many people understand that anyone can make gifts of up to $10,000 per person each year without paying any federal gift tax. Second, people also understand that at death, a person can leave to heirs as much as $600,000 without any federal estate tax. But most people do not understand how these two rules fit together.

The $600,000 federal estate tax credit is also a lifetime gift tax credit. A person who gives away more than $10,000 can avoid a gift tax by using up the $600,000 estate tax credit.

Example 49

You give away $110,000 to your daughter this year. The first $10,000 is always free of any gift tax. You can avoid paying a gift tax on the other $100,000 by reducing your estate tax credit by $100,000. In other words, at death you would then be allowed to leave only $500,000 ($600,000 minus $100,000) free of federal estate tax.

Does this sound complicated? Let me simplify the rule: *As long as your total estate is worth less than $600,000, you can give away the whole thing to anyone at any time with no federal gift tax during life and no federal estate tax at death.*

The recipient of a gift never pays any gift or income tax under any circumstances. The only responsibility of the recipient is to pay income taxes on the income subsequently generated by the gift.

Example 50

Your mother transfers $200,000 to you as part of her Medicaid plan. Neither of you pays any tax on the gift. You invest the $200,000 in CDs paying 5% interest, or $10,000 a year. Your only obligation is to pay income taxes on the $10,000 of interest, just like you pay income taxes on any interest received from investments.

A person who makes a gift of more than $10,000 should file a federal gift tax return, which is pretty simple to do. There won't be any gift tax—Uncle Sam just wants to keep track of the transfer so that he knows whether a person is making gifts of more than $600,000 during his or her lifetime.

CAPITAL GAINS TAXES

While you usually don't have to worry about a gift tax, you may have to think about capital gains taxes if you give away appreciated assets, such as your home. Appreciated assets are those that have gone up in value since you first obtained them, and often include stocks, real estate, paintings, and antiques. Capital gains taxes are charged (at normal income tax rates) on profits made when anything that has increased in value is sold; the initial purchase price (the "basis") is *not* taxed. Giving appreciated assets away to children or others will mean that the recipients will pay these taxes when *they* sell. Depending on the amount of the tax, you may be better off *not* making gifts of appreciated assets. Compare examples 51, 52, and 53.

Example 51

Your mother bought her house thirty years ago for $20,000; today it's worth $120,000. She also bought shares of stock for $2,000, which now are valued at $102,000. Since your mother is worried about the impact of nursing-home costs on her savings, she gives you the home and stock as a present. Remember, there's no gift tax.

After she dies, you sell the house and stock for $222,000. You'd better get out your checkbook. You'll owe Uncle Sam a capital gains tax on the $200,000 profit ($222,000 minus the $22,000 basis). The tax will cost you about $56,000.

Example 52

Same facts as example 51, except that your mother keeps the house and stock until she dies and you receive it under her will. When you sell the assets, you pay no capital gains tax.

Here's why: when your mother leaves the house and stock to you at death, a special tax break eliminates the capital gain. This tax break applies to any type of appreciated assets passing to heirs at death (there's no limit on amount).

Of course, if your mother keeps the house

and stock and then has to go into a nursing home, she may lose everything. Wouldn't planning be easier if we had a crystal ball?

Example 53

Same facts again, except that your mother sells the house and gives you the proceeds. At the time of sale, she can avoid paying a tax on up to $125,000 of profit, thanks to another tax break that applies only to home sales. Since the profit on the sale was only $100,000 ($120,000 minus the $20,000 basis), she'll pay no capital gains tax.

When considering which assets to keep and which to give away, consider the impact of capital gains tax. As example 54 shows, wise planning can avoid a capital gains tax.

Example 54

Your mother has $100,000 of CDs and $100,000 of highly appreciated stock. She has decided to give away $100,000 and to keep the remaining $100,000, which she will use to pay her nursing-home costs for the next thirty-four months (until the ineligibility period runs out). Which assets should she keep and which should she give away?

By keeping the appreciated stock, she should come out ahead. She will sell the stock as she needs cash to pay the nursing home. But the capital gains tax should be offset by the huge medical deduction she will get for paying the nursing-home charges. (See page 66 for further discussion of use of the medical deduction for nursing-home costs.)

If she gave away the stock and kept the CDs, using the CDs to pay her nursing-home bills, the children would lose out. They would have to pay a capital gains tax when they eventually sell the stock, *without* the ability to offset against any big medical deductions.

Before giving away appreciated assets, think about the capital gains tax on the profits. If you want to minimize or eliminate the tax on a home but still give the property away so that you won't lose it to nursing-home costs, you should consider selling first and giving away the cash (example 53) or putting the house into a specialized house preservation trust

,,,er..55555

(see chapter 9). For appreciated assets other than your home, putting them into a specialized irrevocable asset protection trust (see chapter 9) may be your best option.

INCOME TAXES

If parents transfer assets to their children, the children will not pay any income tax on receiving the assets. The only income tax they will eventually pay is on any income produced from the transferred assets.

Example 55

Your parents transfer $100,000 in cash to you. You pay no income tax when you receive the money. You then invest the cash in CDs yielding 5 percent—$5,000 in annual interest. That interest is added to your income and will be taxed, just like any other interest income you receive from investments.

As long as people are aware of the tax rules, they should be able to develop a strategy that protects savings without hiking their taxes.

TAKE ADVANTAGE OF MEDICAL DEDUCTIONS

If your parent gifts assets to you, the assets are yours. If you then use some or all of those funds to care for your parent, you are using *your* money, and you may be able to deduct those costs come tax time.

If your parent is in a nursing home for medical care and you are footing most or all of the bill, all of those costs are deductible (as long as they exceed 7.5 percent of your adjusted gross income). Medical care doesn't have to be the only reason for being in the nursing home, just an important reason. For example, if your father is in a nursing home, at least in part because he's unable to take medications on his own, the entire cost should be deductible. Most people in nursing homes require at least some medical care and attention. Have a doctor state, in writing, the medical reason(s) for the nursing-home stay.

If your tax rate is higher than your parents' rate, then a medical deduction for you will be worth more than for your parents. Paying your parents' nursing-home bills may actually save you money!

Also, don't forget to take a dependency exemption (worth $2,450 in 1994, $2,500 in 1995). If your parents gave you their savings and you are now paying more than one-half of their total support, they may qualify as your dependent. For a parent in a nursing home, payments of the nursing-home bill will almost assuredly get you a dependency exemption.

Giving away assets to children or others can be a wonderful strategy to protect a portion of your life savings from nursing-home costs. As usual, along with the positive, there are a few negatives. You've already learned that the recipients of appreciated gifts may have to pay capital gains taxes. Other risks of gifting arise from the fact that you are losing control of your savings, becoming dependent on children or others to help you.

The next chapter tells how to use specialized trusts to minimize the risks involved when you give assets away.

CHAPTER 8 SUMMARY CHECKLIST

Give Your Money Away

Give Away Part of Your Assets

- ✔ Give away about half of your assets.
- ✔ Keep the rest to protect yourself.
- ✔ Don't put strings on gifted assets.
- ✔ Make "look-back" gifts.
- ✔ Make gifts that do not trigger any ineligibility period.

Pay Children for Their Help

- ✔ Put the agreement in writing.
- ✔ Get an independent estimate to set the price.
- ✔ Set resonable fees for services provided.

Be Aware of the Tax Laws

✔ Don't worry about gift taxes for estates under $600,000.

✔ With gifts of appreciated assets, watch out for capital gains taxes.

✔ Offset capital gains taxes by medical deductions.

✔ Don't worry about income taxes on gifts.

9 Protect Your Savings with Specialized Trusts

As demonstrated in chapter 8, the strategy of making gifts or transfers to protect your life savings while qualifying for Medicaid can work well. But giving away assets does carry certain emotional and financial risks.

If you give your money away hoping the recipient will give you money back as you need it, and the recipient then spends the money, you're in trouble.

Example 56

You give your life savings to your son. You thought he understood that although the money was officially his, he would use it to meet your needs down the road. Well, your son had other ideas. He looked down the road and instead of seeing a nursing home, he pictured paradise.

The next day, your son calls to thank you—from Hawaii! He's taking good care of your money, all right! Looking on the bright side, at least he didn't reverse the charges on the phone call.

The risk that your child (or other recipient of a gift) will spend the money is not the only potential problem. Even if your child is trustworthy, you could run into trouble. What happens to half of the marriages in this country today? They end in divorce. If you give your savings to your child, who subsequently becomes divorced or, worse, dies, some or all of the money you gave up may end up with your child's spouse. Just think—the in-law has your money! Does that make you a little uncomfortable? It should.

Now that I've reviewed the pitfalls, is there any way to minimize the risks involved in giving away assets? The answer is yes. While there is no one perfect solution, a variety of specialized trusts can provide invaluable protection.

What Is a Trust?

A trust is just a contract between one party who creates the trust (the "settlor") and one party who operates the trust (the "trustee").

A trust generally allows a person to give ownership of property (real estate, personal items, or money) to a trustee who will hold and manage the property for the benefit of one or more people. The settlor gets to decide who the trustee will be and how the trust will operate. The trustee can be anyone you choose, including your spouse, your child, a bank, or even yourself.

You set up a trust simply by signing a trust agreement, which looks something like a will. In fact, a trust can even be set up as part of a will. Once the trust is created, you can put any or all of your assets into it—cash, CDs, stocks, bonds, a house, car, furniture, jewelry, and almost anything else can be included. Assets are put into a trust simply by signing title over to the trust. For example, you would go to the bank and change the name on your account from your name, Sam Smith, to the Sam Smith Trust. Important note: don't forget to take this step! If you fail to act, you will be left with an unfunded trust, and your assets, since they were never shifted, won't be protected.

While these are the rules that generally apply to trusts, there are many different types of trusts. The standard revocable living trust, which has become the most popular tool to avoid probate, provides *no* protection from nursing-home costs. As discussed on pages 84–85, a standard revocable living trust can even cost the family a lot of money. A few specially designed trusts *can* protect assets from nursing-home charges. In this chapter we'll look at the old Medicaid trust and the newer family asset protection trust, irrevocable asset protection trust, testamentary trust, special needs trust, and self-care trust. In the next chapter I'll also tell you how a house preservation trust can be used to protect your home from being grabbed by the state.

Medicaid Trust

Prior to OBRA 1993, one of the most useful Medicaid planning tools available was the Medicaid trust. You could put your assets into an irrevocable Medicaid trust and not have those assets count against you when you applied for Medicaid.

There were three primary rules for creating a Medicaid trust:

1. The trust was irrevocable and unchangeable. Once set up, you couldn't change your mind or the terms of the trust.
2. You could have no control over the assets in a Medicaid trust. Neither you nor a spouse, if applicable, could serve as the trustee. You could pick a child or anyone else, but the trustee could not be you or a spouse.
3. You could never touch the principal placed in the trust. You could retain the right to income produced by these assets, and you could provide in the trust that upon your death these assets would go to your children, or other beneficiaries. But you could not remove or receive any of the principal deposited into the trust.

Putting assets into a Medicaid trust required giving up control, just like with gifts directly to children or others. But even if a child was serving as trustee of a Medicaid trust, assets in the trust did not *belong* to the child—he or she could not legally take the funds and run off to Tahiti or spend them on himself or herself. And if a child became divorced or died, the assets remained in the trust—they did not pass to the child's spouse or children. As long as you lived, the assets remained in the trust and the income could be paid to you.

Medicaid trusts were consistent with good public policy. These trusts simply allowed older Americans a legal way to protect assets while avoiding some of the dangers of gift giving.

Why am I talking about Medicaid trusts in the past tense? It is not yet clear if these trusts can still be used as a planning tool since OBRA 1993.

Don't worry if you set up a Medicaid trust before the law changed. Medicaid trusts in effect on or before August 10, 1993, are clearly still valid.

Initially most experts viewed the new laws as prohibiting the creation of new Medicaid trusts. But an interpretation of the law by Sally K. Richardson, director of the Medicaid Bureau of the Health Care Financing Administration (HCFA), breathes new life into the Medicaid trust. Richardson states that the standard Medicaid trust "will not be considered an available resource" by Medicaid when calculating assets. Since HCFA sets the rules for the Medicaid program nationally, her words carry great weight. As a result, it now seems that Medicaid trusts can still be used as a planning tool. To be on the safe side, you should not enter into one without first consulting with an experienced elder law attorney.

While HCFA is saying that Medicaid trusts still work, it is also claiming that a sixty-month look-back period applies to transfers into the trust, not the normal thirty-six–month period (HCFA is also saying that no ineligibility or look-back period applies to subsequent transfers out of the trust).

OBRA 1993 does not seem to me to support HCFA on the look-back period. Instead, the law seems to hold that the standard three-year look-back period applies to assets deposited *into* an irrevocable trust, while a five-year look-back period applies to any distributions *from* an irrevocable trust. States are likely to adopt HCFA's position, unless and until the ambiguities are resolved by the legislature or courts.

Family Asset Protection Trust

A family asset protection trust (FAPT) is a very different kind of trust. Most important, it is a trust created by others—usually children, but not the Medicaid applicant or spouse.

Let's say you give assets to your children. Remember the primary risks: your children could spend the money on themselves, and if they died or became divorced, their spouses or children would end up with the money, making it less likely that the funds would be available for you. An FAPT reduces these risks.

After your children receive the gifted assets, they may choose to get together and make a trust of their own. *They* are the creators of the trust, not you; *they* set the rules of the trust when they make the trust agreement; *they* are in control of the trust as trustees, not you.

Let's say all of your children serve as trustees. A typical setup would provide that any one of the trustees may use funds from the FAPT for the parent's benefit, in the child's complete and unfettered discretion. In other words, if you want to buy a new car or take a trip, you can call your son John and ask for $15,000; under the terms of the trust, he can pull it out and give it to you without consulting with the other children. But if you call John and he "forgets" who you are, you can ask your daughter Mary or any other trustee for the money.

Example 57

You give your four children $100,000—$25,000 each. If you later need $20,000, each child will have to kick in $5,000 (assuming they all still have the funds). If one has spent his or her share, then the other three children would each have to contribute $6,600.

But if the four children had created a FAPT and contributed $25,000 each, then any one of them could pull out the $20,000 from the trust. The effect would be to ensure equal shares from each of the four children.

The typical FAPT also puts severe limits on the children's use of funds in the trust. Some FAPTs absolutely prohibit use of trust funds for anyone other than the parent, until the parent dies. Other FAPTs provide a little more flexibility, allowing the children to use trust funds for themselves, their children, or others, but only if the children (trustees) all agree. By requiring unanimity, the children avoid the risk that any one child will spend his or her share prematurely, while the parent may still need funds. Assets

in the FAPT also should remain there in the event that a child dies or becomes divorced (although this protection may not hold up in community property states).

A FAPT can provide very useful protections, but it must be set up with great care. A FAPT will not work if (1) the parent's assets were given and used for the purpose of forming the trust, and (2) the trust is being set up at the direction or request of the parent (or spouse). To avoid problems, it must be clear that the children are setting up this trust on their own initiative, with their own assets.

Ideally the children should not use assets originally received from parents; instead they should put their own assets into a FAPT before receiving any gift from parents. This would clearly establish that the children are using their own funds for the trust. Unfortunately, in most cases not all of the children will have enough assets to put into a FAPT before receiving a gift.

If assets gifted from parents are to be used, they should not be placed into the FAPT until at least a couple of months after the gift is completed. In the meantime, the assets remain in the children's names; children may even want to spend some of the funds gifted to them, and commingle the funds with their other assets, to further show that they consider the gifted assets to be their own. This should help make it clear that the funds going into the FAPT, even if gifted from the parents, now belong to the children.

The parents also should be careful not to direct or request that the children establish a FAPT. The children should create the FAPT on their own. If the parents have already spoken to an elder law attorney, they may simply ask the children to consult with the attorney; the attorney can then carefully explain, without conveying any request or direction from the parents, the potential use of a FAPT as one of a variety of potential planning options.

Transfers to the children (or others) trigger a thirty-six-month look-back period. Transfers from the children into a FAPT, or by the trustees out of a FAPT, should not create any look-back or ineligibility period.

Two model FAPTs are displayed in appendix B. One allows the trustees to distribute assets only to the parents, prohibiting other uses of the funds; the other allows distributions to others, but only if all trustees agree. These are provided to illustrate the nature and typical terms of this trust. *The forms should* not *be used without first consulting an experienced elder law attorney.*

Irrevocable Asset Protection Trust

This trust looks a lot like the old Medicaid trust (see page 69), with one key difference. Under the old Medicaid trust, the creator (and/or spouse, if applicable) could not touch the principal deposited into the trust but would receive all of the income (interest, dividends, rents). Under an irrevocable asset protection trust, the person setting it up cannot reach income or principal under any circumstances. Income and even principal may be distributed to others, such as children or grandchildren, in the trustee's discretion, but under no circumstances can income or principal ever be paid to the creator of the trust.

Can income or principal be distributed to children (or others), and then can the children make gifts to the parent (or spouse) who established the irrevocable asset protection trust? Yes, but only if done very carefully. You must take steps to ensure that the Medicaid bureaucrats will not be able to claim successfully that the gifts to the parent are really coming from the trust. The best strategy would be for the child to make gifts from his or her own funds well before any distribution is made to the child from the trust. Or at the very least, a long period of time (several months or more) should pass between distribution of trust assets to the child and the child's gift to the parent. Do not develop a routine pattern of distributions from the trust to children followed by gifts from children to parent; trust distributions, if any, should be infrequent and irregular.

In the best case, assets in the trust will not be distributed until the person creating the trust has died. At that time the irrevocable asset protection trust ends and the assets (plus any accumulated income) are distributed to the designated heirs, typically the children. If the children made gifts from their funds to the parent, they'll get a financial benefit when the trust ends.

As with the Medicaid trust, a growing number of experts argue that a five-year look-back period (rather than the typical three-year period), applies to assets placed into an irrevocable trust (see page 69). Again, the language of OBRA 1993 is ambiguous enough to raise questions that may have to be resolved by the legislature or courts.

Why use an irrevocable asset protection trust instead of simply making gifts to heirs, such as children, who might then in turn create a more flexible family asset protection trust? The answer is that the irrevocable asset protection trust can protect against your heirs paying a hefty capital gains tax on appreciated assets. Compare examples 58 and 59.

Example 58

Your father bought shares of stock thirty years ago for $20,000; today they are worth $120,000. If your father gives them to you to get them out of his name for Medicaid purposes, and you later sell them for $120,000, you'll pay a capital gains tax of about $28,000 on the profit.

Example 59

Same facts as in example 58, except that your father puts the stock into an irrevocable asset protection trust instead of giving them to you. The stock is still out of his name for Medicaid purposes. At your father's death, the trust ends and the stock is distributed to you, who sell the stock for $120,000. Because the stock was in the trust, you do not pay any capital gains tax.

As you can see by comparing examples 58 and 59, an irrevocable asset protection trust can save a lot of money by avoiding capital gains taxes on appreciated assets.

A model irrevocable asset protection trust is provided in appendix B. Again, this is for illustration purposes only. No trust should ever be made without first consulting with an experienced elder law attorney.

Testamentary Trust

The biggest drawback of gifts to children or to a family asset protection trust is that you and your spouse must give up control of your savings and then must wait up to thirty-six months for Medicaid eligibility. One possible way around these problems is a testamentary trust.

A testamentary trust will be set up as part of a will, so no money or property goes into the trust until you die. This is the one type of trust that you would not "fund" during your life. As long as you are alive, everything you own remains yours. When you die the assets go into the testamentary trust. The money and property in the trust will be protected in case the surviving spouse must later enter a nursing home. And there will be no Medicaid waiting period, because there is no gift or transfer.

Example 60

Your wife has Parkinson's disease. You have been caring for her at home for the last twenty years, and you expect to continue for the rest of your life. But if you were to die first, she probably would have to go into a nursing home.

You and your wife put everything you own into your name, and you create a testamentary trust. Nothing goes into the trust until your death; as long as you remain alive, the assets are yours. When you die, everything goes into the testamentary trust. Let's say you name your son as trustee. The trust can give your son substantial discretion over the income and principal—he can take out some or all of these funds from the trust to use for your wife.

If your wife needs money to pay for care at home, your son, as trustee, can make it available to her. If she must enter a nursing home, then the trustee has the discretion to provide nothing to her. The trust protects your joint life savings in case your wife must enter a nursing home and can immediately qualify her for Medicaid, because assets passing on death do not trigger any waiting period. None of the principal or income goes to the nursing home, except maybe to pay for things Medicaid won't cover, like a private room. The assets remain in the trust—unaffected by the nursing-home bills—until your wife dies, and then the assets will go to the heirs.

The drawback is that this trust works only after one of you dies. If you or your spouse go into a nursing home while the other is still alive, nothing is protected by the trust.

And you've got to correctly guess which one of you will die first. For that reason, a testamentary trust normally should not be considered until one of you has become ill or been diagnosed with a terminal illness.

NOTE: In some states a surviving spouse may be required to receive an "elective share"—typically one-third to one-half of the estate—when the other spouse dies. In these states, the surviving spouse's elective share would wind up going to the nursing home, and the rest would go into the testamentary trust.

Special Needs Trust

Let's say you have a child, grandchild, brother, sister, or some significant other to whom you'd like to leave an inheritance when you die, but the person has a handicap or illness. For example, maybe your daughter has multiple sclerosis, or perhaps your brother has Alzheimer's disease.

If you leave an inheritance to a family member or friend who is unable to handle the money, who will step in and manage things for him or her? And what if the person is already on or may be eligible in the future for Medicaid benefits? The inheritance you leave will make this individual ineligible for Medicaid until the inheritance is used up. If Medicaid has been paying for nursing-home care, the benefits will be turned off and replaced by the inheritance. Only after the inheritance is gone will the benefits be restarted. In a scenario like this, your attempt to assist a needy family member hasn't done much good.

Here's a better way: instead of leaving an inheritance directly to your handicapped beneficiary at your death, leave the assets in a special needs trust, with instructions that the income, principal, or both be used for that individual's benefit. A trustee named in the trust (perhaps a relative, a friend, or a bank) would manage the funds, handling investments as well as distributions to your loved one.

The key to a special needs trust (also called a supplemental needs trust) is that the inheritance you leave can be used to *supplement*, not supplant, Medicaid and any other public benefits received by your loved one. For example, if your child is receiving Medicaid to cover nursing-home costs, the funds in the trust may be used to pay for a private room, a new television, periodic trips to see other family members, and other expenses not covered by Medicaid.

At the death of the beneficiary of the special needs trust, anything left can pass to other heirs whom you select. For example, if you set up a special needs trust for one child, at the death of that child you may provide that anything left will pass to your other surviving children or grandchildren.

The technical requirements of special needs trusts vary state by state. But generally the primary rule is that the trustee you select must be given broad discretion to determine when and under what circumstances to make distributions to your loved one. If you would like to leave assets at your death to someone with a handicap, again, contact a skilled elder law attorney to discuss this critical document.

Self-Care Trust

I recently met with a client who had about $100,000, and he was suffering from a debilitating muscle disease. He could no longer manage his physical needs and was about to admit himself to a nursing home. His mind was active and alert but the rest of his body was deteriorating steadily.

He had no children or other close relatives that needed his money when he died. His goal was to use his nest egg for his own care, but to stretch it for as long as possible.

If this client simply did what most people do, he would pay privately for the nursing home until his funds ran out, then obtain Medicaid coverage. But at that point he would have no money left to use for improving his lifestyle. Most important, he desired a private room at the nursing home, but a private room costs extra and Medicaid wouldn't cover the added cost. He also had a specially adapted computer, which brought him great personal satisfaction but cost money to equip and operate; so when his money ran out, he would be deprived of one of his few pleasures.

Instead of simply using up his money, I recommended that the client consider a certain type of self-care trust, often called a pooled trust. The trust is actually created and managed by a nonprofit association, such as the Alzheimer's Association or the Muscular Dystrophy Association. It's not necessary that the association a person picks be connected to the disease from which he or she is suffering. The individual's funds are deposited into this trust and the trust maintains a separate account for the individual (although all funds are pooled for purposes of investment). Funds deposited into the trust may be used to supplement, but not replace, Medicaid (and other public benefits) available to the individual. At the individual's death, the funds in the trust go either to the nonprofit association or the state (up to the amount of Medicaid benefits paid by the state). Family members cannot be beneficiaries of the trust.

A self-care trust does not have to be established by a nonprofit association. For a disabled person who is under age sixty-five, a parent, grandparent, legal guardian, or court can set up a self-care trust. Again, the disabled individual's funds can be used to supplement Medicaid benefits during the person's lifetime; at his or her death, anything remaining in the trust will first go to the state to repay any Medicaid benefits previously paid. Only if excess assets remain after repaying the state may they pass to other heirs, such as family members.

One situation in which a self-care trust may be particularly useful is following the receipt of funds from a judgment or settlement for a serious personal injury. A person who is seriously injured, perhaps in an auto accident or on the job, may face huge and continuing medical expenses. If the monetary award had to be used up before the person would qualify for Medicaid, the funds might go fairly quickly, providing little long-term benefit to the injured person. But if the award is placed in a self-care trust, the person would receive Medicaid benefits and the trust funds would be available to supplement the coverage, paying for costs that would otherwise not be covered under any government program.

Who Should Be the Trustee?

Under any of these trusts, a trustee (or more than one trustee) will be taking over control of the assets placed in the trust. In some cases, such as a self-care trust administered by a nonprofit association, you don't have much choice. But in most trusts you can pick the trustee. Obviously, it's crucial that you select the best possible person to serve.

The trustee will be either an individual, typically a close relative or friend, or an institution, typically a local bank. Here are guidelines for choosing either type of trustee:

INDIVIDUAL TRUSTEE

These five questions should be considered when selecting an individual trustee:

1. *Do I trust the person?* This is the most important consideration. You are giving the trustee a great deal of power over, and responsibility for, you and/or your family's well-being. You want someone who will not abuse that power.

2. *Where does the person live?* There is no legal requirement that a trustee live in the same

locale as you. But, all else being equal, you will be better off with a trustee who lives nearby. Convenience is important. For example, you may need quick action by the trustee, and waiting for bills and checks to pass through the mails can prove to be costly. Still, the wonders of modern technology have now made it easier for an out-of-state trustee to handle matters, so pick the person you most trust, even if out of state. But if all things are equal, the closer to home the better.

3. *Is the person willing to accept the job?* You should not just name a trustee without first making sure that he or she will accept the responsibility. Serving as a trustee can be a lot of work, and your choice may decline the "privilege" of serving, especially if there is no compensation.

4. *Can the person handle the job?* If your entire estate is simply savings accounts and CDs, the trustee does not need to be a financial wizard. But if your estate is more complicated, maybe consisting of stocks and bonds that must be sold and bought, real estate that must be managed, or a small business that must be run, it would be wise to select a trustee with the necessary business, financial, or legal experience necessary to handle such affairs.

5. *Is the person a beneficiary of the trust?* If you choose to appoint as a trustee someone who will or could be a beneficiary of the trust, conflicts of interest might arise. Again, if you've picked someone you trust, this should not pose a problem. In addition, there would potentially be some adverse tax consequences to the trustee in situations where the trustee will be making distributions (income and/or principal) of more than $10,000 a year. In those situations the trustee might be considered to be making personal gifts that would be subject to gift tax laws. If your choice for trustee will or could be a trust beneficiary, you should ask a lawyer about the possible gift tax implications.

PROFESSIONAL TRUSTEE

A close family member usually makes the best trustee because the person tends to be more sensitive to the family's needs and wishes. But in situations where there is no appropriate family member, or where there may be conflicts between family members, a professional trustee may be the best choice.

You should shop around at local banks and trust companies and not automatically use the bank that holds your savings account. Although the fact that you have received good service there might be one consideration, bank trust departments generally are completely separate from the rest of the bank; you may receive much different service from the trust department's personnel and administrators.

When you shop around, ask the following questions:

- What was the performance of the bank's trust funds over the last five years? Ten years?
- What fees will be charged?
- Who will manage the account?

NO MATTER WHOM YOU CHOOSE, BE SURE TO PROVIDE COMPLETE INSTRUCTIONS

Although the trustee takes over management of the funds placed in a trust, that doesn't mean a trustee has absolute discretion. You can use the trust agreement to spell out in great detail exactly how the estate should be managed, the funds invested, and (in some trusts) the assets distributed. The trustee can be left with little more than the administrative responsibilities of carrying out your wishes.

For example, you can spell out for the trustee his, her, or its responsibility for:

- *Investments.* Do you want funds invested conservatively in T-bills or would you prefer riskier investments in the stock market? You can specify detailed investment strategies, even specific investments.

- *Distributions.* Do you want the beneficiaries to be paid the entire income from investments annually or quarterly? Do you want a fixed dollar allowance that might be less or more than the income generated? You can specify exactly how disbursements should be made.

- *Reporting and record keeping.* Just because you won't be involved in the daily financial activities doesn't mean the trustee can't provide information about actions taken. You can require that the trustee undertake particular reporting and record-keeping activities.

- *Management.* You may want to give the trustee authority to manage real estate or a business, to buy and sell property, and/or to undertake other specific management responsibilities. All of this can be spelled out in the trust agreement.

- *Tax returns.* Your trustee may have to prepare and file annual tax returns covering the trust activity. Make sure these responsibilities are covered in the trust agreement.

If the trustee is a professional trustee (usually an institution), you may not want to define the investment responsibilities too narrowly. Assuming the trustee has experience and a good track record in managing funds, why mess with success? After all, you are paying the trustee, so let the bank earn its keep by making the investments.

CHAPTER 9 SUMMARY CHECKLIST

Protect Your Savings with Specialized Trusts

Medicaid Trust

- ✔ Create a Medicaid trust to protect assets for heirs and to retain income for yourself.

- ✔ Although OBRA 1993 appeared to have killed this trust, HCFA seems to have given it new life.

- ✔ Watch out for a possible sixty-month look-back period.

Family Asset Protection Trust (FAPT)

- ✔ FAPTs insulate assets from loss or abuse while allowing use for parents.

- ✔ FAPTs must be created by children or others on their own.

Irrevocable Asset Protection Trust

- ✔ Create an irrevocable asset protection trust to protect assets.

- ✔ This trust is similar to the Medicaid trust, but no income or principal can be available to the Medicaid recipient or the spouse.

- ✔ The irrevocable asset protection trust can have special benefit for appreciated assets.

Testamentary Trust

- ✔ This trust protects a surviving spouse.

- ✔ A testamentary trust must be created as part of will and becomes effective only at death.

- ✔ No protection is provided by a testamentary trust while both spouses are alive.

Special Needs Trust

- ✔ Create a special needs trust to protect a handicapped relative.

- ✔ Give the trustee broad discretion.

- ✔ This trust allows the inheritance to supplement, not supplant, Medicaid.

Self-Care Trust

- ✔ Have a nonprofit association create this trust.

- ✔ A Medicaid recipient can stretch his or her own funds by using this trust to supplement benefits.

- ✔ At death, any remaining trust funds go to the nonprofit association or the state.

Selection of Trustee

- ✔ Pick a person who is trustworthy.

- ✔ Select a trustee who is willing to accept and is capable of handling the job.

- ✔ Convenience: will the trustee be able to respond quickly if not living nearby?

- ✔ Consider a professional trustee, such as a bank, if there are no appropriate family members or there may be conflicts between family members.

- ✔ For maximum control, spell out detailed instructions for the trustee to follow.

10 | Your Home Is Your Castle: Defend It

For most people, the home is their largest and most precious asset. I've heard it repeatedly from clients: "I'll pay my fair share for nursing-home charges, but I don't want to have to spend my entire life savings and—most important—I don't want to lose my house."

For married couples, the home has been, and continues to be, protected when it comes to qualifying for Medicaid benefits. As long as one spouse lives there, the house is safe and the other spouse can get Medicaid coverage. For unmarried Medicaid recipients, many states allow the house to remain a protected asset as long as they intend to return home (see table 3.6). At the Medicaid recipient's (and spouse's) death, the house will usually be passed to the heirs.

But OBRA 1993 substantially undercut these protections, requiring that states create estate recovery laws (see chapter 5). Under these new laws, a nursing-home spouse can still keep the home, but at death, the state can send out a "house hit team" to grab the house, sell it, and then use the sale proceeds to recover Medicaid's costs for nursing-home expenses already paid. It can even put a lien on the property while you're still alive as a condition of your receiving benefits (but not while your spouse is living in the house). A lien makes it impossible to sell the property without the state's knowledge or ability to collect.

There are ways to protect your most prized possession. Let's take a look at the best available options.

Transfer Title to the Home

For a married couple, when one spouse enters a nursing home, the home (as well as other assets) should, at the very minimum, be put into the healthy spouse's name. In addition, the healthy spouse should change his or her will, leaving the home to the children or other desired heirs, not to the nursing-home spouse. As discussed in chapter 11, without taking this step, all of your planning will have been useless if the spouse-at-home dies before the nursing-home spouse.

States can recover payments for Medicaid benefits from the estate of a Medicaid recipient, including, most notably (and painfully), the house. But states *cannot* recover assets from the estate of a Medicaid recipient's spouse (unless a lien had been placed on the property while it was still in the nursing-home spouse's name). This is critical: *federal law clearly prohibits states from grabbing the house if it is in the spouse's name.* Unfortunately, it appears that several states are threatening to ignore this key portion of OBRA 1993. If your state refuses to comply with federal law, run—don't walk—to an elder law attorney for help.

In other words, for married couples, protecting the home may be as simple as moving the house into the name of the healthy spouse. The healthy spouse may then put the home into a revocable living trust. This action serves a dual purpose: it protects the house from probate as well as from reverting back to the nursing-home spouse in case the spouse-at-home dies first (see pages 83–85).

What about a house owned by an unmarried Medicaid recipient? One option is simply to put the home into a revocable living trust or into joint ownership with an intended heir. This would have to be done before any lien is put on it. Assets in a revocable living trust or joint ownership avoid probate, and they may avoid the state's house hit team. OBRA 1993 says that states must go after a Medicaid recipient's home if it will pass through probate at death; OBRA 1993 also gives states the *option* to grab homes that avoid probate when passing to heirs. While I anticipate that most states will gladly exercise their option to grab nonprobate assets in revocable trusts or joint ownerships, check your state's rules by contacting your local Medicaid office or an experienced elder law attorney.

Whether married or not, Medicaid recipients may opt to gift or transfer the home to children or others. This gift or transfer works just like other gifts: it typically will trigger an ineligibility period, and once that period passes, the home will be protected. In addition, transferring the home carries with it all of the risks discussed earlier for transferring any assets: you become vulnerable. The children may throw you out, sell the home, and spend the proceeds; if they die or become divorced, the spouse might wind up with everything. (See pages 60–61 and 68 for a detailed discussion about the pros and cons of gifting assets.)

Transfers of the home to certain people, listed on pages 40–41, will not trigger any ineligibility period. For example, the home may be transferred to:

- A child who is under twenty-one, blind, or permanently and totally disabled.
- A child who lived in the home for at least two years immediately before the parent was institutionalized and who provided care to the parent that enabled the parent to remain at home.
- A brother or sister who has an ownership interest in the house and who lived there for at least one year immediately before the sibling was institutionalized.

One special problem for transferring a home that does not apply to transfers of most other assets is that the recipients of the house may have to pay a fat capital gains tax when they sell. Houses typically in-crease in value over the years. If you give your house to your children (or others), they'll pay a capital gains tax on the profit at the time of sale (usually the sale price minus the original purchase price plus the cost of improvements). If you've owned more than one home over the years that has increased in value, the capital gains tax will be on the *combined* profits. (See the general discussion of handling appreciated assets on pages 65–66.)

How can you transfer a home that's gone up in value so that it is out of your name for Medicaid purposes but doesn't cause your family a huge capital gains tax? The next strategy, using a house preservation trust, may do the trick.

House Preservation Trust

If you want to protect your home from the state's grasp without also passing a large capital gains tax on to your children, consider a house preservation trust. This irrevocable trust works a lot like the irrevocable asset protection trust described on page 71.

You cannot be the trustee and your spouse cannot serve, but a child or other person of your choice can. The trust is irrevocable and cannot be changed. The trust cannot give you a legal right to live in the home, and the trustee is permitted to throw you out at any time. But if you pick a trustworthy, sympathetic trustee, that shouldn't be a problem. The state won't be able to grab the house, and at your death it will pass to your heirs. In the meantime, Medicaid will pay your bills (assuming you have spent down or moved around your other assets).

This trust has two major benefits over a transfer to children or other heirs. First, if the house is sold (for example, after you've entered a nursing home), no capital gains tax is paid on the first $125,000 of profit. Second, if the house passes to your heirs at death, the heirs pay no capital gains tax when they sell it.

Transfer the House, Keeping a Life Estate or a Right to Use and Occupancy

You are afraid to give your house to your children (or others) because of the risks. What if your child (or his spouse, if he dies) throws you out or sells the house without your permission? And a house preservation trust seems too restrictive. What can you do?

You may transfer a "remainder interest" in the house, which means that your children will own the home automatically when you die. You then create and keep a "life estate" or a "right to use and occupancy" (with the help of a lawyer), which gives you a legal right to live in the house for as long as you desire. Until you die, your right to the roof over your head is assured.

By giving away a "remainder interest," you are getting rid of much of the value of the house. If you enter a nursing home, at most only the value of the life estate or the right to use and occupancy (which Medicaid will calculate based on your life expectancy and the home value) would be counted against you.

Example 61

You are widowed and your only significant asset is the house, worth $100,000. You give away the remainder interest to your son, but you keep a life estate. According to the Life Estate and Remainder Interest Table provided by HCFA (reprinted here as table 10.1), the life estate is worth $50,000 and the remainder is worth $50,000. Transferring an asset worth $50,000 would create an ineligibility period of about seventeen months, assuming $3,000 a month cost of care for your state. If the transfer is made while you are healthy, the ineligibility period will have expired long before you might ever need nursing-home care.

If you later go into a nursing home, you can transfer the life estate to your son. That transfer would make you ineligible for Medicaid for only about seventeen months. If you had given away the entire $100,000 home when entering a nursing home, you'd be unable to get Medicaid for close to three years.

Note that a few states say that a life estate or a right to use and occupancy has no value because nobody would pay good money to buy it. In those states, retaining a life estate or a right to use and occupancy would not create any additional ineligibility period. But most states use life expectancy tables to put a value on a right to live in the property. Check with your local Medicaid office.

To try to avoid the state placing a value on the life estate or right to use and occupancy, you may limit the right to live in and use the home to the Medicaid recipient only. You then could argue that since no one else could rent the property, the life estate has no market value.

TABLE 10.1

Life Estate and Remainder Table

AGE	LIFE ESTATE	REMAINDER
50	.84743	.15257
51	.83674	.16126
52	.82969	.17031
53	.82028	.17972
54	.81054	.18946
55	.80046	.19954
56	.79006	.20994
57	.77931	.22069
58	.76822	.23178
59	.75675	.24325
60	.74491	.25509
61	.73267	.26733
62	.72002	.27998
63	.70696	.29304
64	.69352	.30648
65	.67970	.32030
66	.66551	.33449
67	.65098	.34902
68	.63610	.36390
69	.62086	.37914
70	.60522	.39478
71	.58914	.41086
72	.57261	.42739
73	.55571	.44429
74	.53862	.46138
75	.52149	.47851
76	.50441	.49559
77	.48742	.51258
78	.47049	.52951
79	.45357	.54643
80	.43659	.56341
81	.41967	.58033
82	.40295	.59705
83	.38642	.61358
84	.36998	.63002
85	.35359	.64641
86	.33764	.66236
87	.32262	.67738
88	.30859	.69141
89	.29526	.70474
90	.28221	.71779
91	.26955	.73045
92	.25771	.74229
93	.24692	.75308
94	.23728	.76272
95	.22887	.77113
96	.22181	.77819
97	.21550	.78450
98	.21000	.79000
99	.20486	.79514
100	.19975	.80025

SOURCE: Health Care Financing Administration Transmittal, No. 64, State Medicaid Manual, November 1994, at 3-3-109, 14, 3-3-109.15.

One more note: the estate recovery rules under OBRA 1993 make a vague reference to states being permitted to seize a life estate at the death of a Medicaid recipient, prompting some concern over the continued use of life estates. But since a life estate ends at a Medicaid recipient's death, the individual's estate has no asset that can be grabbed by the state. In other words, life estates should still serve as a useful planning tool.

Sell Home on a Land Contract or Installment Sale

Back when home mortgage interest rates were running 15 percent and higher, owners were having a tough time finding buyers. To help encourage sales, many owners offered to serve as the bank, providing buyers with financing at lower rates than they could have otherwise obtained from commercial lenders. This process of the seller taking back financing is often called a land contract sale.

Example 62
You sell your home for $100,000. The buyer puts up $10,000 as a down payment and then gives you a note (an IOU) for $90,000. The note states that the buyer must pay you $700 a month for thirty years. To secure the sale, you get a mortgage on the property so that if the buyer fails to make the required payments, you can foreclose and take the house back.

What does a land contract sale have to do with Medicaid qualification? In some states the use of a land contract is a valuable planning tool, as example 63 shows.

Example 63
Your father is a widow and must enter a nursing home. His house is his only significant asset, worth $100,000, and he'd like to protect it. In his state, the house receives no protection, even if he intends to return home.
What if he sells the house to you? If you pay him $100,000, then the cash would make him ineligible for Medicaid coverage and he hasn't accomplished anything. Besides, you don't have $100,000 cash.
Instead you buy the house on a land contract. You give him an IOU for $100,000 and

agree to pay him $500 each month. You then rent out the house (you or another relative might be the renter) for $500 per month, using that money to pay your father. Your father immediately qualifies for Medicaid, because the state doesn't count the IOU against him as an asset; only the monthly payments, which count as your father's income, go to the nursing home.

This planning strategy has worked very well in those states that don't count the land contract as an asset. Check with an elder law attorney about the feasibility of using a land contract as a Medicaid planning tool. One note of caution: under the new estate recovery rules, states may go after the IOU once the Medicaid recipient dies. If that occurs— and it's too early to know if it will—then the state would be entitled to the monthly payments until the amount of Medicaid benefits paid out are recovered.

CHAPTER 10 SUMMARY CHECKLIST

Your Home Is Your Castle: Defend It

Transfer Title to the Home

✔ For married couples, move the home into the name of the healthy spouse.

✔ For unmarried Medicaid recipients, consider a revocable living trust to avoid probate and possibly estate recoveries.

✔ Give the home to children or others, but watch out for capital gains taxes.

✔ Put the home into a house preservation trust to save capital gains taxes.

Transfer the Home While Keeping a Right to Live There

✔ Transfer a remainder interest but keep a life estate.

✔ Transfer a remainder interest but keep a right to use and occupancy.

✔ When applying for Medicaid, argue that the life estate has no value.

Sell Home on a Land Contract

✔ Sell the home and take an IOU instead of cash.

✔ Rent the house to cover the mortgage payments.

✔ When applying for Medicaid, argue that the land contract has no value and should not be counted as an asset.

Use a Revocable Living Trust and Joint Ownership to Protect Retained Assets

The techniques discussed so far can shield money and property from the grasp of a nursing home. I've explained how gifts and transfers can help protect a portion of a person's life savings.

But I rarely recommend transferring everything; I will almost always encourage older people to keep a portion of their assets as a safety net, even if it means those assets might eventually be spent on nursing-home care. Other assets can be kept without worry because they are exempt assets for purposes of determining Medicaid eligibility.

Pauline Thoma explains why she was glad to have retained part of her savings:

> Everything began to fall apart when my husband retired. It's unfortunate, but it happens to many people. He had a heart attack and that's when we learned that diabetes caused it; we didn't even know he had diabetes. Unfortunately he wound up with three heart attacks. . . .
>
> I did things to try to begin to give worldly goods to the family. But you have to keep some money available. Nothing is fully paid for. For example, my husband was in and out of hospitals all the time. Never was a bill fully paid by Blue Cross, by Medicare, or by his insurance from the company he was retired from. There was always money we had to pay of ours. Sometimes it was large sums, and had we not protected some I wouldn't have been able to pay those bills.[1]

With some planning, retained assets that are not spent on ongoing costs might even be protected from a nursing home. Particularly for married couples, several simple steps may enable the family to protect at least a portion of the retained estate while at the same time avoiding probate at death and making life a lot simpler for heirs.

Change Title to Property

Let's start with a common example.

Example 64
> Your father has been diagnosed with Alzheimer's disease. While he's at a very early stage, your mother wants to take precautions to protect at least part of their life savings, which total $200,000.
>
> They gift $100,000 to their children, who put the funds into a family asset protection trust. Your parents keep the rest so that they are not dependent on their children, at least not immediately.

So far this is a pretty common situation. As long as your parents remain reasonably healthy, there's no problem. But let's continue the story:

> Your father has become extremely forgetful, but your mother is able to care for him at home. That is, until she passes away from an

unexpected heart attack. Now your father must be institutionalized.

All of your parents' assets were held jointly with a right of survivorship between them, because they had heard that this was a good way to avoid probate. Unfortunately, at your mother's death, all of the assets pass back to your father and then head on to the nursing home.

How is your or your loved one's home titled? What about checking and savings accounts, stocks, CDs, and money markets? For most married couples, many, if not all, of their assets are jointly held. Although there are a lot of benefits to joint ownership, this startegy can turn out to be the *worst* option when Medicaid looms.

What is joint ownership? Any person together with someone else, usually a spouse or child, may own property jointly with a right of survivorship. This means that while both owners are alive, both own and control the property. When one owner dies, that person's interest in the property is automatically transferred to the surviving co-owner.

For example, if your mother and father have a joint-and-survivorship bank account, when your father dies, the entire account will belong to your mother. Of course, if your mother dies first, the account is your father's.

All sorts of property can be held jointly with a right of survivorship. Homes, bank accounts, CDs, and stocks typically are owned jointly with a right of survivorship.

While joint ownership between spouses may be an easy way to avoid probate when one dies, it can cause the surviving spouse to lose everything to a nursing home, as example 64 showed.

What would have been better? Let's go back to example 64. As soon as your father was diagnosed with Alzheimer's, all of your parents' remaining assets should have been moved into your mother's name, getting rid of all of those joint-and-survivorship accounts!

If older Americans do no other Medicaid planning, once it appears likely that one spouse will require nursing-home care, they should consider moving assets into the name of the healthy spouse. Compare examples 65 and 66.

Example 65

At the time your father enters a nursing home, he and your mother have jointly held assets of $170,000. Your father and mother will be able to protect a total of $74,820 under the Medicaid rules for married individuals.

Two years after your father enters the nursing home, they have $110,000 left; the rest has been spent on the nursing home and on your mother's living expenses. Then your mother dies. Since the assets were held jointly, your father automatically owns the entire remaining $110,000. And since your father is no longer married, the Medicaid rules for unmarried individuals take over. Now your father is allowed to keep only about $2,000. Kiss the rest of your parents' life savings good-bye.

Example 66

At the time your father enters a nursing home, he and your mother have total assets of $170,000; your father doesn't qualify for Medicaid. As soon as he enters, he transfers everything into your mother's name. That transfer won't help him qualify for Medicaid immediately, but it will help later, as you'll soon see. Your mother also changes her will, removing your dad's name as a beneficiary.

Two years after he enters the nursing home, your mother has $110,000 left in her name; the rest went to pay bills. Then she dies. Under her will, all $110,000 would pass to the children (or other named beneficiaries); your father would then qualify for Medicaid, which would pick up the remaining nursing-home costs.

As you can see from these two examples, changing the names on assets, coupled with the next step, changing the will, can change a family's financial future.

Change the Will and Insurance Beneficiaries

Shifting assets from one spouse to another, in and of itself, won't protect a couple's life savings while both spouses are living. If your spouse enters a nursing home, all you'll be allowed to keep is half of the total amount (up to $74,820), regardless of whether the assets are in your name, your spouse's name, or held jointly.

Transferring assets from a spouse who enters a nursing home to the spouse still at home can be very useful in the event that the spouse-at-home dies first, as examples 65 and 66 just showed. This works, though, only if coupled with a change in the will by the spouse-at-home.

The spouse-at-home *must* change his or her will, deleting as a beneficiary the spouse that has already entered, or is likely to enter, a nursing home. The spouse-at-home will leave everything to other heirs, such as children. The beneficiary on the life insurance policy and IRAs should also be changed so that those assets will not end up with the nursing-home spouse.

If the spouse-at-home dies first, the assets will pass under the will to the heirs rather than to the spouse in the nursing home. The nursing-home spouse will immediately qualify for Medicaid, because he or she has nothing; passing assets at death under a will should not be considered a gift or transfer that would make anyone ineligible for Medicaid. Everything should go to the heirs and would be fully protected. Assets in the name of the spouse-at-home, not the Medicaid recipient, should not be subject to the estate recovery rules.

There's one big hitch: in most states, the surviving spouse in the nursing home will have the right to an "elective share," even if cut out of the will. That share is usually one-third to one-half of the total estate. If the surviving spouse refuses to take the elective share, that is likely to be considered a gift or transfer of assets, triggering a Medicaid ineligibility period. And if the spouse in the nursing home is incompetent at the time the spouse-at-home dies, he or she may be forced by the probate court to take the elective share. In other words, changing the will will probably not be enough to cut out a surviving spouse completely—part of the estate will get to the heirs designated in the will, but part will still go to the nursing-home spouse, and then to the nursing home.

How can you get around this risk? Instead of changing the will, the spouse-at-home can leave assets to heirs (other than a spouse) in a revocable living trust or by joint ownership with the heirs. These avoid probate and should be able to get assets directly into the hands of the desired heirs rather than the open arms of the nursing home.

Create a Revocable Living Trust or Joint Ownership with Heirs, to Avoid Probate and a Spouse's Elective Share

If you look forward to going to the dentist or paying taxes, you'll love probate. Seriously, lots of people today want to avoid probate for lots of good reasons. But what exactly is it, and why does it have such a bad name?

In a nutshell, probate is the system designed to facilitate the passing of a person's money and property at his or her death—at least that's the nice way to describe it. It involves filing and verifying a will with the local courts, appraising existing property, paying debts (including death taxes), and distributing remaining property to the rightful heirs. If you leave assets to pass under a will, you'll go through probate.

In his classic book *How to Avoid Probate!* Norman Dacey offers his own view of the process: "Probate . . . is essentially a form of private taxation levied by the legal profession upon the rest of the population."[2]

A 1990 study of probate by the AARP concludes that probate is "costly, slow, and outmoded . . . [a] sad state of affairs." The report first focuses on costs, finding that "for the estates of the middle class . . . fees can deplete the assets by as much as 10 percent even in uncomplicated cases."[3]

Costs are only part of the problem. The same AARP study found that probate of estates under $100,000 took, on average, well over a year. Why so long? Most of the delay lies in the mountain of paperwork that must be completed in order to comply with state laws that have multiple deadlines and requirements.

What's all this have to do with Medicaid planning? Avoiding probate can have two benefits when it comes to protecting assets from nursing homes:

1. A surviving spouse in a nursing home is likely to have to take an elective share of the assets passing under a will, through probate, to heirs. This means that the nursing home, not the intended heirs, receives at least part of the couple's hard-earned nest egg. A strategy to avoid probate typically also invalidates the surviving spouse's right to any share, allowing all assets to pass to the intended beneficiaries.

2. Under a state's estate recovery program, assets passing from a Medicaid recipient to heirs through probate must be grabbed by the state as a reimbursement for Medicaid benefits paid. Some states are threatening to grab assets in the estate of a Medicaid recipient's spouse as well. But states do *not* have to go after nonprobate assets. So in at least some states, avoiding probate may avoid the

state's estate recovery program as well (see chapter 5).

In other words, avoiding probate means that your heirs have a better chance of recovering the estate you want them to receive.

The two primary ways to avoid probate are through joint ownership and living trusts. Let's look at each of these strategies.

As discussed earlier, you can hold almost any asset with someone else jointly with rights of survivorship. While both owners are alive, both own and control the property. When one dies, the survivor owns the asset automatically, without having to go through probate.

This is the simplest way to avoid probate, but it is also the most dangerous. When you add a child to your house deed, for example, the child becomes an equal co-owner. You have transferred half of the value of the house, creating a Medicaid ineligibility period (see pages 35 and 41–42) and possibly costing your child capital gains taxes down the road (see page 65). You can't sell the house without the co-owner's approval and signature, which can create big problems.

A revocable living trust is far less risky and in most cases is the best way to avoid probate. A revocable living trust is simply a contract between you and a trustee. In the trust agreement, you appoint someone of your choice (a trustee) to manage and distribute assets in the trust. You may give the trustee very specific instructions about how to handle the trust or you can allow him or her broad discretion. You may put some or all of your money and property into the trust—including bank accounts, CDs, real estate, stocks, and so forth—just by putting them into the name of the trustee. You may find this trust particularly attractive because you can retain control during your lifetime over assets placed in the trust. You can make yourself the trustee; you can name yourself as a beneficiary of the trust so that you can continue to receive the benefit of your money and property during your lifetime; and you can change or cancel the trust at any time. In other words, you can continue to conduct your financial affairs under a revocable living trust just as you always have.

Even if you choose to serve as your own trustee—as most people do—you will need a backup to take over should you become incapacitated or when you die. Pick someone who is capable, trustworthy, and willing to serve—usually a relative, close friend, or professional trustee. To find a professional, shop

around at local banks and trust companies; compare the results of their investments over the last one, five, and ten years. And remember, just because you select a particular person now doesn't mean you're stuck forever. As long as you remain competent, you can change your trustee at any time.

Beneficiaries named in the trust will immediately receive your assets when you die, without going through probate and without additional cost. And, most important, a spouse can legally be cut out, avoiding the risk of assets going to a nursing home rather than to the intended heirs.

Remember, a revocable living trust does nothing to protect assets from a nursing home while the creator of the trust is alive. Other types of trusts, such as the irrevocable asset protection trust, can insulate savings deposited into that trust from a nursing home, but a standard revocable living trust will not.

Yet a revocable living trust can still be extremely valuable to protect assets retained by a nursing-home patient's spouse; if the spouse dies before the nurs-

---

WARNING

A revocable living trust can cost your family a lot of money if you are not careful. Under OBRA 1993, distributions from a revocable living trust to third parties (other than the person who created the trust) create a sixty-month look-back period, rather than the usual thirty-six months.

Let's say your father set up a revocable living trust, and fifty months ago he gave the children a large gift of $200,000 directly from the trust. Now he is going into a nursing home. Since a gift from the trust triggered a sixty-month look-back period instead of a thirty-six-month period, the gift makes him ineligible for Medicaid.

If your father had taken the $200,000 from the trust, put it into his own checking account, and then written a check to the children for the same amount, there would have been only a thirty-six-month look-back period, and he would now qualify for Medicaid!

The moral of the story: never make gifts to third parties from a revocable living trust. Instead take the money out of the trust first, and then make gifts.

ing-home patient, assets should pass to heirs, not the nursing home. In a state that does not apply the estate recovery rules to nonprobate assets, even an unmarried nursing-home resident may benefit from a revocable living trust.

CHAPTER 11 SUMMARY CHECKLIST

Use a Revocable Living Trust and Joint Ownership to Protect Retained Assets

Change Title to Property and Update the Will

- ✔ Move assets into the name of the healthy spouse.

- ✔ Change the will of the healthy spouse to eliminate the nursing-home spouse as a beneficiary of any assets.

- ✔ Remove the nursing-home spouse as beneficiary of the healthy spouse's life insurance and retirement funds.

Create a Revocable Living Trust or Joint Ownership

- ✔ Create joint ownership to avoid probate, but be aware of the risks.

- ✔ Move assets into a revocable living trust to avoid probate and the spouse's "elective share."

- ✔ Don't make distributions directly from a revocable living trust to third parties; instead return assets to the trust's creator so that he or she can make distributions.

12 | Durable Power of Attorney: The Most Important Planning Tool

Preparing a durable power of attorney is the single most important thing most people can do to avoid the Medicaid trap and protect their savings. Yet most people have never even heard of this simple tool.

A durable power of attorney allows you to retain control of your assets—and your life—for as long as possible. Once it's clear that you must go into a nursing home, the assets can be transferred. If you can give them away yourself, fine, but if you can't, the durable power of attorney assures that someone you trust will be able to get rid of them for you. And until you clearly need nursing-home care, you can keep your life savings for yourself.

A durable power of attorney can guarantee that you and your loved ones will not spend any more than about $100,000 to $150,000 of the accumulated nest egg on nursing-home care. While that's certainly a lot, a durable power of attorney will enable most middle-class Americans to keep a portion of their life savings. *No one should ever lose everything.*

Example 67

Your father is incapacitated in an auto accident and must be admitted to a nursing home. At the time of his accident, he has assets worth $150,000.

As soon as he enters the nursing home, he transfers $75,000 to you and keeps $75,000. Coupled with his income, he should have enough to pay the nursing home during the twenty-five-month period of ineligibility triggered by the transfer ($75,000 divided by $3,000 a month).

Twenty-five months later, when the ineligibility period has passed, he qualifies for Medicaid. He was able to protect $75,000 of his assets.

This example, drawing on techniques already discussed, demonstrates how people can preserve their nest egg even if they haven't started shifting assets before entering a nursing home. By transferring assets upon entering an institution and then waiting for the ineligibility period to expire, a person should be able to avoid losing any more than the costs incurred during that period.

This sounds great, except that many people aren't able to transfer property when they enter a nursing home. Maybe they're so physically or mentally impaired that they can't legally make a valid transfer. The law in every state bars someone who is incompetent from making a legal transfer. If a person can't understand the significance of what he or she is doing, he or she won't be permitted to give away assets.

Example 68

Your father, who always seemed quite healthy, never did any Medicaid planning. Suddenly he suffers a stroke and becomes incapacitated. He must be admitted to a nursing home, and he is not likely to return home.

Because the stroke damaged his brain, he is now mentally incompetent. As a result, he can't transfer his bank accounts, CDs, or stocks. Within a short time, his life savings will all be paid to the nursing home.

This sad tale is repeated every day in this country. People who fail to plan ahead will lose their entire life savings to nursing homes. And often the family is unable to help manage the financial affairs because they lack the authorization.

A nursing-home resident's spouse cannot transfer assets simply because he or she is the spouse; the same holds true for children. *No* person is entitled to act for a nursing-home patient to transfer assets from his or her name, just because that individual is related by blood or marriage.

When someone had become incapacitated and can't handle his or her own affairs, how is a transfer usually handled? There are three primary vehicles: withdrawing funds from joint assets, establishing a guardianship, or using a durable power of attorney. Withdrawals from joint assets are often of only limited use. A guardianship is worthless for Medicaid purposes, for reasons explained below. But a durable power of attorney can be invaluable.

What Are Withdrawals from Joint Assets?

Let's go back to example 68. Your father is unable to transfer his bank accounts, CDs, or stocks. If you are named as a joint co-owner of those assets, can you transfer the assets for him?

In most cases, co-owners on bank accounts or CDs are named "either/or," which allows either co-owner to withdraw the entier amount on his or her own. As a co-owner, you could then take your father's name off the accounts and transfer to yourself or others. While this withdrawal triggers a Medicaid ineligibility period, at least the transfer can be made. But the stock is a different story. Typically co-owners of stock are named "and," requiring all co-owners to sign in order to sell or transfer shares. If your father can't sign, the stock cannot be transferred by anyone other than a court-appointed guardian; it's locked in his name.

Withdrawals of joint assets by a co-owner are often of limited use. Many assets, such as stock and real estate, typically require the signing of all co-owners for a transfer. And, of course, assets in the name of the nursing-home resident alone cannot be withdrawn by another person because there's no joint ownership.

What Is a Guardianship?

A guardian (sometimes known as a "conservator," "curator," "committee," "tutor," or "fiduciary") can be appointed by a probate judge for someone (often called a "ward") who cannot conduct his or her own affairs. Once appointed, a guardian may take any steps necessary, under the probate court's supervision, to manage the finances of the person for whom the guardian is appointed. The guardian must act for the benefit of the ward and must report regularly to the probate court.

Could a guardian appointed for your parent transfer his or her assets after your parent enters a nursing home, so that your parent would qualify for Medicaid? After all, isn't that what your parent would do if he or she were competent?

To my knowledge, no judge has ever allowed a guardian to get rid of someone's assets in order to qualify that person for Medicaid. This is because a guardian's job is to protect and promote the best interests of one person: the ward. Taking actions that would benefit the ward's *family* is not part of a guardianship's job description. A judge is not likely to conclude that it's in a person's best interest to become impoverished (even though that may have been consistent with the person's wishes in order to leave an inheritance to heirs). There are additional disadvantages when the court must appoint a guardian—emotional and financial. To have a loved one publicly labeled "incompetent" can be traumatic for the family. And the costs generally run at least $1,000, and often much higher.

A less common alternative, appointment of a representative payee, has the same limitations. A representative payee may be appointed under certain public programs (such as Social Security or veterans' programs) to receive and spend benefits on behalf of a beneficiary who is unable to manage his or her benefits alone. Again, an elderly person's representative payee can make expenditures only in the best interest of that person, and he or she probably will not be permitted to transfer assets from a nursing-home patient in order to qualify the patient for Medicaid.

The *only* way an older person can avoid appointment of a guardian or representative payee should he or she become incompetent is to plan ahead. Giving someone a durable power of attorney while you are still able to do so can mean the difference between losing or retaining control over your nest egg.

What Is a Durable Power of Attorney?

Let's start by talking about a regular power of attorney, because you may already be familiar with that. A regular power of attorney authorizes someone else to act for the maker of the document. The maker is often called the "principle"; the person authorized to act for the principal is called an "attorney-in-fact" or an "agent."

A regular power of attorney can give someone very specific, limited powers. For example, it can authorize someone to sign the deed to sell your house while you are out of town. Or a power of attorney can give someone very broad powers. For example, it may authorize someone to do anything you could do—endorse checks, pay bills, or have access to bank accounts.

A durable power of attorney is almost exactly the same as a regular power of attorney, but with one key difference: A regular *power of attorney becomes ineffective and stops working the moment the maker becomes incompetent;* durable *power of attorney remains valid even after the maker becomes incompetent.*

Since the time an individual may really need a power of attorney is when he or she becomes incompetent, this is no small difference. An older person should have a *durable* power of attorney for his or her protection.

Example 69

Your widowed father suffers a stroke and becomes incapacitated. As a result, he is admitted to a nursing home.

He is incompetent and can't transfer his own assets. But he did give you a durable power of attorney authorizing you to transfer assets. You use that durable power of attorney to transfer assets from your father to you and your brothers and sisters. This triggers a thirty-six-month ineligibility period.

Three years later, your father's nursing-home tab can be covered by Medicaid, and the rest of his assets will be protected. If at a later date his condition improves and he's able to leave the nursing home, his assets can be transferred back to him.

A durable power of attorney may be crucial to the planning techniques discussed in chapters 7, 8, 10, and 11. For example, I discussed how a nursing-home patient can protect assets by moving them into exemptions or transferring them to children or a spouse. The success of these techniques may depend on whether the nursing-home resident previously gave someone a durable power of attorney, so that the agent would then be authorized to shift the assets. Not including a durable power of attorney as part of your planning strategy would be like buying a car without a fuel tank.

Example 70

Your father is suddenly incapacitated by a stroke and becomes incompetent. Your mother has no choice but to admit him to a nursing home. Since your father is incompetent, he can't transfer the bank accounts, CDs, and stocks from his name. Your mother dies shortly after that, and all but $2,000 of your father's savings will be turned over to the nursing home.

Had your father given your mother a durable power of attorney, she could have used it to transfer assets from your father's name into her name and/or the names of their children. Then when she died, the financial disaster described in example 70 would have been averted.

If a person becomes incompetent and has not given anyone a durable power of attorney, his or her financial affairs typically will be carried on by a guardian appointed by the court. And the incompetent person will probably then lose his or her savings to a nursing home.

Can a Person Prepare His or Her Own Durable Power of Attorney?

A durable power of attorney does not have to be complicated, but I generally wouldn't recommend preparing your own. It must be in writing, signed by the principal, and it must state the name of the person who is being authorized to act for the principal and the scope of his or her powers.

Every state has its own rules governing the use of a durable power of attorney. Because laws differ significantly concerning the use, execution, and recording of durable powers of attorney, and because the laws are constantly changing, it is always good procedure to consult a lawyer. Since durable powers of attorney are relatively simple to prepare, you shouldn't have to pay any more than $100, and often $25 to $50. Note that if a durable power of attorney does not clearly authorize gifts or transfers, then someone might later challenge any transfers made using it. However, spelling out a right to make gifts in the durable power of attorney may create tax problems for the person named as agent.

You will find sample durable power of attorney forms for various states at the back of the book, in appendix A.

How to Avoid Abuse by the Holder of a Durable Power of Attorney

When you draw up a durable power of attorney, you are giving someone else the right to go into your bank accounts, cash checks, sell stocks, and do anything you could do with respect to your own finances. If that makes you uncomfortable, it should!

As soon as you give someone a durable power of attorney, that person can use it—unless you limit its use, the durable power of attorney is effective immediately, not just when you become incapacitated.

Legally the person to whom you give a durable power of attorney can act only in your best interest. If he or she decides to sell your car or house, you are entitled to the money; he or she can't legally raid your accounts and take the money to Tahiti. But as a practical matter, if someone does abuse your trust and misuse the durable power of attorney, you will have a legal nightmare.

Here are four options that can minimize your risks:

1. Give a durable power of attorney only to someone who is trustworthy.
2. Give it to a third party to hold until it must be used.
3. Make a "springing" durable power of attorney.
4. Name more than one person as agent in the durable power of attorney and designate that they must act jointly.

GIVE A DURABLE POWER OF ATTORNEY ONLY TO SOMEONE YOU TRUST

You shouldn't give just anyone a durable power of attorney. Give this document only to a trustworthy individual. Normally this means your spouse, a child, or a very close friend.

The person to whom you give a durable power of attorney does not, under the laws of most states, have to live in the same state. But for convenience and speed of action, it is always better to give it to someone who lives reasonably close by.

Although the person you choose is called an "attorney-in-fact," he or she does not have to be a lawyer; the attorney-in-fact also need not be a financial planner, businessperson, accountant, or in any other particular profession. Sure, it's helpful if the recipient of a durable power of attorney has some understanding of finances and the legal impact of a durable power of attorney, but it's not required. The only requirement is that you trust the person to whom you give a durable power of attorney.

GIVE A DURABLE POWER OF ATTORNEY TO A THIRD PARTY TO HOLD

Another way to reduce the risks is to give the durable power of attorney to a third person to hold until you need it. For example, you may name your son in the durable power of attorney and then hand it to a third party, say another relative, a friend, or a lawyer, to hold, with instructions not to give it to your son until you become incapacitated and are unable to handle your own affairs. The person holding the durable power of attorney can't use it because he or she is not named in it. And your son won't have access to and be able to use the durable power of attorney unless and until the person holding it gives it to him. So you'd better give it to a very trustworthy person to hold, too!

MAKE A SPRINGING DURABLE POWER OF ATTORNEY

In some states, a durable power of attorney can be written so that it doesn't become effective until you become incapacitated—at that time it "springs" into effect. However, this type of power of attorney has not yet been accepted in all states, and even where it is used, it often invites legal challenges over the issue of defining the actual onset of someone's incapacity.

NAME MORE THAN ONE PERSON IN THE
DURABLE POWER OF ATTORNEY

You may choose to give a single durable power of attorney jointly to two people. (The forms provided in
appendix A will illustrate how to do this.) The benefit of naming two people jointly in one document is
that both would have to agree before acting on your
behalf. That gives you an added degree of protection—one person can't steal you blind.

But naming two people in the same durable
power of attorney may also create problems. Sometimes actions must be taken quickly under a durable
power of attorney. Delays will be more likely if two
people must act together.

Although there are risks involved in making a
durable power of attorney, the benefits usually out-
weigh the risks. And if you follow these tips, you can
minimize the dangers involved.

Can You Give Durable Powers of Attorney to More than One Person?

You can give durable powers of attorney to as many
people as you like. You could give one to each of your
three kids, one to Aunt Macey, and one to your
lawyer. But I don't advise it.

As I've said, these are powerful documents. If it's
risky giving a durable power of attorney to one person, it's more risky to give two or three people
durable powers of attorney. Each person you give
one to has full powers to act for you.

There are very few occasions when I'd recommend giving out more than one durable power of attorney. In the case of elderly parents, each may want
to give one durable power of attorney to the other
and another durable power of attorney to a child (so
that there will be a greater likelihood that at least the
child will be available, should both parents become
incapacitated or either die). If you have two children
and don't want to show favoritism, you may want to
give each child a durable power of attorney. Still, you
are best off minimizing the number of durable powers of attorney that you hand around.

Can You Cancel a Durable Power of Attorney?

In most states, you can easily cancel a durable power
of attorney. In theory, all you need to do is declare

that it's canceled. You usually aren't even required to
put the cancellation in writing; just announce it to
the holder, preferably in the presence of witnesses.
That's in theory; now let's talk reality. Effectively
canceling a durable power of attorney may be much
harder.

Let's say that you announce that a durable power
of attorney you granted to a friend is canceled. Your
friend immediately goes to the bank with his durable
power of attorney and tries to take out your savings.
The bank personnel won't know that you have canceled the power of attorney; they'll see a document
that looks valid, and your friend (some friend!) can
take the money and run.

In practice, you would have to try to get back all
copies of the durable power of attorney. But that's
not easy, since the friend could have made any number of copies, and many financial institutions will accept photocopies.

Of course, you could also give notice of the cancellation, in writing, not only to the holder but also to
all those people and institutions (like your bank) you
believe might be asked to honor the durable power
of attorney. But it's usually impossible to predict
everyone who may be asked to take some action
based on a durable power of attorney.

If worse comes to worst, you could go to court and
have a judge order that all copies be returned. But
that's a hassle and expense you don't need. Better to
minimize the risk in the first place by giving a
durable power of attorney only to someone you
trust.

CHAPTER 12 SUMMARY CHECKLIST

**Durable Power of Attorney:
The Most Important Planning Tool**

Make a Durable Power of Attorney

✔ Prepare a durable power of attorney for
   your spouse.

✔ Prepare durable powers of attorney for one
   or more of your children.

✔ Have an experienced lawyer prepare the
   documents.

✔ Name as agent someone you trust.

✔ Give the durable powers of attorney to a third person to hold until it becomes necessary for them to be used.

✔ Tell your children who is holding the durable power of attorney and/or where the document is located.

Make Withdrawals from Joint Accounts

✔ If you haven't obtained a durable power of attorney, you may still make withdrawals from certain joint assets.

✔ Unfortunately, one co-owner cannot make withdrawals or transfers from many joint assets, such as real estate.

Obtain a Guardianship as a Last Resort

✔ Get a guardianship to help manage the affairs of a person who's become incompetent.

✔ Don't expect a guardian to engage in Medicaid planning; that's not his or her responsibility.

$\boxed{13}$ More Aggressive Planning Strategies

I've already described dozens of planning strategies and opportunities that can help you avoid the Medicaid trap and protect at least part of your and your loved ones' savings. But we're not done yet. Here are a few additional, more aggressive planning techniques. By aggressive I mean that the strategies involve an interpretation of the Medicaid rules that may or may not be accepted by Uncle Sam. The higher risk for denial makes it more likely to require appeals and litigation, possibly in court, in order to receive benefits. But they all have reasonable legal bases and might prove beneficial. This information is being presented to provide you with the full range of options available. Because of the increased risks, each person will need to decide for himself or herself the level of aggressiveness that he or she feels comfortable pursuing.

Keep Assets to Generate Income

When describing the amount of income you may keep (pages 30–32), I explained that the law guarantees the spouse-at-home a minimum amount of income—at least $1,230 a month, and in some states as much as $1,870.50 a month. If the spouse-at-home doesn't have enough income to reach the minimum, the difference generally is made up from the income of the spouse in the nursing home. For example, if you receive $300 a month in your name and your spouse, who is in a nursing home, has an income of $1,500 a month, you should be entitled to an addi-

tional $930 a month, which generally will come from the institutionalized person's income.

But there's another—and often much better—way to gain the minimum income: keep enough assets to generate sufficient income for the spouse-at-home.

Example 71

Your income from Social Security is $430 a month; your husband, who has just entered a nursing home, gets $900 a month from a pension. In addition, the two of you have assets of $150,000. You could spend down your assets to $74,820, generating interest income of $300 a month. At that point your husband would qualify for Medicaid. Your husband would give you $500 a month from his income to bring your monthly income up to $1,230.

But here's a better idea. You choose to keep more *assets* to generate more income, rather than taking income from your husband, or your husband refuses to give you anything from his income (which he has a legal right to do). Since you still need an additional $500 of income each month to bring you up to the minimum of $1,230, you can keep sufficient assets to generate that income. At 5 percent interest, you would need all of your $150,000. In other words, your husband would qualify for Medicaid immediately, without spending down assets, and you can keep the entire $150,000!

This strategy makes a lot of sense from a public policy perspective. Let's take the facts in example 71. If you had to spend down to $74,820 and supplement your income with $500 from your husband, you'd have $1,230 per month of income—which our legislators have said is the minimum amount a person needs to live. But when your spouse in the nursing home dies, his income disappears. You will be stuck with a monthly income of only $730, clearly not enough to live on and likely to create a great hardship. But if you had been permitted to keep the $150,000 to generate income, then your financial future would remain secure even after your institutionalized spouse died.

Some states are allowing a spouse-at-home to choose to retain enough assets to generate income rather than to supplement income from the nursing-home spouse; other states are not. At this writing, several major class action lawsuits are pending that should clarify the usefulness of this strategy in the near future. The federal Health Care Financing Administration is saying that states *should* approve this planning tool.

Refuse to Make Assets Available to the Spouse in a Nursing Home

The following technique requires developing a thick skin, because it sounds heartless.

Let's say your spouse has entered a nursing home. Together you have total assets of $150,000, mostly in your name, which is well over the limit of $74,820. Do you have to spend down the balance?

You may decide to refuse to support your spouse. If your spouse then assigns to the state his legal rights to support from you, your spouse should become entitled to Medicaid benefits, without you spending a dime. If your spouse is incompetent and unable to assign his support rights, the state has the right to step in and pursue your spouse's support rights anyhow. What this means is that while the state provides Medicaid coverage for your spouse, it can sue you for the money, at least until your assets are spent down to the proper Medicaid eligibility limits.

If the state can sue you for the Medicaid benefits, what have you gained? If the state really does take you to court, you've gained nothing. But the experience in many states is that state Medicaid agencies are lax or don't have the staff to pursue support rights. In many cases the spouse-at-home has been able to protect his or her savings using this technique.

Purchase an Annuity

I've already explained how harsh the Medicaid laws can be on one spouse when the other must enter a nursing home. Spending down half of the assets, to no more than $74,820, often leaves the at-home spouse without enough funds to live on. Purchasing an annuity might make life a lot easier.

Example 72

On the day your spouse goes into a nursing home, you jointly have $100,000. Your spouse won't qualify for Medicaid until you've spent down to $50,000.

You take $50,000 and purchase an annuity that pays you, say, $600 a month for life. The income is yours because it comes in your name, and so it won't be used to pay your spouse's nursing-home costs. With an annuity you'll be getting more income than you ever were before, and your husband immediately qualifies for Medicaid because you've spent down to $50,000. Since no transfer to any third person occurred, there should be no Medicaid ineligibility period.

To take advantage of this planning tool, the annuity generally must meet three requirements: It must be immediate, irrevocable, and nonassignable. Irrevocable and nonassignable mean that you can't cash it in or sell it—under those circumstances it has no market value as a resource, and so it doesn't count as part of your assets. Immediate means that it starts paying you a monthly payment immediately rather than on a deferred basis. If some or all of the payments were deferred, the state would probably argue that the annuity is really a gimmick to leave assets to heirs after you pass away.

When you die, the annuity payments should end. Again, by setting up the annuity payments in this way, the state can't argue that this is simply a trick to pass assets to heirs.

An annuity, as described above, can allow a spouse-at-home to increase income while quickly qualifying a spouse in a nursing home for Medicaid benefits. The primary drawback is that heirs may end up with nothing.

If the healthy spouse lives for a number of years, that won't necessarily be so. Since the spouse-at-home will have increased his or her income by the annuity, there should be enough to allow the spouse to begin to accumulate additional savings. Once the nursing-home spouse is receiving Medicaid, savings accruing in the name of the spouse-at-home should be protected. Depending on how long the spouse-at-home lives, the heirs may receive as much as or more than they would have received otherwise.

Example 73

Your wife has just entered a nursing home. Your combined assets are $100,000, and you're allowed to keep only half that amount. You move the assets into your name and purchase an annuity with $50,000. Since your combined assets have now dropped to half, your wife qualifies for Medicaid.

The annuity generates about $350 a month, which is double the interest previously generated by the $50,000 investment you previously had in CDs. You spend $175 a month and invest the other $175 a month. In about fifteen years, you should accumulate more than $50,000 from this investment, and if you live longer, your heirs would get even more.

What if you die the day after buying an immediate annuity? All your money would be gone and your heirs would get nothing. To avoid this financial disaster, most people obtain a guarantee from the insurance company that payments will continue for a fixed number of years. For example, if you arranged for a ten-year guarantee period and died after three years, payments would be made to your heirs for seven more years.

To prevent people from using unreasonably long guarantees to pass assets to heirs, the federal HCFA is telling states to limit the guarantee period to a person's life expectancy. Purchasing an annuity with a guarantee longer than your life expectancy would be considered a transfer of assets to your heirs and would trigger an ineligibility period.

Tables 13.1 and 13.2 show life expectancies used by HCFA.

TABLE 13.1

Life Expectancy for Males

AGE	LIFE EXPECTANCY (YEARS)
50	26.32
51	25.48
52	24.65
53	23.82
54	23.01
55	22.21
56	21.43
57	20.66
58	19.90
59	19.15
60	18.42
61	17.70
62	16.99
63	16.30
64	15.62
65	14.96
66	14.32
67	13.70
68	13.09
69	12.50
70	11.92
71	11.35
72	10.80
73	10.27
74	9.27
75	9.24
76	8.76
77	8.29
78	7.83
79	7.40
80	6.98
81	6.59
82	6.21
83	5.81
84	5.51
85	5.19
86	4.89
87	4.61
88	4.34
89	4.09
90	3.86
91	3.64
92	3.43
93	3.24
94	3.06
95	2.90
96	2.74
97	2.60
98	2.47
99	2.34
100	2.22

NOTE: Health Care Financing Administration Transmittal, No. 64, State Medicaid Manual, November 1994, at 3-3-109.17.

TABLE 13.2

Life Expectancy For Females

Age	Life Expectancy (years)
50	31.37
51	30.48
52	29.60
53	28.72
54	27.86
55	27.00
56	26.15
57	25.31
58	24.48
59	23.67
60	22.86
61	22.06
62	21.27
63	20.49
64	19.72
65	18.96
66	18.21
67	17.48
68	16.76
69	16.04
70	15.35
71	14.66
72	13.99
73	13.33
74	12.68
75	12.05
76	11.43
77	10.83
78	10.24
79	9.67
80	9.11
81	8.58
82	8.06
83	7.56
84	7.08
85	6.63
86	6.20
87	5.79
88	5.41
89	5.05
90	4.71
91	4.40
92	4.11
93	3.84
94	3.59
95	3.36
96	3.16
97	2.97
98	2.80
99	2.64
100	2.48

NOTE: Health Care Financing Administration Transmittal, No. 64, State Medicaid Manual, November 1994, at 3-3-109.18.

The use of annuities as a planning tool, particularly by the spouse-at-home after the other spouse entered a nursing home, has been gaining acceptance over recent years. But many states have not yet decided whether or not to permit the purchase of annuities as a tool to shelter assets.

Put Assets into a Limited Liability Company or a Family Limited Partnership

Limited liability companies (LLCs) are the newest and one of the most exciting estate planning tools available. At this writing, about forty-five states have adopted laws allowing LLCs. The key benefit of an LLC is that it protects assets from creditors. In this lawsuit-crazy world, the risk of losing your entire life savings to creditors is very real.

Let's say you are laid off from work, and while the paychecks have ended, the bills keep coming. Creditors are threatening to seize your home and bank accounts. Or maybe you hit a car carrying three kids and your insurance coverage may not be anywhere near enough to pay a judgment. If your assets are in an LLC, creditors will be unable to touch them.

Here's how LLCs work: You first create an LLC under the rules of your state; it's not that difficult, although you should have a lawyer's help. Once created, you will place assets in the LLC. Just as you would do with a trust, you would change the names on every asset being transferred to the name of the LLC. Once that's done, your assets are protected. A family limited partnership works in much the same way, providing the same creditor protection, although it's usually more burdensome to set up and operate.

How can an LLC or family limited partnership help when it comes to Medicaid planning? That's not yet clear. But it seems that these two tools should be effective.

The concept is similar to that used in the old Medicaid trust (see page 69). Assets put into this specialized irrevocable trust were protected from nursing-home costs (after an ineligibility period). All of the income generated by the trust assets would be paid to you, but you could not touch the principal.

The same basis results can be achieved with an LLC (or with a family limited partnership). You would create and place assets into an LLC. Your children or others would receive all or almost all of the income. If set up properly, your children would ultimately receive your assets at your death.

Will this work for Medicaid planning? It should, but I can't give any assurance that it will. It is simply too early to tell; LLCs have not been tested as Medicaid tools.

If LLCs can be used as Medicaid planning tools, they may even allow the Medicaid recipient to keep control of the assets. For example, if you took your assets (say $100,000) and gave them to your children, the assets would belong to them. You lose control. Even under the old Medicaid trust, you could not retain control of your assets if you wanted to protect them from nursing-home costs.

But let's say you took your $100,000 of assets and put them into an LLC or a family limited partnership, then gave ninety-nine of the one hundred shares to your children. Your share has almost no value; the bulk of your assets have gone to your children. However, you can make your share the only voting share. You remain in complete control; your children have no role in decisions dealing with the LLC. (Alternatively, you could give your children the voting share and they could hire you under a separate management agreement.)

And there's another benefit. If you gave $100,000 of bank accounts, CDs, and other assets to your children, you would create a Medicaid ineligibility period based on a gift or transfer of $100,000. Assuming an average cost of care for your state of $3,000 a month, you would have triggered an ineligibility period of about thirty-four months.

But if you create an LLC or a family limited partnership, put $100,000 into the LLC or partnership, and then give away ninety-nine out of one hundred shares, what have you given away? For tax purposes, the IRS has determined that the value of the gifts to the children is significantly less than $100,000—after all, the children have very limited ability to market or sell their units, and they may not have control. As a result, the gift to the children may be valued at only $60,000 or $70,000. If the same principles are applied in the Medicaid context, that would create a much lesser ineligibility period, perhaps only about twenty to twenty-four months. And the market value of the one share you retained still has negligible value.

Will an LLC or family limited partnership in which you keep control work for purposes of Medicaid planning? Again, this has not yet been tested. The primary risk is that the Medicaid bureaucrats will argue that an LLC is similar to a trust. They

might go on to say that since you couldn't create a trust that worked like an LLC or partnership (with you in control), then an LLC or partnership shouldn't work to insulate assets, either. If you keep control, it is even more likely that the state will challenge the LLC or partnership. Under any circumstances, at this point, the use of an LLC or family limited partnership would probably involve appeals and eventual court litigation.

CHAPTER 13 SUMMARY CHECKLIST

More Aggressive Planning Strategies

Keep Assets to Generate Income

✔ Instead of spending down assets, keep enough to generate the income for the spousal allowance.

Refuse to Make Assets Available to the Spouse in a Nursing Home

✔ Refuse to support the spouse in a nursing home, so that he or she can qualify for Medicaid.

✔ Hope the state won't sue you for support.

Purchase an Annuity

✔ Move assets into the name of the spouse who's at home, then purchase an immediate, nontransferable annuity.

✔ Set aside part of the added income to accumulate savings for the healthy spouse.

✔ Arrange for a reasonable payment guarantee period, based on the owner's life expectancy.

Put Assets into a Limited Liability Company or Family Limited Partnership

✔ Give away principal but keep the present income stream.

✔ Maybe even keep control.

✔ Reduce the Medicaid ineligibility period by discounting gifts.

✔ Be prepared for appeals and court litigation.

14 Avoid Harsh Income Limits

Each state is permitted to decide how much income an individual is entitled to keep and still be eligible for Medicaid benefits. Some states impose severe, unbending income limits (see tables 3.1 and 3.2) that can lead to disastrous financial consequences, as example 74 shows.

Example 74

Your father is in a nursing home. He gets $1,000 a month from Social Security and a $500-a-month pension. The $1,500-a-month total income is not enough to pay the $4,000 monthly nursing-home bill, but it exceeds the $1,374-a-month income cap for Medicaid eligibility. Under the rules, your father will have to learn to sleep on a park bench.

But by taking a few critical steps, the onerous effect of a state's income cap can be avoided.

Transfer Income-Producing Assets

If income generated by assets is causing you or a loved one to exceed the state's income cap, transferring assets may bring down the income.

Example 75

Your father is in a nursing home. He gets $1,300 a month from Social Security and $250 a month in interest from $60,000 of funds (CDs and bank accounts) in his name. Your mother also gets some income, but this money doesn't affect your father's Medicaid qualification.

Although they have spent down enough of their assets to qualify for Medicaid, your father's income is slightly over the $1,374 monthly limit imposed by the state. As long as his income is too high, he can't get Medicaid.

Your parents simply have to shift the $60,000 to your mother, so that the interest and dividend checks will come in her name. Now Dad is below the income limit and immediately qualifies for Medicaid.

Get QDRO to Shift Pension Income

QDRO stands for qualified domestic relations order. You might need to learn this acronym when it is pension income that is putting a nursing-home spouse over the income cap. The couple may be able to get a domestic relations judge to order the income paid to the spouse-at-home. Since the income of the spouse-at-home doesn't count against the income of the spouse in the nursing home, the court order, called a QDRO, can enable the nursing-home patient to qualify for Medicaid.

Create a Miller Trust

Shifting assets, as described above, works fine if the excess income is generated by assets. And a QDRO works fine for pension income when the nursing-home resident is married. But what if the income comes from Social Security or other sources, and/or the nursing home resident is not married? How can you reduce the income? You can't just give this income away. You can't even get the government or pension plan to stop payments.

Prior to OBRA 1993, judges in many states recognized the unfairness of income caps and allowed the creation of what have become known as Qualifying Income Miller trusts (named after the individual involved in the first major case approving the use of these trusts). Judges would direct Social Security, pension, and other income into a Miller trust, removing it from the Medicaid applicant. The excess income in the trust generally would be paid to the state, and the Medicaid applicant could qualify for Medicaid. This process was complicated and required involvement of lawyers and courts.

In response to the problems created by state income caps, OBRA 1993 attempted to ease Medicaid eligibility. The best approach would simply have been to prohibit the use of income caps, but that would have been too easy. Instead OBRA 1993 specifically authorized the creation of Miller-type trusts.

Under the law, income from pensions, Social Security, and other sources can be directed into this type of trust. The trust must provide that at the death of the Medicaid recipient, its assets must be used to repay the state for any Medicaid benefits previously paid out. After this obligation is met, any remaining assets can go to the Medicaid recipient's heirs.

This trust, permitted under OBRA 1993, should be a little easier to use than the previous Miller trusts. Before OBRA 1993, Miller trusts had to go through the courts; now it should be possible to create them without court involvement.

Pack Up and Move

This is no joke. Many states do not impose income caps. You may find that the best strategy is simply to move to a state without an income cap.

CHAPTER 14 SUMMARY CHECKLIST

Avoid Harsh Income Limits

✔ Transfer income-producing assets.

✔ Get a qualified domestic relations order to shift pension income to a spouse-at-home.

✔ Move income into a Miller trust.

✔ Relocate to a state that does not impose an income cap.

15 As a Last Resort, Get a Divorce

This is really sad. An older couple may be blissfully happy, but if they want to look out for their best interests, they may need to get divorced! Although it sounds crazy, for some folks this strategy might be the only option for assuring financial survival.

Divorce Can Protect a Couple's Assets

Our country is supposed to be pro-family, and the laws are supposed to encourage family values. Yet when it comes to long-term care, the law penalizes marriage and encourages divorce.

Consider the following real-life situation: George and Mary have been happily married for fifty years. George has a degenerative muscle disease. Mary has been caring for him for years at home, but it is becoming clear that pretty soon a nursing home will be needed.

They have about $200,000 in cash, stocks, CDs, and T-bills. Mary doesn't want to give the money to the children because she'd lose control of the assets; but even if she did give away the funds, they'd have to pay the nursing home costs for thirty-six months. In the area where they live, a good nursing home runs $45,000 a year. In three years they'd spend $135,000 or more.

Their best plan is to get divorced. They can file for an uncontested divorce, providing that Mary gets all of the savings. If the judge grants the divorce, George will immediately qualify for Medicaid when he goes into a nursing home, because assets divided under a divorce decree do not cause any Medicaid waiting period.

There is some risk that a judge would not approve a settlement giving all of the assets to the spouse-at-home and nothing to the spouse who is ill and may need nursing-home care. But if both parties are mentally competent and know what they are doing, the judge is likely to approve their agreement.

If one spouse is not competent, then there is a greater risk that the divorce will not be granted on terms weighted heavily in favor of the healthy spouse. The incompetent spouse will need to have the court appoint someone (not the divorcing spouse) to represent the incompetent spouse's best interests. In most divorces, marital property will be split evenly between the two spouses, although divorce judges do have flexibility.

In some cases, a judge may award a larger portion to the spouse who is ill, feeling that he or she needs more, owing to higher medical and nursing-care expenses. But on the other hand, a divorce judge may tilt toward the spouse-at-home, recognizing that the institutionalized spouse will have Medicaid available. Even if a judge splits the assets evenly, the spouse-at-home may come out ahead.

Example 76

A couple has been married for forty years. They have combined assets of $200,000. The husband is extremely ill, not competent, and will probably have to enter a nursing home.

The wife files for divorce, and the judge grants it after a full hearing. The assets are split

99

down the middle, $100,000 to the husband and $100,000 to the wife. The husband's half will be paid to the nursing home, but the wife's portion is protected.

If the couple in example 76 had not obtained a divorce, they would have been able to keep only $74,820. In other words, the divorce saved $25,180. Although a divorce is certainly a drastic step, especially after a long and happy marriage, the savings can be significant.

Divorce Can Protect Income

A divorce can be crucial to protecting assets. It is usually much less important to protect income for the spouse-at-home, although in some cases it may be helpful here, too.

Example 77

A couple is living on the modest amount of $1,575 a month—the husband's pension payments of $375 and Social Security benefits of $800, and the wife's Social Security benefits of $400. Then the husband enters a nursing home.

A case with the same facts went before a court in New York a number of years ago. A woman designated in the court papers as Rose Septuagenarian asked the court to grant support payments from her institutionalized husband after Medicaid insisted that his entire income of $1,175 a month should be used to pay his nursing costs, leaving Rose to live on just $400 a month. Rose was devoted to her husband and visited him regularly at the nursing home; she was seeking reasonable support payments only to allow her to maintain a modest standard of living.

The New York Medicaid officials argued that no support should be allowed. They pointed out that Rose's husband was receiving Medicaid, a form of public assistance, and so could not support himself, let alone his spouse. Her husband's medical and living expenses far exceeded his income, so they argued that all of his income should be applied to those expenses before any deduction for Rose's support.

The divorce judge, Jeffrey H. Gallet, disagreed, displaying compassion and uncommon common sense. Judge Gallet said:

To deprive women, and particularly women of [Rose's] generation who, in many cases, were denied an equal opportunity to fulfill their potential in the employment market and are, therefore, dependent on their husbands for support, access to their husbands' pension and assets in their later years effectively sentences many of them to tremendous hardship and a complete disruption of their lives at a time when they are extremely vulnerable.

We must note that an overwhelming majority of married women are younger than their husbands. In addition, actuarial tables tell us that women live longer than men . . . (for example, a woman of 70 will outlive her 75-year-old husband by more than 11 years . . .) From those facts, together with the common knowledge that medical costs for many illnesses of old age are beyond the financial means of most American families, we can reasonably draw the conclusion that husbands are more likely to require care which will deplete the marital assets than their wives, who are likely to be the economically weaker spouse. So in cases such as this, where the petitioner is 72 years old and infirm, women will be forced from their homes, deprived of even their modest life-styles and relegated to a life of grinding poverty.[1]

Judge Gallet ended up awarding Rose support from her husband of $1,125 a month; only $50 a month was paid to the nursing home, with Medicaid picking up the rest of the tab.

The law has changed since the case of Rose Septuagenarian. Under the Medicaid law now, the spouse-at-home is entitled to an allowance from the nursing-home spouse based on a complicated formula discussed in chapter 3, to bring him or her up to a minimal level of income. Although the amount permitted is not huge, at least the spouse-at-home won't be left with virtually no income, as Rose almost was. Still, a divorce may enhance the spouse-at-home's income. (In some states, including New York, support can be awarded without a divorce.)

Don't Wait Too Long to Divorce

A divorce can be a very helpful planning tool, especially to protect assets for the spouse-at-home. But there's a hitch: the couple can't wait too long. While divorce should be the planning tool of last resort, if a couple puts the decision off too long, they may lose the opportunity to take advantage of this technique.

Why the time crunch? Should the nursing-home spouse become incompetent, a divorce might then be impossible. Many divorce judges are reluctant to grant a divorce from an incompetent spouse. And even if the couple should obtain a divorce, it would likely be only at great legal and emotional costs.

Once a nursing-home spouse becomes incompetent, the path to divorce court becomes more circuitous. The first stop now might have to be at probate court before a divorce can proceed. A probate judge will declare your spouse incompetent and name a guardian who will represent your spouse in the divorce case.

A guardian has a legal duty to act in your incompetent spouse's best interest, which may not be the same as your own best interest or those of any children you may have. The guardian may even have a legal obligation to oppose the divorce on the grounds that, given your spouse's high medical costs, no assets should be given away—even if Medicaid could pick up those same costs!

In other words, once one spouse becomes incompetent, divorce becomes far less attractive as a planning tool. If an elderly couple is considering a divorce as the way to protect their savings, they shouldn't put off the decision too long.

Spouses who find themselves facing tremendous nursing-home costs may have to consider a divorce. However unpleasant the prospect is for a happily married couple, the financial devastation resulting from staying together could prove to be even more unpleasant.

Don't Get Married: When You Say Yes, Medicaid Says No!

With increased frequency, older persons are getting married or remarried later in life. Finding a loving companion is wonderful. But if your new spouse becomes ill, watch out!

Example 78

You have just remarried, and you are looking forward to a new life together. To protect your savings for your children from a prior marriage, you and your husband signed a premarital contract. Your will leaves everything to the kids. You feel peaceful knowing that they'll be protected in case anything happens to you. No problem, right? Wrong! The honeymoon was too much for your husband; he suffered a stroke and must go into a nursing home.

You have $150,000 in savings and your husband has nothing—you were marrying him for love and companionship, not money. All of the savings were yours, the marriage is only two weeks old, and you both signed a premarital agreement. Too bad, none of those facts matter. He won't be eligible for Medicaid until *your* savings are spent down to $74,820. The moment you said "I do," all of your assets were put at risk. The premarital agreement does not protect your assets from his nursing-home costs.

Before getting married, think long and hard about the risk to your life savings. Marriage may be hazardous to your financial health.

CHAPTER 15 SUMMARY CHECKLIST

As a Last Resort, Get a Divorce

✔ Get a divorce to protect assets.

✔ Get a divorce or support order to add to a healthy spouse's income.

✔ If divorce looks like the best option, don't delay. Once a spouse becomes incompetent, divorce becomes a far less viable option.

✔ Consider "living in sin" rather than getting married later in life. Even a prenuptial agreement will not shelter your assets from a spouse's nursing-home costs.

✔ Ask the judge to approve a distribution of most or all assets to the healthy spouse.

16 Private Insurance for Long-Term Care

Many older Americans receive a rude awakening when they discover that the costs of the long-term care they need will not be paid by Medicare or Medicare supplemental insurance. What's happened? Surely these essential services must be covered? Sorry! Right now, no one is covered for long-term nursing-home care under Medicare or standard Medigap policies, and don't assume that your expensive insurance plan will pay either, because very few older Americans are actually covered for this under any health care policy.

This is not to say that there is no insurance available to cover long-term care costs. A growing number of long-term care policies are being offered, and if you are willing to do a lot of homework, it is possible to find some affordable policies. The Long-Term Care Questionnaire in this chapter will help guide you through the morass of long-term care insurance products. Unfortunately, the costs of the policies continue to be outside the budgets of most older Americans.

Is there any good way to cut the premium cost while maintaining adequate coverage? Using long-term care insurance together with other planning techniques can be an effective solution. In this chapter I'll explain how these strategies can work for you.

First, let's take a look at the private insurance options currently available.

Medigap Policies Won't Cover Long-Term Care Needs

Surely anyone who watches TV has seen commercials starring famous television personalities who extol the virtues of Medigap insurance policies for the elderly. Many of the ads give the impression that these policies will fill all of the gaps left by Medicare coverage. As a result, millions of Americans have purchased private supplemental health care coverage believing that these policies will take care of any future long-term care needs. Although the TV stars are reassuring, the reality is not.

Even the best Medigap policies will cover very little of a person's nursing-home costs. As discussed in chapter 1, Medicare generally pays for part of the costs of a *skilled* nursing home for only the first one hundred days; most Medigap policies will pay the difference not paid by Medicare for just those first one hundred days. *No* standard Medigap policy provides coverage for custodial (nonskilled) long-term care.

Long-Term Care Insurance May Be the Answer

There is one type of private insurance, commonly called long-term care insurance, that will cover long-term custodial care, the type of nursing-home care needed most often. Today about a hundred private insurance companies, including many of the largest, such as Bankers United Life, UNUM, American Express, John Hancock, The Travelers, and CNA, offer long-term care policies. These policies vary widely as to coverage and cost. So far they have proved of limited utility because of their expense, restrictions, limitations, and eligibility requirements.

Still, for some families, a well-chosen policy may be a worthwhile alternative to losing their savings to a nursing home, particularly if they are still healthy. This insurance allows you to protect your life savings and still keep control of your money without having to pursue other planning strategies, such as gifts to children.

So how do you track down a suitable private long-term care insurance policy? Before even beginning your search, take a second look at your existing coverage; you might be pleasantly surprised to find good news buried in the fine print. Although the chances are extremely slim, it's worth the investment of time. If you are covered by a group health insurance plan sponsored by an employer, union, trade association, or some other organization, you should ask the benefits representative about what benefits are included, particularly after retirement.

Also, it might be worthwhile for you to check with any health maintenance organizations in your area. Sometimes HMOs offer a good long-term care package at a more reasonable price than that for long-term care insurance.

But most likely you will find that no coverage is provided and that no HMO offers a reasonable option. Once you have exhausted all potential sources for coverage, it will be time to begin your search for long-term care insurance.

What You Should Look for in a Long-Term Care Policy

Long-term care policies currently on the market very greatly in cost and coverage. The following pages offer information to use and questions to address when investigating the available options.

THE COST OF THE POLICY

What is the Annual Premium?

The major reason long-term policies haven't caught fire is simple: the premium costs are extremely high.

Families USA Foundation looked at the costs of long-term care insurance in a report entitled "Nursing Home Insurance: Who Can Afford It?" The conclusion was unequivocal:

> Private nursing home insurance is not likely to offer most Americans a viable means of financing nursing home care in the foreseeable future. Except for the wealthiest individuals, private nursing home insurance fails to make nursing home care affordable for the vast majority of today's elderly and middle-aged Americans. This generation and future generations of elderly persons will continue to face the daunting specter of poverty should they need nursing home care. Alternatives to the present system of financing nursing home care will have to come from outside the private insurance market.[1]

Pretty depressing, isn't it?

Premiums vary depending on a number of factors, including the company, the insuree's age and health, the amount and type of benefits provided, and the length of time the insuree has to cover the nursing-home tab himself or herself before insurance coverage begins (as with a deductible).

Age is the most significant element; the exact same policy may cost a sixty-year-old $1,500 a year, a seventy-year-old $3,000 a year, and an eighty-year-old $8,000 annually. Premium rates can range widely, from a few hundred dollars to more than $10,000 a year.

Tables 16.1 and 16.2 provide a comparison of premiums for several companies to give you an idea of what to expect. These are provided as examples only; policies and premiums are constantly changing, so you must contact the insurance companies for current information.

Can the Company Raise the Premium?

You should check to make sure the policy is renewable at the same rates as you first pay. If the rates can be increased, you could eventually be priced out of the market and forced to give up the coverage. Note that even a guaranteed rate may not always remain unchanged; the law allows an insurer to increase the premiums on a policy of it's an across-the-board increase and affects not just you but everyone in the state.

TABLE 16.1

Premium Comparison of Long-Term Care Insurance with Home Health Care Rider

Age	Bankers United Life[1] (0-Day Wait)	CNA[2] (0-Day Wait) Preferred	CNA[2] (0-Day Wait) Standard	John Alden[3] (0-Day Wait) Preferred	John Alden[3] (0-Day Wait) Standard	AMEX[4] (20-Day Wait)	John Hancock[5] (20-Day Wait)	The Travelers[6] (20-Day Wait)	UNUM[7] (20-Day Wait) Pro-HHC	UNUM[7] (20-Day Wait) TOT-HHC
18–39	$ 640.00	—	—						—	—
40	640.00	—	—	$ 1,183.40	$1,690.50	$ 1,390.00	$ 1,381.00	$ 854.00	—	—
45	800.00	$1,005.00	$1,261.00	1,479.30	2,113.10	1,390.00	1,551.00	1,019.00	—	—
50	1,020.00	1,244.00	1,555.00	1,775.00	2,535.80	1,580.00	1,615.00	1,212.00	—	—
55	1,360.00	1,619.00	2,028.00	1,992.30	2,846.40	2,100.00	2,044.00	1,561.00	$1,755.60	$ 2,603.70
60	1,880.00	2,167.00	2,713.00	2,535.80	3,622.60	2,870.00	2,661.00	2,046.00	2,258.70	3,343.50
65	2,720.00	2,566.00	3,206.00	3,586.30	5,123.30	4,300.00	3,662.00	2,681.00	3,100.50	4,493.70
70	4,020.00	3,649.00	4,569.00	5,977.10	8,538.80	6,100.00	5,266.00	4,046.00	4,255.50	5,930.70
75	6,030.00	5,443.00	6,804.00	10,414.70	14,878.20	7,660.00	7,791.00	6,453.00	6,337.80	8,633.40
79	8,990.00	7,417.00	9,278.00	14,580.50	20,829.40	13,610.00	12,269.00	10,338.00	8,422.20	11,283.60
80	—[8]	—[8]	—[8]	15,486.30	22,123.10	—[8]	—[8]	—[8]	9,062.70	12,069.00
84	—[8]	—[8]	—[8]	18,268.30	26,097.50	—[8]	—[8]	—[8]	—	—

NOTE: Table is based on a $100-a-day daily benefit and a lifetime benefit period, with a 5.0 percent compound benefit increase option. Note that premiums are always changing. Contact individual insurance companies for up-to-date information.

[1]Bankers United Life: Protector (1993).
[2]CNA: Classic LTC (1993); Premier LTC (1993).
[3]John Alden: Independent Life Plan (1993).
[4]AMEX: Nursing Home and Alternate Care Coverage/Home and Community Care Rider (1992); Privileged Care Select (1994).
[5]John Hancock: Protectcare Advantage Plus (1994).
[6]The Travelers: LTC III Plus (1994).
[7]UNUM: Advantage II (1994), Pro-HHC (a 5-year home health care plan) and TOT-HHC.
[8]Limited benefit periods are available from ages 80 to 84.

Premium Comparison of Long-Term Care Insurance with No Home Health Care

AGE	BANKERS UNITED LIFE[1] (0-DAY WAIT)	CNA[2] (0-DAY WAIT) PREFERRED	STANDARD	JOHN ALDEN[3] (0-DAY WAIT) PREFERRED	STANDARD	AMEX[4] (20-DAY WAIT)	JOHN HANCOCK[5] (20-DAY WAIT)	THE TRAVELERS[6] (20-DAY WAIT)	UNUM[7] (20-DAY WAIT) PRO-HHC TOT-HHC
18–39	$ 470.00	—	—	—	—	—	—	—	—
40	470.00	—	—	$ 514.50	$ 735.00	$ 540.00	$ 991.00	$ 611.00	—
45	590.00	$ 550.00	$690.00	643.10	918.80	540.00	1,091.00	734.00	—
50	750.00	730.00	910.00	771.80	1,102.50	610.00	1,125.00	881.00	—
55	1,000.00	980.00	1,230.00	866.40	1,237.50	810.00	1,444.00	1,163.00	$1,046.10
60	1,390.00	1,380.00	1,730.00	1,102.60	1,575.00	1,270.00	1,911.00	1,537.00	1,370.40
65	2,010.00	1,680.00	2,100.00	1,559.30	2,227.50	2,180.00	2,712.00	2,031.00	1,983.30
70	2,980.00	2,460.00	3,080.00	2,598.80	3,712.50	3,370.00	4,036.00	2,900.00	2,947.80
75	4,430.00	3,770.00	4,710.00	4,528.20	6,468.80	4,910.00	6,111.00	4,600.00	4,513.80
79	6,620.00	5,260.00	6,580.00	6,339.40	9,056.30	6,630.00	9,949.00	7,034.00	6,161.40
80	—[8]	—[8]	—[8]	6,733.10	9,618.80	—[8]	—[8]	—[8]	6,689.40
84	—[8]	—[8]	—[8]	7,942.70	11,346.80	—[8]	—[8]	—[8]	—

NOTE: Table is based on a $100-a-day daily benefit and a lifetime benefit period, with a 5.0 percent compound benefit increase option. Note that because premiums are always changing, insurance companies should be contacted for up-to-date information.

[1]Bankers United Life: Protector (1993).
[2]CNA: Classic LTC (1993); Premier LTC (1993).
[3]John Alden: Independent Life Plan (1993).
[4]AMEX: Nursing Home and Alternate Care Coverage/Home and Community Care Rider (1992); Privileged Care Select (1994).
[5]John Hancock: Protectcare Advantage Plus (1994).
[6]The Travelers: LTC III Plus (1994).
[7]UNUM: Advantage II (1994).
[8]Limited benefit periods are available from ages 80 to 84.

WHAT THE POLICY PAYS

How Are Benefits Calculated and Paid?

Insurance companies use either of two different methods of paying claimants their benefits: indemnification and reimbursement. Each method has its pluses and minuses. Neither offers any distinct financial advantage over the other in the long run.

Indemnification pays a fixed daily (or monthly) benefit amount directly to the insuree, regardless of the actual cost of care. It operates essentially in the same manner as a disability income policy.

For example, if the insuree chose a $150-a-day indemnification benefit and the daily nursing-home cost is $100 a day, the policy will still pay the insuree $150 per day. The extra $50 can be spent for other medical costs, for a haircut, or on bubble gum, or put into a bank account—the insurance company doesn't care. Its obligation is to pay the promised daily dollar benefit as long as the insuree qualifies for long-term care.

The second method, *reimbursement*, pays the insuree only for actual covered expenses. Typically these policies coordinate benefits with Medicare and any other insurance coverage in order to conserve long-term care policy benefit dollars. This method is similar to the approach followed by most medical insurance policies.

Using the example above, had the insuree chosen a $150-a-day reimbursement benefit and the nursing-home cost was $100 a day, the policy would reimburse the $100. The remaining $50 of "unused" benefit would remain in the insuree's "bank of dollars," to be available for use at some time in the future.

Both methods have their strengths and weaknesses. If the insuree prefers having more dollars of benefit available up front, then indemnification is the better choice. (How the IRS will eventually decide to treat those excess dollars received that were not spent on bona fide long-term care expenses is not known.) And the premiums for these policies tend to be higher than for reimbursement policies.

On the other hand, if the insuree wants to maximize coverage for actual long-term care expenses and accepts the notion that the policy exists to cover actual expenses only, then the reimbursement method makes more sense. One positive feature is that at the $100-a-day nursing-home cost, the $150-a-day benefit will last much longer. The negative is that any extra, noncovered expenses, such as medications and trips to the hairdresser, will have to be paid by other insurance or out of pocket.

How Much Is the Daily Benefit Payment?

Most policies let the insuree choose the amount of coverage, usually running from $30 to $300 a day for skilled nursing care, less for more typical custodial care. Of course, the higher the benefit provided, the more costly the premium. You should check the cost for nursing homes in your community—experts recommend that an insuree try to obtain a benefit amount that will cover at least one-half to two-thirds of the average daily cost for nursing homes in his or her area, with the insuree's income (Social Security, pension, and other income) covering the rest. Any lesser benefit won't be very helpful. If the policy pays $50 a day and nursing homes in your area charge $130 a day, a lifetime of savings could quickly be depleted *despite* the insurance.

THE BENEFITS

What Types of Long-Term Care Expenses Are Covered?

You should check to see what levels of care are included in the coverage. Any policy should cover all of these types of care: skilled, intermediate, and custodial. Otherwise the person may discover, when it's too late, that the policy won't pay for the level of care he or she needs. Most long-term care insurance does provide coverage for all three levels of care.

It is wise, particularly if you live in a rural area where the choices of long-term care facilities are limited, to obtain and read a sample policy before purchasing insurance. Make certain the policy definitions correspond to the care actually available to you locally.

Other levels of care have also been emerging. Terms like "continuing care facility," "alternate care facility," and "assisted living facility" are now commonplace—and these are often ambiguously defined in policies. If you are particularly interested in coverage for a specific type of care, you must choose a policy in which that type of coverage is available.

Is Home Health Coverage Available?

Nobody wants to go into a nursing home; just about everyone would prefer to stay at home. Home health insurance might help make this option possible. So should everyone purchase this coverage? Not necessarily. And in fact many people who obtain long-term care insurance policies do not opt for home care coverage. According to a 1992 study by the Health Insurance Association of America (HIAA), "Who Buys Long-Term Care Insurance?" only 39 percent of long-term care policy purchasers chose a home care option.

Home health coverage can be very useful for people who need only minimal assistance. If a family member is available to provide primary care, a home health aide might be useful to provide supplementary help. The United Seniors Health Cooperative (a nonprofit organization in Washington, D.C.) recommends that a person without a family member to count on as a primary caregiver would be wise to pass on home health care. Without a "free" family caregiver, home care riders simply cannot provide enough dollars to cover all of the costs of most long stays in the home. These situations are more practically handled in an institutional environment.

For example, a private-duty nurse in a major city will typically cost $20 to $35 an hour. Even a less skilled companion or home health aide will cost $8 to $20 an hour, meaning a twenty-four-hour shift will run between $192 and $840 a day. Since the most generous daily home care insurance benefit currently available is about $250 a day, there are simply not enough benefit dollars available in most policies to adequately cover the cost. In addition, home care premiums can be very expensive, in some cases equaling or exceeding the cost of the nursing-home portion of the policy. Compare the premiums listed in tables 16.1 (with home care) and 16.2 (without home care).

Home care makes sense when a loved one is recovering from an acute illness and will not need lifetime care. Home care may also be practical to provide assistance to a primary caregiver for an individual with early dementia or Alzheimer's disease. For these situations, you probably would not need home care coverage for longer than about two years.

Note that most insurance companies require that home care be administered by professionals working for a recognized health care organization. But a few companies will also pay for friends or relatives who are providing care at home. Unfortunately, the added premium for this type of care can be pricey (see table 16.1, UNUM Advantage II with TOT-HHC—total home care coverage).

When Do Benefits Start?

Some policies begin paying benefits on the first day a person enters a nursing home, while others wait a certain period, up to 365 days, before starting to pay benefits. During the waiting ("elimination") period, the nursing-home resident pays privately.

How long should the waiting period be? While a shorter waiting period costs more than a longer one, a longer waiting period may not be the best choice. Let's compare what happened to two sixty-five-year-old twin brothers. Brother One buys nursing-home insurance with a ninety-day waiting period and pays $1,100 a year; Brother Two buys the same policy but with no waiting period and pays $1,310 a year—$210 a year more.

While driving back from the mall together, and arguing over who would be foolish enough to pay $210 extra for a policy, they are involved in an auto accident that results in broken legs for both of them. They both enter the hospital, are treated, and are released to a nursing facility to recover. They both spend ninety days in the facility for physical therapy and are released, fully recovered.

The facility's fee was $100 a day, so both brothers accumulated charges totaling $9,000. Brother One, with the ninety-day waiting period, must pay the $9,000 out of pocket. His "foolish" brother, with the zero-day waiting period and the slightly larger premium, pays nothing. The extra $210 annual premium, equal to the cost of about two days in the nursing facility, was money well spent in this example.

Younger people are more apt to experience more frequent, relatively short stays in nursing homes, while older individuals are more likely to experience fewer but longer stays. Since the difference in cost between shorter and longer waiting periods at younger ages is substantially less than it is after the early-to-mid-seventies and beyond, a good rule of thumb is to purchase the shortest waiting period offered by the policy at younger ages and look to longer waiting periods at older ages.

The shortest waiting periods range from zero to thirty days, depending on the carrier. The longest waiting periods you should consider are sixty to one hundred days, but they are not very practical on a cost-benefit basis.

According to HIAA's "Who Buys Long-Term Care Insurance?" Sixty-five percent of purchasers chose waiting periods of twenty days or less and about 28 percent chose a zero-day wait. They found that older purchasers (ages seventy-five and up) bought an average forty-six-day waiting period while younger purchasers (ages fifty-five to sixty-four) bought an average twenty-eight-day wait.

How Long Will the Benefits Last?

How many years should benefits cover a nursing-home stay? While older Americans (ages sixty-five and up) face a 40 to 50 percent chance (lower for men, higher for women) that they will spend some time in a nursing home only 10 to 20 percent will stay more than five years.[2] Genuine "lifetime" benefits are necessary in only 3 to 5 percent of the cases.

According to the HIAA study, 96 percent of all policies sold in 1990 covered at least two years of nursing-home care, a little more than half exceeded five years, and 38 percent were issued with lifetime benefits.

People generally choose lifetime benefits to buy peace of mind. Some legitimately purchase it because some type of chronically debilitating disease or condition "runs in the family" or because the family is genetically predisposed to longevity. But most people's needs are met by a three-to-five-year benefit period; most people who buy lifetime benefits are wasting their money.

Even at that, the premium will be expensive. As mentioned earlier, a report by Families USA determined that "except for the wealthiest individuals, private nursing home insurance fails to make nursing home care affordable for the vast majority of today's elderly and middle-aged Americans."[3]

Reducing the benefit period to four years, three years, or even two years can cut the premium cost significantly, often 30 to 50 percent off the cost of the same policy providing lifetime benefits. Compare the simple premiums listed in table 16.3, for policies covering only a fixed number of years, with table 16.1 lifetime benefits, and you'll see a tremendous difference. But doesn't shorter coverage leave consumers at risk? If they do need a longer stay, won't they risk losing their entire savings? Not if they combine the purchase of insurance with the wise use of the Medicaid planning strategies discussed in this book.

In order to try to reduce reliance on Medicaid, four states—California, Connecticut, Indiana, and New York—have instituted programs that encourage their residents to purchase some basic long-term care insurance coverage. Here's how this incentive plan works: A resident buys a long-term care policy from an approved insurance carrier with a fixed minimum benefit amount, say $50,000. If the person enters a nursing home and uses the $50,000 of insurance benefit, the person may still keep an additional $50,000 of assets allowed under the state's Medicaid law. Only the four states mentioned above had adopted these insurance incentive programs prior to OBRA 1993, which prohibited other states from adopting this type of program.

Finally, when purchasing less than a lifetime benefit, a person should consider a policy with a "restoration of benefits" clause. After a stay in a nursing home and a subsequent release, the provision restores the policy benefit to the original level after the insured is certified "treatment-free" for a period of at least six months. This benefit helps prevent short stays from eating up the coverage, making the choice of a lifetime benefit less important.

Does the Plan Offer Inflation Protection?

Long-term care plans typically pay a fixed daily amount. But while benefits are fixed, you can be sure that nursing-home costs won't remain level. Inflation will cause costs to rise, and nursing-home charges have been far outpacing the rate of inflation. For example, using a conservative 5 percent annual increase in costs, a $120 daily charge in 1995 will go up to more than $150 in five years and to more than $195 in ten years.

There are three basic ways to cover this inevitable coverage shortfall:

1. Pay the difference out of savings or income.
2. Buy a higher-than-needed daily benefit.
3. Buy an inflation protection rider (commonly referred to as a benefit increase option, or BIO) when first purchasing the policy.

The most common form of inflation rider is 5 percent compound benefit increase option (CBIO), which increases the daily benefit annually on the policy anniversary by 5 percent of the previous year's benefit. Some companies offer a 5 percent simple benefit increase option (SBIO), which works simi-

Premium Comparison of Long-Term Care Insurance with Limited Years of Coverage

Type of Care	Bankers United Life[1] (0-Day Wait)	CNA[2] (0-Day Wait) Preferred	CNA[2] (0-Day Wait) Standard	AMEX[3] (20-Day Wait)	John Hancock[4] (20-Day Wait)	The Travelers[5] (20-Day Wait)	UNUM[6] (20-Day Wait)
Nursing-Home Care	4-year benefit ($150,000) +	4-year benefit ($146,000) +	4-year benefit ($146,000) +	4-year benefit ($146,000) +	3-year benefit ($109,500) +	3-year benefit ($109,500) +	6-year benefit ($216,000) +
Home Health Care	w/750 days of benefit	w/2 years of benefit	w/2 years of benefit	w/2 years of benefit	w/3 years of benefit	w/3 year of benefit	w/3 years of benefit (Procare)
Age							
55	$ 760.00/ 1,020.00	$ 760.00/ 1,113.00	$ 950.00/ 1,390.00	$ 600.00/ 1,450.00	$ 824.00/ 1,314.00	$ 662.00/ 949.00	$ 887.70/ 1,494.60
65	$1,630.00/ 2,190.00	$1,320.00/ 1,810.00	$1,650.00/ 2,263.00	$1,600.00/ 2,990.00	$1,471.00/ 2,241.00	$1,167.00/ 1,627.00	$1,172.70/ 2,663.60
75	$3,730.00/ 5,050.00	$3,030.00/ 3,955.00	$3,790.00/ 4,946.00	$3,600.00/ 6,420.00	$3,268.00/ 4,638.00	$2,835.00/ 3,922.00	$3,936.60/ 5,600.40

NOTE: Table is based on a $100-a-day daily benefit with a 5.0 percent compound benefit increase option. Because rates are always changing, check with companies for up-to-date information.

[1]Bankers United Life: Protector (1993).
[2]CNA: Classic LTC (1993); Premier LTC (1993).
[3]AMEX: Nursing Home and Alternate Care Coverage/Home and Community Care Rider (1992); Privileged Care Select (1994).
[4]John Hancock: Protectcare Advantage Plus (1994).
[5]The Travelers: LTC III Plus (1994).
[6]UNUM: Advantage II (1994).

larly but is based on an annual increase of 5 percent of the original daily benefit. Because some states have mandated that only CBIOs be sold to their residents, SBIOs seem to be on the way out.

Some companies have BIOs that cap benefits when the insuree reaches a certain age, typically eighty-five to eighty-six. Competitive market pressure has favored policies with no caps, so most major carriers have no caps or are planning to lift their caps on their next generation of policies.

Inflation protection is nice because it increases benefits at a level premium cost—your premium will start higher if you buy inflation protection, but the premium won't increase in future years.

A small number of companies offer another alternative: the right to purchase additional coverage in the future, usually based on some sort of published inflation index. The downside to this is that additional coverage will be calculated at rates based on the insuree's age when the added coverage is purchased. Although this method has its merits, it can be a very expensive way to increase benefits.

In general, younger purchasers, up to age seventy-five or so, should probably consider a "level premium" BIO of one type or another. Older purchasers would probably be best served by initially buying a higher-than-necessary fixed daily benefit, using a policy option (if available) to purchase additional coverage in the future, paying any increase in cost out of pocket, or some combination of the above. The decision should be based on age, health, attitude, and ability to pay.

Does the Policy Contain a Premium Waiver Option?

Most policies include a premium waiver for nursing-home care as part of the basic policy. This means that an insuree won't have to continue paying premiums and the policy will remain in force once a person enters a nursing home. A premium waiver is important because once a nursing-home resident has begun an extended stay, he or she may no longer be able to afford premiums.

Waiver clauses vary considerably from one company to the next, but there are two basic types—one in which the waiver starts as soon as the insuree starts receiving benefits, and one in which the waiver is activated after a certain time, normally sixty to one hundred days after benefits have begun.

The second type can be misleading. For example, if the policy has a waiver that is activated after a "covered nursing-home stay of ninety consecutive days" and you have chosen a ninety-day waiting period, how many days after entry into a nursing home will you be eligible for the waiver? Ninety days, right? Wrong!

The answer is 180, because a "covered nursing-home stay" is typically defined as that period of time during which the *policy* is paying benefits. The fact that you have already paid a bundle with a ninety-day waiting period does not count. This policy starts paying benefits on day ninety-one of your *covered* nursing-home stay; then at that point the waiver "clock" starts ticking off another ninety days before activating.

A few companies include a waiver-of-premium clause that applies to both nursing-home care and home or community care. Remember that most waivers currently apply only to the nursing-home portion of the policy. Policy brochures and agents can sometimes be misleading.

Is There a Grace Period for Late Payment?

Policies usually provide a grace period (typically a week to a month) during which the policy continues even if the insuree is late with the premium. Without any grace period, a policy could be canceled immediately. Some provide an extended grace period if the insuree is cognitively impaired.

Does the Insurer Give the Insuree a "Free Look"?

Almost all policies allow the insuree to cancel and obtain a full refund within a specified period after he or she signs up—typically ten to thirty days. In fact, most states require the insurer to provide this money-back guarantee.

Can the Policy Be Upgraded?

Long-term care insurance is still fairly new on the market, and products are constantly changing. You should look to see if the insurance company that issues a policy gives the right to switch to an improved version of the policy as upgrades or improvements are made.

What Extra Bells and Whistles Are Included?

To attract consumers, companies often offer one or more extra "goodies" in a long-term care policy package. These may include:

- Hospice care: care for the terminally ill.
- Respite care: allows for care for the insuree while the primary caregiver takes a brief rest.
- Return of premium/reduced paid-up option: allows for some level of value to be built up within the policy. An additional premium is required.
- Bed reservation benefit: pays for an unoccupied nursing-home bed in the event that you must enter the hospital, so the bed is available upon hospital discharge.
- No modal fees: policy charges no additional fees if less than an annual payment mode is chosen (for example, monthly or quarterly).
- Postconfinement benefit: includes a small home care benefit in the base policy. This benefit is paid in addition to any home care rider benefits received.
- Restoration of benefits: restores nursing-home benefit to original level after being treatment-free for six months following a nursing-home stay.
- Medical equipment purchase or lease: enables the insuree to obtain necessary devices to accommodate care being given in the home.
- Survivorship benefit for married couples: provides for paid-up policy for a surviving spouse once you have paid premiums for a specified number of years (usually four to ten).

This is merely a partial list. There are almost innumerable benefits available in today's long-term care insurance policies. And they are not unimportant. The right combination of bells and whistles can be a major determinant in the decision to go with policy A or policy B. But remember that without a solid base policy from a reputable company, the luster of these extra goodies will quickly tarnish.

LIMITS OF THE POLICY

Does the Policy Contain Health- or Age-Eligibility Requirements?

Policies impose health- and age-eligibility requirements, typically excluding applicants who are over a specified age (usually eighty-four) or who, owing to poor health, may no longer be able to care for themselves.

Just because a person may not be healthy enough to qualify for life insurance doesn't mean he or she won't qualify for long-term care insurance. For example, cancer may disqualify a person for life insurance, since his or her life expectancy is shortened, but if the condition is under control, that same person might still be a good risk for long-term care insurance.

How Does a Person Qualify for Benefits?

Knowing the eligibility requirements ahead of time alleviates any surprises at the time of a claim—a time when surprises are seldom appreciated.

To qualify for benefits, insurees must meet one of the two or three "tests" for coverage. Generally the insuree can qualify by (1) being cognitively impaired, (2) being unable to perform a certain number of "activities of daily living" (ADLs), or, with some policies, (3) requiring care that is deemed medically necessary.

Most policies contain the first two qualifiers. Be sure to determine the policy's definition of ADLs. Most policies require that the insuree be unable to perform two out of five ADLs before honoring a claim. Others recognize six ADLs and may require the inability to perform either two or three of them to be eligible. Common ADLs include dressing, eating, toileting, transferring from bed or chair, maintaining continence, and taking medications.

In addition, check the policy for the degree to which an insuree must be "nonperforming" in any ADL to be able to trigger a claim. For example, if the insuree can chew and swallow food but cannot lift it to his mouth without some assistance, will that trigger the "eating" ADL?

The old saying "actions speak louder than words" says it all when it comes to assessing policies. Make sure you understand exactly how the insurer interprets and applies the terms of coverage.

How Does the Policy Treat Existing Medical Conditions?

Even if one is eligible to buy insurance, policies typically either exclude preexisting conditions or impose a waiting period before coverage goes into effect for those conditions.

Preexisting conditions are generally defined as medical conditions that were diagnosed or treated, or which should have been diagnosed or treated based on their symptoms, prior to purchasing the policy. Insurers will typically look back at your health record up to five years prior to your application for coverage; if a condition existed more than five years before application and is no longer giving you problems, you shouldn't have trouble obtaining coverage. If you do have a preexisting condition and are issued a policy, you may have to wait for up to six months before that condition is eligible for coverage.

If you think you can slip one by the insurer just because the company does not require a medical examination, forget it. Insurees are required to provide accurate information about their health; if it is later discovered that you were not truthful, you can kiss your coverage good-bye. You may even open yourself up to criminal charges for insurance fraud.

Does the Policy Restrict Coverage by Requiring a Prior Hospital or Skilled Nursing Stay?

These undesirable restrictions were common at one time but are not any longer. You want to avoid any policy with these restrictions.

Are Any Injuries or Diseases Not Covered?

Check to see whether the policy excludes any injuries or diseases. At one time policies often excluded Alzheimer's, Parkinson's, and senility, but this is no longer the case.

Is There a Total Dollar Limitation?

The policy may place a dollar limitation on the total lifetime benefit payment that will be made. Obvi-

ously, the amount at which this limit is set can affect the value of the policy.

Can the Company Cancel or Refuse to Renew the Policy?

A policy should be guaranteed renewable, which means that its coverage can't be canceled just because the insuree's health has become poor or because of increased age. Under a guaranteed renewable policy, a person can retain coverage as long as he or she pays the premiums.

Also watch out for a policy that is "renewable at the option of the insurer"—not the same as a guaranteed renewable policy. Without a guaranteed renewable policy, you are at the mercy of the insurer and could lose coverage at the very time you need it most.

COMPARING THE COMPANIES

How Can the Safety and Stability of a Company Be Checked?

You will want to pick an insurance company in the same way you would select a stock or bond—do your homework.

Check out the financial security of the company by reviewing its A.M. Best and Company's rating as well as the opinion of at least one other rating service, such as Moody's, Standard and Poor's, or Duff and Phelps. These resources are available at your local library. I also suggest requesting a copy of the company's annual report, particularly if the firm has had large holdings in commercial real estate. Most of the larger companies have toll-free numbers; try calling to request a copy of the annual report. Remember, the carrier needs to be solvent in the event that a claim is made in ten, twenty, or thirty years. Given today's financial climate, consumers need to be a little fussy. The variety of companies offering long-term care policies gives consumers the chance to be choosy.

On the following pages is a questionnaire based on the above discussion, to use for comparing policies.

LONG-TERM CARE INSURANCE QUESTIONNAIRE

How Much Does the Policy Cost?

1. What is the annual premium? $ _____

2. Can the company raise the premium over time or under other circumstances?
   yes _____ no _____
   If so, under what circumstances? _____
   _____

How Much Does the Policy Pay?

3. How are benefits calculated and paid?
   indemnification _____ reimbursement _____

4. What is the maximum amount the policy will pay?
   - skilled nursing care $ _____ per day
   - intermediate nursing care $ _____ per day
   - custodial nursing care $ _____ per day
   - home health care $ _____ per day

What Are the Benefits?

5. What types of long-term care expenses are covered?
   - skilled nursing care   yes _____ no _____
   - intermediate nursing care   yes _____ no _____
   - custodial nursing care   yes _____ no _____

6. Is home health care coverage available?
   yes _____ no _____

7. How much does home health coverage add to the premium cost? $ _____

8. Who will home health coverage pay for?
   - professionals only   yes _____ no _____
   - family and friends   yes _____ no _____

9. When do benefits start?
   - skilled nursing care   _____ days after entering nursing home
   - intermediate nursing care   _____ days after entering nursing home
   - custodial nursing care   _____ days after entering nursing home
   - home health care   _____ days after entering nursing home
   - all of the above services   _____ days after entering nursing home

10. How long will the benefits last?
    - skilled nursing care   _____ days
    - intermediate nursing care   _____ days
    - custodial nursing care   _____ days
    - home health care   _____ days
    - all of the above   _____ days

11. Does the plan offer inflation protection?
    yes _____ no _____

12. What is the inflation protection?
    _____ % compound benefit increase
    _____ % simple benefit increase

13. Can additional coverage be purchased in the future?
    yes _____   no _____

14. Does the policy contain a premium waiver option?
    yes _____   no _____

15. When does the premium waiver begin?
    _____ days after benefits start

16. Is there a grace period for late payments?
    yes _____   no _____
    If so: _____ days

17. Does the insurer offer a "free look"?
    yes _____   no _____
    If so: _____ days

18. Can the policy be upgraded?
    yes _____   no _____

19. What additional bells and whistles are provided?
    - hospice care   yes _____   no _____
    - respite care   yes _____   no _____
    - return of premiums/reduced premium   yes _____   no _____
    - bed reservation   yes _____   no _____
    - no modal fees   yes _____   no _____
    - postconfinement benefit   yes _____   no _____
    - restoration of benefits   yes _____   no _____
    - medical equipment purchase or lease   yes _____   no _____
    - survivorship benefit for married couple   yes _____   no _____
    - others: _____   yes _____   no _____
      _____   yes _____   no _____
      _____   yes _____   no _____
      _____   yes _____   no _____
      _____   yes _____   no _____

What Are the Limits?

20. Does the policy contain health- or age-eligibility requirements?
    yes _____   no _____
    If so, are you eligible for coverage?
    yes _____   no _____

21. How does a person qualify for benefits?
    - must be cognitively impaired   yes _____   no _____
    - must be unable to perform ADLs   yes _____   no _____
    - must require medically necessary care   yes _____   no _____

22. What ADLs are recognized?
    - dressing   yes _____   no _____
    - eating   yes _____   no _____
    - toileting   yes _____   no _____

- transferring from bed or chair   yes _____   no _____
- maintaining continence   yes _____   no _____
- taking medication   yes _____   no _____
- other: _____ yes _____   no _____
            _____ yes _____   no _____
            _____ yes _____   no _____

23. To be eligible for benefits, how many ADLs must the insuree be unable to perform?
    _____ ADLs

24. a. Does the policy exclude coverage for any conditions you presently have?
       yes   _____   no _____

    b. Will the company look for preexisting conditions?
       yes   _____   no _____
       If so:_____ years

    c. Does the company impose a waiting period?
       yes   _____   no _____
       If so:_____ months

25. Is a prior hospital stay required before the policy will pay for:
    - skilled care   yes_____ no _____ If so: _____ days
    - intermediate care   yes_____ no _____ If so: _____ days
    - custodial care   yes_____ no _____ If so: _____ days

26. Is a prior skilled nursing-home stay required before the policy will pay for:
    - intermediate care   yes_____ no _____ If so: _____ days
    - custodial care   yes_____ no _____ If so: _____ days

27. Are any injuries or diseases not covered?
    _____
    _____
    _____

28. Is there a total dollar limitation for benefits?
    yes   _____   no _____
    If so: $ _____

29. Can the company cancel or refuse to renew a policy?
    yes   _____   no _____
    If there are conditions, what are they? _____
    _____

How Does the Company Compare to Others?

30. What is the company's rating by:
    Best   _____
    Moody's   _____
    Standard and Poor's _____
    Duff and Phelps   _____

Note: Adapted, with permission, from *The Consumer's Guide to Long-Term Care Insurance* (Washington, D.C.: Health Insurance Association of America, 1988).

More Information About Long-Term Care Insurance

For more information about long-term care insurance, contact your state insurance department (listed below). Your state department of aging services may also be a good source. The National Asso-ciation of Insurance Commissioners publishes an information pamphlet called the *Shopper's Guide to Long-Term Care Insurance,* which you can obtain by writing that nonprofit organization at 120 West Twelfth Street, Suite 1100, Kansas City, Missouri 64105-1925, or calling (816) 842-3600.

STATE INSURANCE DEPARTMENTS, AGENCIES ON AGING, AND INSURANCE COUNSELING PROGRAMS

Each state has its own laws and regulations governing all types of insurance. The insurance departments, listed in the left-hand column for each state, are responsible for enforcing these laws as well as providing the public with information about insurance. The agencies on aging, listed on the right-hand column, are responsible for coordinating services for older Americans. Centered below each state listing, where available, is the telephone number for the insurance counseling program. Please note that calls to 800 numbers listed here can be made only from within the respective state.

Alabama

Insurance Department
135 S. Union St.
Montgomery, AL
  36130-3401
(205) 269-3500

Commission on Aging
770 Washington Ave., Suite 470
Montgomery, AL
  36130-1851
(800) 243-5463
(205) 242-5743

Insurance counseling
  program: (800) 243-5463

Alaska

Division of Insurance
800 E. Dimond, Suite 560
Anchorage, AK 99515
(907) 349-1230

Older Alaskans Commission
P.O. Box 110209
Juneau, AK 99811-0209
(907) 465-3250

Insurance counseling   (800) 478-6065
  program: (907) 562-7249

Arizona

Insurance Department
Consumer Affairs and
  Investigation Division
3030 N. Third St.,
Suite 1100
Phoenix, AZ 85012
(602) 912-8400

Department of Economic
  Security
Aging and Adult
  Administration
1789 W. Jefferson St.
Phoenix, AZ 85007
(602) 542-4446

Insurance counseling
  program: (800) 432-4040

Arkansas

Insurance Department
Seniors Insurance
  Network
1123 S. University Ave.
400 University Tower
  Bldg.
Little Rock, AR
  72204-1699
(800) 852-5494
(501) 686-2900

Division of Aging and Adult
  Services
1471 Donaghey Plaza South
P.O. Box 1437, Slot 1412
Little Rock, AR 72203-1437
(501) 682-2441

Insurance counseling   (800) 852-5494
  program: (501) 686-2939

California

Insurance Department
Consumer Service
  Division
Ronald Reagan Bldg.
300 S. Spring St.
Los Angeles, CA 90013
(213) 927-4357

Department of Aging
1600 K St.
Sacramento, CA 95814
(916) 322-3887

Insurance counseling   (800) 927-4357
  program: (213) 383-4519

Colorado

Insurance Division
1560 Broadway, Suite 850
Denver, CO 80202
(303) 894-7499

Aging and Adult Services
Department of Social
  Services
1575 Sherman St., 4th Floor
Denver, CO 80203-1714
(303) 866-3851

Insurance counseling
  program: (303) 894-7499

Connecticut

Insurance Department
153 Market St.
P.O. Box 816
Hartford, CT 06142-0816
(203) 297-3802

Department on Aging
175 Main St.
Hartford, CT 06106
(203) 424-5025

Delaware

Insurance Department
Rodney Bldg.
841 Silver Lake Blvd.
Dover, DE 19901
(800) 282-8611
(302) 739-4251

Division of Aging
Department of Health and
  Social Services
1901 N. Dupont Highway
Administration Building,
  2nd Floor Annex
New Castle, DE 19720
(302) 577-4791

Insurance counseling
  program: (800) 223-9074

District of Columbia

Insurance Department
613 G Street NW, Room
  638
P.O. Box 37200

Office on Aging
1424 K Street NW, 2nd Floor
Washington, DC 20005

Washington, DC (202) 724-5626
20001-7200 (202) 724-5622
(202) 727-8009

Insurance counseling
program: (202) 676-3900

Florida

Department of Insurance   Department of Elder Affairs
State Capitol, Plaza   1317 Winewood Blvd.
Eleven   Bldg. 1, Room 317
Tallahassee, FL   Tallahassee, FL 32301
32399-0300   (904) 922-5297
(800) 342-2762
(904) 922-3100

Insurance counseling
program: (904) 922-2073

Georgia

Insurance Department   Office of Aging
2 Martin Luther King, Jr.,   Department of Human
Drive   Resources
716 W. Tower   878 Peachtree St. NE,
Atlanta, GA 30334   Room 632
(404) 656-2056   Atlanta, GA 30309
(404) 657-5258

Hawaii

Department of Commerce   Executive Office on Aging
and Consumer Affairs   335 Merchant St., Room 241
Insurance Division   Honolulu, HI 96813
P.O. Box 3614   (808) 586-0100
Honolulu, HI 96811
(808) 586-2790

Insurance counseling
program: (808) 586-0100

Idaho

Insurance Department   Office on Aging
Public Service   Statehouse, Room 108
Department   Boise, ID 83720
700 W. State St., 3rd Floor   (208) 334-3833
Boise, ID 83720
(208) 334-4200

Insurance counseling
program: (800) 247-4422

Illinois

Insurance Department   Department on Aging
320 W. Washington St.,   421 E. Capitol Ave.
4th Floor   Springfield, IL 62701
Springfield, IL 62767   (217) 785-3356
(217) 782-4515

Insurance counseling
program: (800) 252-8966

Indiana

Insurance Department   Division of Aging and Home
311 W. Washington St.,   Services
Suite 300   402 W. Washington St.
Indianapolis, IN 46204   P.O. Box 7083
(800) 622-4461   Indianapolis, IN 46207-7083
(317) 232-2395   (800) 545-7763
(317) 232-7020

Insurance counseling
program: (800) 452-4800

Iowa

Insurance Division   Department of Elder Affairs
Lucas State Office Bldg.   Jewett Bldg., Suite 236
E. 12th and Grand Sts.,   914 Grand Ave.
6th Floor   Des Moines, IA 50319
Des Moines, IA 50319   (515) 281-5187
(515) 281-5705

Insurance counseling
program: (515) 281-5705

Kansas

Insurance Department   Department on Aging
420 9th St. SW   122-S Docking State Office Bldg.
Topeka, KS 66612   915 Harrison SW
(800) 432-2484   Topeka, KS 66612-1500
(913) 296-3071   (913) 296-4986
Insurance counseling   (800) 432-3535
program:

Kentucky

Insurance Department   Division of Aging Services
229 W. Main St.   Cabinet for Human
P.O. Box 517   Resources
Frankfort, KY 40602   275 E. Main St.
(502) 564-3630   Frankfort, KY 40621
(502) 564-6930

Insurance counseling
program: (800) 372-2973

Louisiana

Insurance Department   Governor's Office of Elderly
P.O. Box 94214   Affairs
Baton Rouge, LA   4550 N. Boulevard
70804-9214   P.O. Box 80374
(800) 259-5301   Baton Rouge, LA 70898-0374
(504) 342-5900   (504) 925-1700

Insurance counseling
program: (800) 259-5301

Maine

Bureau of Insurance
  Consumer Division
State House, Station 34
Augusta, ME 04333
(207) 582-8707

Insurance counseling
program:

Bureau of Elder and Adult
  Services
State House, Station 11
Augusta, ME 04333
(207) 624-5335

(800) 750-5353
(207) 624-5335

Maryland

Insurance Department
Complaints and Investi-
  gation Unit
501 St. Paul Pl.
Baltimore, MD
  21202-2272
(410) 333-6300

Insurance counseling
program:

Office on Aging
301 W. Preston St.,
  Room 1004
Baltimore, MD 21201
(410) 255-1100
(410) 225-1100

(410) 225-1100

Massachusetts

Insurance Division
Consumer Services
  Section
280 Friend St.
Boston, MA 02114
(617) 521-7794

Insurance counseling
program:

Executive Office of
  Elder Affairs
1 Ashburton Pl., 5th Floor
Boston, MA 02108
(800) 882-2003
(617) 727-7750

(617) 727-7750

Michigan

Insurance Department
P.O. Box 30220
Lansing, MI 48909
(517) 373-0220

Insurance counseling
program:

Office of Services to the Aging
611 W. Ottawa St.
P.O. Box 30026
Lansing, MI 48909
(517) 373-8230

(517) 373-8230

Minnesota

Insurance Department
Department of Commerce
133 E. 7th St.
St. Paul, MN 55101-2362
(612) 296-4026

Insurance counseling
program:

Board on Aging
Human Services Bldg.,
  4th Floor
444 Lafayette Rd.
St. Paul, MN 55155-3843
(612) 296-2770

(800) 882-6262

Mississippi

Insurance Department
Consumer Assistance
  Division
P.O. Box 79
Jackson, MS 39205
(601) 359-3569

Division of Aging and Adult
  Services
455 N. Lamar St.
Jackson, MS 39202
(800) 345-6347/(800) 948-3090
(601) 359-4929

Missouri

Department of Insurance
Consumer Services
  Section
301 W. High St., 6 North
Jefferson City, MO
  65102-0690
(800) 726-7390
(314) 751-2640

Insurance counseling
program:

Division of Aging
Department of Social
  Services
P.O. Box 1337
615 Howerton Ct.
Jefferson City, MO
  65102-1337
(314) 751-3082

(800) 735-6776

Montana

Insurance Department
126 N. Sanders
Mitchell Bldg., Room 270
Helena, MT 59601
(406) 444-2040

Insurance counseling
program:

Governor's Office on Aging
State Capitol Bldg., Room 219
Helena, MT 59620
(406) 444-5900

(800) 332-6148

Nebraska

Insurance Department
Terminal Bldg.
941 O St., Suite 400
Lincoln, NE 68508
(402) 471-2201

Insurance counseling
program:

Department on Aging
State Office Bldg.
301 Centennial Mall South
Lincoln, NE 68509-5044
(402) 471-2306

(402) 471-4506

Nevada

Department of Insurance
Consumer Services
1665 Hot Springs Rd.
Carson City, NV 89710
(800) 992-0900
(702) 687-4270

Insurance counseling
program:

Department of Human
  Resources
Division for Aging Services
340 N. 11th St., Suite 114
Las Vegas, NV 89101
(702) 486-3545

(702) 687-4270

New Hampshire

Insurance Department
Life and Health Division
69 Manchester St.
Concord, NH 03301
(800) 852-3416
(603) 271-2261

Insurance counseling
program:

Department of Health and
  Human Services
Division of Elderly and Adult
  Services
State Office Park South
115 Pleasant St.
Annex Bldg. No. 1
Concord, NH 03301
(603) 271-4680

(603) 271-4642

New Jersey

Insurance Department
20 W. State St.
Roebling Bldg.
CN325
Trenton, NJ 08625
(609) 292-5363

Department of Community
  Affairs
Division on Aging
101 S. Broad and Front Sts.
CN807
Trenton, NJ 08625-0807
(800) 792-8820
(609) 984-3951

Insurance counseling
program: (800) 792-8820

New Mexico

Insurance Department
P.O. Box 1269
Santa Fe, NM 87504-1269
(505) 827-4500

State Agency on Aging
La Villa Rivera Bldg.
224 E. Palace Ave.
Santa Fe, NM 87501
(800) 432-2080
(505) 827-7640

Insurance counseling
program: (800) 432-2080

New York

Insurance Department
160 W. Broadway
New York, NY 10013
(800) 342-3736 outside of
  New York City
(212) 602-0429

State Office for the Aging
2 Empire State Plaza
Albany, NY 12223-0001
(800) 342-9871
(518) 474-7012

Insurance counseling
program: (800) 342-9871

North Carolina

Insurance Department
Seniors Health Insurance
  Information Program
P.O. Box 26387
Raleigh, NC 27611
(800) 662-7777
(919) 733-0111

Division of Aging
693 Palmer Dr.
Caller Box 29531
Raleigh, NC 27626-0531
(919) 733-8390

Insurance counseling
program: (800) 443-9354

North Dakota

Insurance Department
Capitol Bldg., 5th Floor
600 E. Boulevard
Bismarck, ND 58505-0320
(800) 247-0560
(701) 328-2440

Department of Human Services
Aging Services Division
P.O. Box 7070
Bismarck, ND 58507-7070
(701) 328-2577

Insurance counseling
program: (800) 247-0560

Ohio

Insurance Department
Consumer Services
  Division

Department of Aging
50 W. Broad St., 8th Floor
Columbus, OH 43266-0501

2100 Stella Ct.
Columbus, OH
  43266-0566
(800) 686-1526
(614) 644-2673

(614) 466-1221

Insurance counseling
program: (800) 686-1578

Oklahoma

Insurance Department
P.O. Box 53408
Oklahoma City, OK
  73152-3408
(405) 521-2828

Department of Human Services
Aging Services Division
312 28th St. NE
Oklahoma City, OK 73125
(405) 521-2327

Insurance counseling
program: (405) 521-6628

Oregon

Department of Insurance
  and Finance
Insurance Division
Consumer Advocacy
200 Labor and Industries
  Bldg.
Salem, OR 97310
(503) 378-4484

Department of Human
  Resources
Senior and Disabled Services
  Division
500 Summer St. NE, 2nd Floor
Salem, OR 97310-1015
(800) 282-8096
(503) 945-5811

Insurance counseling
program: (503) 378-4484

Pennsylvania

Insurance Department
Consumer Services Bureau
1321 Strawberry Sq.
Harrisburg, PA 17120
(717) 787-2317

Department of Aging
231 State St.
Barto Bldg.
Harrisburg, PA 17101
(717) 783-1550

Insurance counseling
program: (717) 783-8975

Rhode Island

Insurance Division
233 Richmond St.,
  Suite 233
Providence, RI 02903-4233
(401) 277-2223

Department of Elderly
  Affairs
160 Pine St.
Providence, RI 02903
(401) 277-2858

Insurance counseling
program: (800) 322-2880

South Carolina

Insurance Department
Consumer Assistance
  Section
P.O. Box 100105
Columbia, SC 29202-3105
(800) 768-3467
(803) 737-6140

Commission on Aging
400 Arbor Lake Dr.,
  Suite B-500
Columbia, SC 29223
non published

Insurance counseling
program: (800) 868-9095

South Dakota

Insurance Department
500 E. Capitol Ave.
Pierre, SD 57501-5070
(605) 773-3563

Insurance counseling
program:

Office of Adult Services and
    Aging
700 Governors Dr.
Pierre, SD 57501-2291
(605) 773-3656

(605) 773-3656

Tennessee

Department of Commerce
    and Insurance
Insurance Assistance Office
500 James Robertson
    Pkwy., 4th Floor
Nashville, TN 37243
(800) 525-2816
(615) 741-4955

Insurance counseling
program:

Commission on Aging
706 Church St.,
    Suite 201
Nashville, TN 37243-0860
(615) 741-2056

(800) 525-2816

Texas

Department of Insurance
Complaints Resolution,
    MC 111-1A
333 Guadalupe St.
P.O. Box 149091
Austin, TX 78714-9091
(800) 252-3439
(512) 463-6515

Insurance counseling
program:

Department on Aging
P.O. Box 12786
Austin, TX 78711
(212) 444-2727

(800) 252-9240

Utah

Insurance Department
Consumer Services
3110 State Office Bldg.
Salt Lake City, UT
    84114-1201
(800) 439-3805
(801) 538-3805

Insurance counseling
program:

Division of Aging and Adult
    Services
120 N. 200 West, Room 401
P.O. Box 45500
Salt Lake City, UT 84103
(801) 538-3910

(801) 538-3910

Vermont

Department of Banking
    and Insurance
Consumer Complaint
    Division
89 Main St., Drawer 20
Montpelier, VT
    05620-3101
(802) 828-3301

Insurance counseling
program:

Department of Aging
    and Disabilities
Waterbury Complex
103 S. Main St.
Waterbury, VT 05671-2301
(802) 241-2400

(800) 642-5119

Virginia

Bureau of Insurance
Consumer Services
    Division
1300 E. Main St.
P.O. Box 1157
Richmond, VA 23209
(804) 371-9694

Insurance counseling
program:

Department for the Aging
700 Centre, 10th Floor
700 E. Franklin St.
Richmond, VA 23219-2327
(800) 552-3402
(804) 225-2271

(800) 552-3402

Washington

Insurance Department
Insurance Bldg., AQ21
P.O. Box 40255
Olympia, WA 98504-0255
(800) 562-6900
(206) 753-7300

Insurance counseling
program:

Aging and Adult Services
    Administration
Department of Social
    and Health Services
P.O. Box 45050
Olympia, WA 98504-5050
(206) 586-3768

(800) 562-6900
(206) 753-3613

West Virginia

Insurance Department
2019 Washington St. East
Charleston, WV 25305
(800) 642-9004
(304) 558-3386
For hearing impaired:
(800) 558-1296

Insurance counseling
program:

Commission on Aging
State Capitol Complex
Holly Grove
1900 Kanawha Blvd. East
Charleston, WV 25305-0160
(304) 558-3317

(304) 558-3317

Wisconsin

Insurance Department
Complaints Department
P.O. Box 7873
Madison, WI 53707
(800) 236-8517
(608) 266-0103

Insurance counseling
program:

Bureau on Aging
Department of Health
    and Social Services
P.O. Box 7851
1 W. Wilson St.
Madison, WI 53707-7851
(608) 266-2536

(800) 242-1060

Wyoming

Insurance Department
Herschler Bldg.
122 W. 25th St.
Cheyenne, WY 82002
(800) 438-5768
(307) 777-7401

Insurance counseling
program:

Commission on Aging
Hathaway Bldg.
2300 Capitol Ave., Room 139
Cheyenne, WY 82002
(800) 442-2766
(307) 777-7986

(800) 438-5768

NOTE: *A Shopper's Guide to Long-Term Care Insurance,* National Association of Insurers Commissioners, revised 1993, reprinted with permission.

Using Long-Term Care Insurance Together with Other Planning Strategies

Is there any way to combine good-quality coverage with a reasonable premium? The answer for many is yes—by limiting the benefits to three or four years. With that limitation, the insurance company is able to offer reduced premium rates because the company's risks are cut.

But what good is a policy that will pay for only three or four years in a nursing home when your parent may remain there for a much longer period? Read on and you'll see.

Example 79

Your elderly mother's assets consist of $150,000 in CDs. She has held on to these funds as long as possible, hoping she would be one of the lucky ones who will not require nursing-home care. However, she did purchase nursing-home insurance limited to three years of coverage.

Unfortunately, her condition deteriorates and she will need to be institutionalized. To protect her savings from catastrophic costs, she transfers everything to you. The transfer triggers a thirty-six-month period in which she will not qualify for Medicaid; during that time, the insurance policy (not your parent or you) pays the daily cost. After thirty-six months has passed, the insurance runs out and Medicaid coverage begins.

In other words, by combining the purchase of insurance with one of the other planning tools (gifting), your mother was able to retain her assets as long as possible and yet keep them protected from devastating nursing-home charges for the cost of a reasonable insurance premium.

Private Insurance Rip-offs

Many Americans have been tricked into purchasing unnecessary private insurance coverage (whether Medigap or long-term care coverage) by deceptive advertising and high-pressure sales. Some salespeople have even taken money from elderly citizens and disappeared without providing any insurance coverage at all.

Here are some tips for protecting yourself from insurance deception:

- Don't buy insurance just because a TV star says it's the right thing to do. Stars are paid to endorse products, and their advice to consumers is not necessarily based on experience or conviction.

- Don't assume that any insurance policy is sponsored or endorsed by the federal or state government or an established senior advocacy organization. Some policies use deceptive names, and some salespeople even falsely tell consumers that their policy is offered under government auspices. No Medigap or long-term care policy is offered by a state or the federal government, and only a very few group policies are sold by legitimate senior advocacy organizations like the AARP.

- Stay away from insurance for specific illnesses, such as cancer. These policies are often sold by using scare tactics. Their protection is narrow, applying only to certain terrifying diseases. Such policies also tend to duplicate existing coverage under Medicare and standard Medigap policies.

- Don't duplicate coverage. Although it is now illegal for a salesperson to sell more than one Medigap policy, most states have not yet adopted laws regulating long-term care insurance. Remember, you don't need to buy more than one policy.

- Just because a policy does not require a medical exam does not mean that it provides coverage for preexisting illnesses. Insurers will ask about an applicant's health; if the questions aren't answered fully and honestly, you risk cancellation of a previously granted policy.

- Don't be misled by glittering generalities about the policy costs, such as "low weekly rates." Look closely at the monthly and annual costs and then use these bottom-line totals to compare policies.

- If you decide to buy private insurance, write the check out to the insurance company, *not* the agent.

- Don't rely on oral promises made by a salesperson. If it's not in writing, it's not in the policy.

Conclusion

Long-term care insurance can be an extremely useful asset protection tool. This insurance gives one the peace of mind that comes from knowing that your life savings will not be sacrificed in the event that care is needed by either you or your spouse. To reduce premium costs, insurance can be used in conjunction with Medicaid planning.

Each person's needs are unique. There is no one best policy for everyone. The market is filled with policy and benefit options. Use common sense and your eyeglasses to obtain a policy that best suits your particular circumstances at the lowest available premium.

CHAPTER 16 SUMMARY CHECKLIST

Private Insurance for Long-Term Care

✔ Consider long-term care insurance for peace of mind, while retaining control of your savings.

✔ Purchase a shorter benefit period, of three to four years, to reduce premium costs.

✔ Combine the purchase of long-term care insurance with Medicaid planning strategies.

✔ Shop carefully and pick the best policy for you by using the questionnaire on pages 113–15.

✔ Get a policy that is guaranteed renewable at fixed rates; pays a daily benefit of at least half the cost of nursing homes in your area; covers skilled, intermediate, and custodial care; provides inflation protection; and halves the premium once you've been admitted to a nursing home.

✔ Take a look at a home health care rider and determine if the benefits are worth the added costs for you.

✔ Watch out for high-pressure insurance rip-offs.

17 | A Living Will and Health Care Power of Attorney Can Protect Peace of Mind and Savings

On the night of January 11, 1983, a young woman named Nancy Cruzan was in a serious car accident. Paramedics were able to restore her breathing and heartbeat at the accident site, and Nancy was taken to a hospital. Although she was unconscious, Nancy's husband and parents were relieved to know that she was alive. They held out hope that Nancy would recover. To sustain her, feeding and water tubes were implanted.

After the days turned to months and the months turned to years, the doctors determined that Nancy would never recover. She was in what the doctors called a persistent vegetative state, which meant that her brain no longer processed information and she would never regain an awareness of her surroundings. Given this hopeless diagnosis, her parents asked the hospital to "pull the plug"—to stop supplying nutrition and hydration by artificial means. They felt that a "life without life" is not what Nancy would have wanted, and so she was entitled to "die with dignity."

But the hospital refused, setting the family on a long, emotionally draining trip through the courts, ending at the United States Supreme Court. The Supreme Court issued a landmark ruling, critical in at least two respects: First, the Court recognized that Americans have a constitutional right to refuse lifesaving treatment, including feeding and water tubes. Second, the Court decided that a person's wishes concerning life support should be carried out, even if the person has become incompetent, *if* those wishes can be shown by clear and convincing

evidence. Based on these rules, Nancy finally was allowed to die.

In other words, if you wish to be allowed to "die with dignity" rather than to be kept alive on life support machinery, you must express these preferences clearly and convincingly. How? By preparing a living will and/or a durable power of attorney for health care.

What Exactly Is a Living Will?

A living will is a piece of paper that tells your family, doctors, and friends what medical treatment is desired in the event that you become terminally ill or seriously injured and cannot make or communicate decisions regarding treatment. Although these documents are not designed primarily to save money, they can protect and relieve a family of the terrible emotional burden and financial devastation of unwanted long-term care.

Don't be confused. A living will is *not* the same as a will or a living trust. A will deals with the distribution of money and property after a person dies; a living trust can be used to hold and manage money and property during a person's lifetime or after his or her death. Both are completely different from a living will, and neither addresses the issue of withholding or terminating medical treatment.

Why Have a Living Will?

All but three states—Massachusetts, Michigan, and New York—have passed living will laws designed to protect a patient's right to refuse medical treatment. In the vast majority of states, a living will is recognized as a legally enforceable document and can ensure that a doctor who abides by a patient's wishes not to be kept alive on life supports will be protected from any liability.

Even in those three states without living will laws, a living will can still be useful. Without state legislation, judges are often left to determine what an unconscious patient would want if he or she could speak. In making such a decision, a judge is likely to give weight to a living will, even though it is not legally recognized by specific legislation.

If your parent (or you) wants to exercise his or her right to make choices concerning health care in the event of incapacity and at the same time spare the rest of the family the terrible trauma of making life-and-death decisions, a living will is essential.

When Should a Living Will Be Made?

Your parents (and you, too) should prepare separate living wills now, while they are still of sound mind and capable of communicating. If a parent is later diagnosed with a terminal illness, another living will should be prepared. The purpose of this is to avoid challenges to the first living will's validity. No one can then say that it was executed while your parent was healthy and that his or her feelings may have changed after becoming ill.

Once the living will is signed, copies should be given to family, doctors, clergy, and very close friends. The document should also be carried in the glove compartment of the car. If your parent goes into the hospital, give copies to the doctors and nurses and other staff who might be involved with decisions concerning critical care. Taking this initiative will enhance the chance that your parent's living will will be considered when actually needed.

In the event that someone has a change of heart, it is always possible to cancel a living will. An oral revocation is legally sufficient in most states. Still, to avoid any mix-ups, all copies of that living will previously given out should be returned and destroyed. A statement explaining that the living will is canceled should be written and signed in the presence of two people. This should eliminate any possible confusion over anyone's true wishes.

A sample living will declaration form, prepared by the nonprofit organization Choice in Dying, an be found on pages 126–27. The form is helpful because it includes instructions and it clarifies the sometimes confusing terms of these documents.

In those states that have living will laws, the living will forms are prescribed by the state. You can get a free copy of suitable state forms prepared by Choice in Dying by calling (800) 989-9455 (toll-free) or (212) 366-5540, or by writing to them at 200 Varick Street, Tenth Floor, New York, New York 10014-4810. Choice in Dying also has additional publishing information and resources available for answering any further questions you might have about living wills.

The AARP Legal Counsel for the Elderly has published a forty-page booklet called *Planning for Incapacity: A Self-Help Guide,* for each state and the District of Columbia. The booklets include living will and durable power of attorney forms for your state. To obtain a copy, send five dollars to Legal Counsel for the Elderly, P.O. Box 96474, Washington, D.C. 10090-6474, and specify your state of residence.

What Is a Durable Power of Attorney for Health Care?

Generally speaking, a power of attorney authorizes another person to make decisions and/or act for the maker; many people have used powers of attorney at some time or another. A *durable* power of attorney is the same thing, except it continues to be valid even if the maker becomes incapacitated. Use of durable powers of attorney in connection with management of a person's financial affairs is discussed in chapter 12.

Most states now allow specialized durable powers of attorney for health care decisions—including decisions about life support machines. Only Alabama and Alaska do not. These durable health care powers of attorney allow your parent (or you) to appoint an agent (or "surrogate" or "proxy")—a trusted relative or friend—to make decisions about medical care. The document is effective only if and when your parent cannot make his or her own health care decisions.

If you already have a living will, do you need a durable power of attorney for health care too? Ab-

INSTRUCTIONS	# CHOICE IN DYING LIVING WILL
PRINT YOUR NAME	I, _____, being of sound mind, make this statement as a directive to be followed if I become permanently unable to participate in decisions regarding my medical care. These instructions reflect my firm and settled commitment to decline medical treatment under the circumstances indicated below:
	I direct my attending physician to withhold or withdraw treatment if I should be in an **incurable or irreversible mental or physical condition with no reasonable expectation of recovery.**
	These instructions apply if I am a) **in a terminal condition;** b) **permanently unconscious;** or c) **if I am minimally conscious but have irreversible brain damage and will never regain the ability to make decisions and express my wishes.**
	I direct that treatment be limited to measures to keep me comfortable and to relieve pain, including any pain that might occur by withholding or withdrawing treatment.
CROSS OUT ANY STATEMENTS THAT DO NOT REFLECT YOUR WISHES	While I understand that I am not legally required to be specific about future treatments, **if I am in the condition(s) described above I feel especially strongly about the following forms of treatment:**
	I do not want cardiac resuscitation (CPR).
	I do not want mechanical respiration.
	I do not want tube feeding.
	I do not want antibiotics.
	However, I **do want** maximum pain relief, even if it may hasten my death.
ADD PERSONAL INSTRUCTIONS (IF ANY)	Other directions (insert personal instructions):

SIGN AND DATE THE DOCUMENT AND PRINT YOUR ADDRESS

These directions express my legal right to refuse treatment, under federal and state law. I intend my instructions to be carried out, unless I have rescinded them in a new writing or by clearly indicating that I have changed my mind.

Signed: _____ Date: _____

Address: _____

_____

WITNESSING PROCEDURE

I declare that the person who signed this document is personally known to me and appears to be of sound mind and acting of his or her own free will. He or she signed (or asked another to sign for him or her) this document in my presence.

Witness: _____

Address: _____

_____

TWO WITNESSES MUST SIGN AND PRINT THEIR ADDRESSES

Witness: _____

Address: _____

_____

solutely! Because these documents enable your agent to make decisions about a wide range of health care issues, not just life-and-death decisions, they offer more flexibility than living wills.

The laws dealing with the "right to die with dignity" are still evolving. They reflect the fact that health care issues are complex and emotionally charged. One area that has been especially difficult for state legislatures to resolve is the withholding or withdrawal of artificial nutrition and hydration (food and water). Tables 17.1 and 17.2 show the status of each state's laws concerning nutrition and hydration.

Can a Person Help Another to Commit Suicide?

Living wills and durable health care powers of attorney generally involve the withholding or withdrawal of life support machinery when a person is no longer competent or able to communicate. But what if a competent individual wishes to end his or her own life? That's a different story.

There's not much any state can do to a person who decides to commit suicide. In fact, a best-selling book entitled *Final Exit* (Dell, 1991), by Derek Hemphrey, founder of the National Hemlock Society, gives readers step-by-step instructions on how to end their lives.

But in many instances, people are physically incapable of taking their own lives and need assistance. Can a state criminally punish someone for assisting a suicide? The state of Michigan has been trying to prevent Dr. Kevorkian from using his infamous "death machine" to help desperate individuals commit suicide, but so far the state has been unsuccessful.

Obviously, if a loved one wishes to take his or her life, you will be faced with an emotionally and ethically wrenching decision. You could also be faced with a jail term, because many states have explicitly criminalized assisted suicide. Those states are listed in table 17.3. Before coming to any final conclusion, it would be wise to check with a criminal or elder law attorney.

CHAPTER 17 SUMMARY CHECKLIST

A Living Will and Health Care Power of Attorney Can Protect Peace of Mind and Savings

✔ If you don't want to be kept alive by "heroic measures," sign and distribute copies of a living will.

✔ Get a free living will from Choice in Dying, (800) 989-9455.

✔ Distribute copies widely, to family, doctors, clergy, and close friends.

✔ Prepare a durable power of attorney for health care, to enable others to make health care decisions for you in case of your incapacity.

TABLE 17.1

Artificial Nutrition and Hydration Rules for Living Wills

STATE LAWS PERMITTING REFUSAL OF ARTIFICIAL NUTRITION AND HYDRATION		STATE LAWS REQUIRING PROVISION OF NUTRITION AND HYDRATION	STATE LAWS NOT ADDRESSING ARTIFICIAL NUTRITION AND HYDRATION
Alaska	New Hampshire	Missouri	Alabama
Arizona[1]	New Jersey		Arkansas
California	North Carolina		Delaware
Colorado	North Dakota		District of Columbia
Connecticut	Ohio		Florida
Georgia	Oklahoma		Kansas
Hawaii	Oregon		Mississippi
Idaho	Pennsylvania		Montana
Illinois[2]	Rhode Island		Nebraska
Indiana	South Carolina		New Mexico
Iowa	South Dakota		Texas
Kentucky	Tennessee		Vermont
Louisiana	Utah		West Virginia
Maine	Virginia		
Maryland	Washington		
Minnesota	Wisconsin		
Nevada	Wyoming		

NOTE: "Artificial Nutrition and Hydration in Living Will Statutes," reprinted, with permission, from Choice in Dying (New York: Choice in Dying, 1994).

[1]The authority to withhold or withdraw artificial nutrition and hydration is explicitly mentioned only in the sample document, not in the text of the law.

[2]Artificial nutrition and hydration cannot be withheld or withdrawn if the resulting death is due to starvation or dehydration.

TABLE 17.2

Artificial Nutrition and Hydration Rules for Durable Powers of Attorney for Health Care

STATE LAWS PERMITTING AGENTS TO ORDER WITHHOLDING OR WITHDRAWAL OF ARTIFICIAL NUTRITION AND HYDRATION		STATE LAWS NOT ADDRESSING ARTIFICIAL NUTRITION AND HYDRATION
Arizona	New Jersey	Arkansas
Colorado	New York	California
Connecticut	North Carolina	Delaware
Georgia	Ohio	District of Columbia
Hawaii	Oklahoma	Florida
Idaho	Oregon	Kansas
Illinois	Pennsylvania	Maine
Indiana	South Carolina	Massachusetts
Iowa	South Dakota	Michigan
Kentucky	Tennessee	Mississippi
Louisiana	Utah	Montana
Maryland	Virginia	New Mexico
Minnesota	Washington	North Dakota
Missouri	Wisconsin	Rhode Island
Nebraska		Texas
Nevada		West Virginia
New Hampshire		Wyoming

NOTE: "Artificial Nutrition and Hydration in States Authorizing Health Care Agents," reprinted, with permission, from Choice in Dying (New York: Choice in Dying, 1994).

TABLE 17.3

Assisted Suicide Laws

STATES WITH LAWS CRIMINALIZING ASSISTED SUICIDE		STATES THAT EITHER ALLOW ASSISTED SUICIDE OR IN WHICH THE LAW IS UNCLEAR
Alabama	Mississippi	Iowa
Alaska	Missouri	Louisiana[2]
Arizona	Montana	North Carolina[3]
Arkansas	Nebraska	Ohio
California	Nevada	Utah[3]
Colorado	New Hampshire	Virginia
Connecticut	New Jersey	Wyoming[3]
Delaware	New Mexico	
District of Columbia	New York	
Florida	North Dakota	
Georgia	Oklahoma	
Hawaii	Oregon	
Idaho	Pennsylvania	
Illinois	Rhode Island	
Indiana	South Carolina	
Kansas	South Dakota	
Kentucky	Tennessee	
Maine	Texas	
Maryland	Vermont	
Massachusetts	Washington[1]	
Michigan	West Virginia	
Minnesota	Wisconsin	

NOTE: "Assisted Suicide Laws in the United States," reprinted, with permission, from Choice in Dying (New York: Choice in Dying, 1994).
[1]Washington's law criminalizing assisted suicide has been declared unconstitutional by a federal court.
[2]State constitution stipulates that "no law shall subject any person to euthanasia."
[3]State has abolished the common law of crimes and therefore does not explicitly prohibit assisted suicide.

18

How to Handle the Nursing-Home and Medicaid Applications

Applying for Medicaid will never make the top-ten list of what to do for fun. There are actually two separate applications to deal with, and neither one is a picnic. But if you know your rights and proceed with caution, you should be able to get over these painful hassles.

Nursing-Home Application

Each nursing home has its own application that must be filled out in order to be accepted as a resident. Since many nursing homes have long waiting lists, these forms often must be completed months in advance.

You will find that nursing-home applications vary widely. Take time to read through the forms before you begin. Remember the saying "honesty is the best policy"? When it comes to filling out the nursing-home application, that rule is wise advice.

Before applying, if you anticipate using Medicaid benefits now or in the future, check to make sure the nursing home takes Medicaid patients. Most, but not all, do. If the nursing home does not accept any resident with Medicaid and is not licensed by the state to receive Medicaid, then save your ink, don't even file the application unless you are committed to paying privately. Admitting a loved one to a non-Medicaid facility and then moving once the money has run out can be disruptive and harmful, and it may severely limit the resident's nursing-home options.

Nursing homes prefer patients who are not Med-icaid recipients, because Uncle Sam is cheap and they can charge private-pay patients higher fees (in part this is done to compensate for the government's lower payments). Since nursing homes are businesses, their profit motive is understandable. (Even with Medicaid, though, nursing homes do make money.) Some applicants are afraid to list all of their assets, especially when they are planning to move assets into exemptions or to transfer assets out of their names. But in this case, the more assets shown on the application the better. Since nursing homes like private-pay patients, an application showing lots of assets should reduce the risk that the home will discriminate against the applicant because he or she is or looks poor. And if the assets are later transferred by the applicant, that will be OK too as long as everything is done legally.

Can nursing homes legally discriminate against applicants who are currently on or likely to go on Medicaid in favor of private-pay patients? The answer is no. Let me say this as clearly as possible: nursing homes cannot *legally* treat Medicaid applicants or recipients any differently than they do private-pay patients. Do they discriminate? Unfortunately, the answer increasingly seems to be yes, at least when it comes to admission to the nursing facilities.

Many nursing facilities are requesting full disclosure of applicants' financial records and then are using this information to delay or refuse admission to applicants who do not have the resources to pay privately for some extended period of time (usually at least four to six months, and sometimes longer).

As the population ages and more people require nursing-home care, and as states freeze the number of nursing-home beds (by refusing to license new facilities eligible for Medicaid benefits), the problem worsens. Waiting lists at nursing homes get longer and nursing-home administrators can become more selective in admission.

Although nursing homes cannot legally refuse to accept applicants because they are on or likely to go on Medicaid, their practice of requiring detailed financial records can have only one purpose: to unlawfully weed out those individuals who lack substantial assets. The Federal Affairs Health Team of the AARP states:

> In our view, this practice violates the federal Nursing Home Reform law because it is equivalent to the prohibited practice of requiring "oral or written assistance that such individuals are not eligible for, or will not apply for, benefits under" Medicaid. These forms of financial discrimination have also been shown to have a disparate impact on minorities' access to nursing facilities. In general, the practice gives nursing homes yet another way to close their doors to all but those with substantial financial resources, relegating middle and lower income applicants to undesirable and possibly distant facilities. AARP will continue to seek redress on this issue.[1]

While the government has toughened the Medicaid eligibility rules and attempted to strike back against so-called Medicaid planning by changes made in OBRA 1993, the new law does not entitle nursing homes to treat people who qualify for Medicaid benefits worse than nursing-home residents who pay privately for their care. If a nursing home accepts Medicaid reimbursement from the government, as most do, it must comply with the government's antidiscrimination rules as well.

Some facilities claim to have only a certain number of Medicaid beds; the rest are for private-pay patients. In some cases the state actually has approved and participated in this practice. However, several courts have ruled that this practice is unlawful. If a nursing home takes even one Medicaid patient, it cannot discriminate by limiting the number of admittees on Medicaid or imposing a Medicaid patient quota.

Nursing homes cannot require patients to turn over all or much of their savings in order to get in, particularly where such a contribution would cause the applicant to pay more than would otherwise be required under the Medicaid rules. The federal Health Care Financing Administration says that nursing homes may not require an up-front payment of any more than two months' costs. And residents cannot be forced to pay privately for a fixed time period or up to a fixed amount; when a resident is eligible for Medicaid, he or she must be free to go on Medicaid.

Many nursing homes also require family members to sign a statement that will make them responsible for the resident's bills. Some try to use this to coerce family members to pay private-pay rates for a resident who would otherwise qualify for Medicaid.

Again, this practice is illegal. A nursing home cannot force anyone to pay privately for a resident who qualifies for Medicaid benefits. Children, siblings, and others cannot be forced to pay for a loved one's nursing-home charges.

How can you protect yourself? First, a nursing-home applicant is less likely to meet with discrimination if he or she has at least enough cash to pay for four to six months of nursing-home care privately. As part of your planning, try to reserve enough money to cover at least this much time, if not longer.

Second, family members should try to avoid signing any contract agreeing to guarantee nursing-home payments. At most, sign a contract that clearly limits family members' payment obligations to situations in which the resident does not otherwise qualify for Medicaid.

If the nursing home insists on your signing a broad payment guarantee and refuses to admit your loved one if you don't, can you sign it? Yes, because the contract is illegal, and if a nursing home ever tried to enforce this type of contract, it should be voided by a court. But again, you're always better off if you can avoid litigation.

Medicaid Application

After a person has taken steps to protect his or her assets, and following the expiration of any transfer-ineligibility period, the person will be ready to apply for Medicaid.

The first step down the Medicaid application path is to complete a form that in most states can be procured from a local welfare, public health, or Social

Security office. Many hospitals and nursing homes have a social worker on staff who can help direct you to the right place for an application and who will even give advice about how to complete the form.

The application forms differ in each state. Often they look complicated and involved. *Don't be scared off by the application.* Fill out as much as you can and submit it as quickly as possible. The sooner you get the application in, the sooner the patient may begin to collect.

But don't apply before any pertinent ineligibility period has passed. Nursing homes have a tendency to push residents to apply too early, and after OBRA 1993, that can have disastrous results. As explained on pages 38–40, following a significant gift or transfer, an application made within the three-year lookback period could trigger an ineligiblity period of many years. Let me repeat: *apply only when you are sure you qualify.* If there's any doubt, talk to an elder law attorney.

The Medicaid application forms generally seek information concerning a nursing-home patient's age, income, assets, citizenship, residency, personal circumstances (such as employment and family members), disability (if any), and medical expenses. The form will also ask about any gifts made within the last three years. Again, this application must be filled out accurately and honestly.

After the person has submitted the application form, someone from Medicaid generally will interview the person, his or her spouse, and/or any children. Proof of the information requested in the application should be brought to the interview. For example, to show income, pay stubs, W-2s, or similar information will be required; to show assets, copies of items like bank and money market statements may be necessary. All information provided in the application and the interview is strictly confidential.

Can you handle the application yourself, possibly with the help of a social worker at the nursing home, or should you get the help of a lawyer? This is a tough question. I don't like to promote lawyers too much, because they charge for their services; since the Medicaid application process typically is time-consuming, the legal costs can be significant. And the application process really isn't brain surgery.

On the other hand, I have seen and heard of *many* instances in which consumers acting without lawyers have been wrongfully turned down by Medicaid bureaucrats. In one of my own cases, for example, I submitted an application for a client that should have been approved easily. The client had made a gift of assets of about $60,000, but the ineligibility period had long since passed. All other funds had been spent on nursing-home care; nothing else presented any questions.

Yet in the interview the Medicaid bureaucrat told me she was going to deny the application. When I asked why, she responded, "I don't like the large transfer that was made. People shouldn't be allowed to get away with that." I explained politely that her personal views were irrelevant and that under the law, she had to approve the application. When she still refused to change her view, I got up and spoke with a supervisor. In a few minutes, the matter was resolved and the application was approved. But had I not been there, the applicant would have been wrongfully denied. Unfortunately, these kinds of incidents occur regularly.

The social worker at the nursing home is no substitute for an elder law attorney. While the nursing-home representative may be very nice, chances are good that this person does not have the same level of legal knowledge or experience that a good elder law attorney would have. And keep in mind that it is often not in the nursing home's best interest to help residents get onto Medicaid.

After reviewing the application and considering the interview, Medicaid will decide whether the applicant needs nursing-home care and is eligible for Medicaid. The state sets a time limit—usually forty-five to sixty days—within which the Medicaid bureaucrats must make a decision. Of course, the quicker Medicaid receives the necessary information, the faster the applicant should get a response.

If the application is approved, Medicaid funding should begin promptly. In fact, if someone has entered a nursing home while waiting for Medicaid's decision and has paid out of pocket for a period of time, the patient might even be able to get a refund from the nursing home for part or all of those prior payments. Not surprisingly, reimbursements are hard to get, so while a Medicaid application is being reviewed, you'll be better off refusing to pay the nursing home and advising the home that you've applied for Medicaid. Medicaid benefits can actually be paid back three months prior to the application.

If Medicaid denies a person's application, that person has a right to appeal. The denial notice must disclose the reason for the denial and the law on which the decision was based. Depending on the rules in the state, the applicant may appeal to a state hearing office, a state medical board, or a state court. In the case of an appeal, Medicaid must provide a form and will help the applicant fill it out. But if a person has been denied, he or she should probably get legal help with the appeal. Don't delay. Ask Medicaid how much time you or your loved one has to appeal. If you miss the deadline (this varies from state to state but is usually from ten to ninety days), you may lose your right to appeal.

Before the appeal hearing, take the time to stop by the Medicaid office and review the state's file on your case. You are legally entitled to review any information in the file, and the information there might enable you to better present your case.

The appeal hearing will be decided by a Medicaid employee who was not involved in the previous denial of your application. The applicant may be represented by a person of his or her choice and may introduce evidence and witnesses.

If you lose the appeal, you'll still get another chance to fight back, and you can take your case to court. Often the fairest decision will be made by an impartial judge, who is *not* an employee of the Medicaid office.

After approval, don't rest too easy. The state must reexamine your file every twelve months to make sure you remain eligible. If circumstances change during the year (for example, you inherit a bundle of money), you cannot wait until the redetermination. Instead you must promptly notify the state Medicaid bureaucrats of your new financial status.

CHAPTER 18 SUMMARY CHECKLIST

How to Handle the Nursing-Home and Medicaid Applications

Nursing-Home Application

- ✔ Find a Medicaid-qualified nursing home.

- ✔ Fill out the application completely and honestly.

- ✔ If the nursing home takes any Medicaid patients, don't let them delay or refuse admission just because you are on or likely to go on Medicaid.

- ✔ Try to keep enough cash to pay four to six months of nursing-home care privately.

- ✔ Don't pay more than Medicaid requires.

- ✔ Family members should try to avoid signing illegal guarantee contracts.

Medicaid Application

- ✔ Fill out the application completely and honestly.

- ✔ Don't apply too early or too late—apply at the earliest eligibility date.

- ✔ Consider getting a lawyer to help you through the application process.

- ✔ Don't pay the nursing home while the Medicaid application is pending.

- ✔ Appeal a wrongful denial, and do so promptly.

19 A Lawyer Can Be Helpful if You Pick the Right One

An elderly woman went to see her lawyer about a will. After she nervously went through the list of gifts she wanted to make, the lawyer said, "Don't worry, just leave it all to me." She immediately responded, "I guess you're right—you'll get it all anyway." For many of us, this joke has more than a ring of truth to it.

No one wants to spend a fortune on legal fees, but a lawyer experienced in Medicaid matters, often called an elder law attorney, can be helpful, particularly if you (or a loved one) would like personalized guidance concerning planning techniques. The right lawyer can offer invaluable assistance and save you money in the long run.

How Do You Find the Right Lawyer?

Finding a lawyer is rarely a problem. The challenge is finding the *right* lawyer—ideally an individual who's experienced in Medicaid planning and sensitive to the needs of the elderly. Here are nine tips to consider when shopping for an attorney:

1. Ask your friends; perhaps they've already used a lawyer for estate or Medicaid planning advice. If they recommend their personal injury lawyer, that lawyer is probably *not* the right attorney to advise you about Medicaid matters, although he or she might be able to recommend someone who can.

2. Ask other professionals whom you trust for any suggestions. Your doctor, clergyman or -woman, or banker might know an experienced Medicaid lawyer. These people often work with such lawyers and may know a good one.

3. Contact the local chapter of the Alzheimer's Association, the Arthritis Foundation, the Diabetes Association, or one of the other nonprofit organizations that regularly deal with older persons. Personnel in these organizations often know the attorneys who are experienced in Medicaid matters; some of these organizations even have referral lists. A growing number of hospitals have instituted gerontology units, and doctors or other personnel in these units may be able to recommend an experienced elder law attorney.

4. If there's a law school nearby, ask for a professor who handles probate or estate planning. Some professors will be happy to recommend a lawyer to you.

5. If you or your parent works for a company that hires outside lawyers, call one of those lawyers and ask for a referral. Because a member of your family works for one of his clients, he is likely to want to make you happy and may help find an experienced Medicaid lawyer if he doesn't already know one.

6. Local bar associations often offer referral services that can provide names of attorneys.

These should be used only as a last resort. Lawyers generally get on such lists by paying a small fee—bar associations rarely do any screening at all—so you have no assurance about the competency or expertise of a lawyer recommended through a referral service.

7. Don't pick a lawyer at random from the telephone book unless you like playing Russian roulette.

8. Don't rely on general advertising. Anyone can advertise, regardless of ability or experience.

9. Be wary of recommendations from anyone who stands to benefit from a referral. For example, a real estate agent, an accountant, or a financial planner may work with one or two lawyers; they refer business to the lawyer and the lawyer refers business to them. Sometimes these referrals are fine, because the referrer can benefit from your satisfaction; however, your needs may not be the primary concern in such a situation.

How Do You Choose a Lawyer?

Once you have a list of names, how do you pick the right one for you? First, try to narrow the field by finding out as much as possible about each lawyer's reputation and experience. Ask lawyers you know if they are familiar with the names recommended to you. You can also check the *Martindale-Hubbell Directory,* available in most libraries.

The *Martindale-Hubbell Directory* lists most lawyers in the country and gives some helpful information about them. Unfortunately, it is not the easiest book to decipher. Here's how to read it:

1. Choose the volume that includes the state in which the lawyer practices.

2. Find the roster of lawyers in the state near the beginning of the volume.

3. Find the city in which the lawyer practices and locate his or her name.

4. Immediately following the attorney's name are his or her date of birth and date of first admission to the bar.

5. Sometimes a rating, indicated by one or two lowercase letters, will be next. An explanation of this rating can be found below.

6. Next is a "C." followed by a number and an "L." followed by a number; respectively, these indicate the lawyer's college and law school. Now turn to the beginning of the volume to find the list showing what school is represented by each number. The degrees received are also usually included (i.e., B.A., J.D.)

7. Finally, some names are followed by the name of a law firm in brackets. If an "A" precedes the firm's name, that indicates the lawyer is an associate (an employee of the office, not a partner). If a firm's name is listed in brackets, there may be additional information about its attorneys in the biographical section later in the volume.

Here's an example of how the listing works:

Smith, John . . . '53'77 a v C.821 B.A. L.569 J.D. [Hahn L. & P.]

John Smith was born in 1953 and graduated from law school in 1977. "C.821 B.A." means that he earned his bachelor's degree at Swarthmore College; "L.569 J.D." means that he received his law degree at New York University. "[Hahn L. & P.]" is shorthand for Hahn Loeser & Parks, his law firm.

Since there is a law firm listed, you can look to the biographical section of the volume for additional information. For John Smith you might find:

JOHN D. SMITH, born Cleveland, Ohio, June 2, 1953; admitted to bar, 1977, Maryland; 1979, District of Columbia, Ohio, U.S. District Court for the District of Columbia and U.S. Court of Appeals for the District of Columbia Circuit. Education: Swarthmore College (B.A., cum laude, 1974); New York University (J.D., cum laude, 1977). Order of the Coif. Root-Tilden Scholar. Associate Editor, New York University Law Review, 1976–1977. Law Clerk to Honorable Aubrey E. Robinson, Jr., Chief Judge, U.S. District Court for the District of Columbia. Author: "You and the Law," columns in the Cleveland Plain Dealer, 1982–, and Columbus Dispatch, 1985–, Member Cleveland (Chairman, Young Lawyers Section, 1983–1984; Member, Board of Trustees, 1983–1984), Ohio State and American (Member, Executive Council, Young Lawyers Division, 1986–1987) Bar Association.

The *Martindale-Hubbell Directory* also rates lawyers, based on their legal ability and ethical standards, by surveying lawyers and judges in the area where the lawyer practices. These are the only nationally recognized lawyer ratings.

The legal ability ratings are "a" (very high), "b" (high), and "c" (fair). These ratings are supposedly based on the lawyer's ability, experience, and nature and length of practice. The ethical rating is a "v" (very high). There is no other ethical rating available; a lawyer receives either a "v" or nothing. So if the lawyer you are considering has an "a v" rating, like John Smith does, take that as a major plus. Of course, many lawyers, good and bad, are not rated by the *Martindale-Hubbell Directory*. The absence of a rating doesn't necessarily mean that a lawyer is unqualified.

Interviewing and Comparison Shopping

Once you have narrowed the field, you should interview the lawyers remaining on your list. Most lawyers will meet without charging a fee for an initial "get to know you" conference.

Upon arriving at a lawyer's office, you should try not to let the surroundings affect your judgment. A beautiful office might mean that the lawyer got rich from doing great work for clients, but it might also mean that the lawyer's mother is wealthy and decorated the office for him or that the lawyer made a lot of money by overcharging clients.

Nor should you be misled by fancy-looking certificates on the walls. Some of the worst lawyers have the most impressive wall coverings. For example, the lawyer may prominently display a certificate stating that he or she has been admitted to practice before the local federal court or even the United States Supreme Court. Don't be fooled—any lawyer can get one of those with a minimal fee and a few references from lawyers in town. Diplomas may be a little more helpful as they show what schools the lawyer has attended. A certificate from the Order of the Coif means that the lawyer graduated at the top of his or her law school class.

Following is a questionnaire that you can use for guidance when interviewing prospective lawyers.

How the lawyer answers the questions is as important as *what* is said. You should feel comfortable with the lawyer, confident in his or her abilities, and satisfied that he or she understands your or your parent's needs and will never answer your questions clearly and without making you feel that you are wasting his or her time.

CHAPTER 19 SUMMARY CHECKLIST

A Lawyer Can Be Helpful if You Pick the Right One

Get the Names of Elder Law Attorneys

✔ Ask friends for names of elder law attorneys they may have used.

✔ Contact trusted professionals for names of elder law attorneys.

✔ Call the local Alzheimer's Association and other nonprofit organizations that work with older persons and ask for the names of experienced elder law attorneys.

Check Out Attorneys' Credentials.

Interview and Comparison Shop

✔ Ask about the lawyer's experience in handling elder law matters generally and Medicaid matters specifically.

✔ Get references and call them.

✔ Find out if the lawyer is familiar with OBRA 1993. Ask questions and compare the answers with what you have learned from this book.

✔ Ask the lawyer how he or she charges.

✔ Make sure you feel comfortable.

✔ Use the Lawyer Interview Questionnaire, page 139.

LAWYER INTERVIEW QUESTIONNAIRE

1. How many people have you counseled on Medicaid matters in the past five years?

   Answer: _____

2. How many Medicaid-related trusts and/or durable powers of attorney have you prepared, and how many Medicaid applications have you filed, in the past five years?

   Answer: _____

3. Will you give me a list of references—clients whom you've counseled on Medicaid matters? (Then call them, just as you would if you were hiring a painter. If the lawyer refuses to provide references, look elsewhere.)

   Answer: _____

4. Are you familiar with the Medicaid rules as changed by OBRA 1993?

   Answer: _____

5. What outside activities do you participate in? (If the lawyer teaches estate and probate law at a law school, that is a positive recommendation. The fact that he might be active in his church is nice, but it's not pertinent to you.)

   Answer: _____

6. With whom do you consult on legal questions you're not sure about? (A lawyer should have other experienced attorneys, either in the office or in the community, with whom he or she consults when necessary. No lawyer knows everything; if a lawyer tells you otherwise, look elsewhere.)

   Answer: _____

7. Are you the person who will handle my matter, or will you pass it off to someone else? (You may actually be better off if a younger, lower-priced attorney in the office handles the matter, as long as he or she will be well supervised.)

   Answer: _____

8. Wil you keep me informed about the progress of my matter (preparation of trusts, etc.) on a regular basis?

   Answer: _____

9. What will your fee be?

   Answer: _____

10. Will you provide me with regular, detailed billings?

   Answer: _____

20 | Conclusion

A variety of tools to safeguard family nest eggs, within the existing laws, have been presented in this book. To summarize and exemplify these tools, here are two final series of guidelines that draw on the full range of this book's various alternatives:

Master Checklist to Protect Assets

The following steps can help an elderly person protect his or her assets from being wiped out by catastrophic long-term care costs.

OPTIONS AVAILABLE BEFORE ONE REQUIRES LONG-TERM CARE

While you are healthy and not in need of long-term care, you should:

- Prepare a durable power of attorney for a spouse and/or a child, giving it to a third person to hold, if possible. This allows you maximum planning flexibility and should guarantee that you incur no loss of principal greater than about $100,000 to $150,000 (three years of nursing-home costs).

- Consider making a large gift to children (or others), which will trigger a penalty of up to three years. After the three years have passed, the transferred funds are protected from nursing-home costs. Your children may decide to place the funds into a family asset protection trust to further insulate the funds.

- If you decide not to make a large gift, make small look-back gifts, which can allow you to make a large gift just prior to entry into a nursing home without jeopardizing Medicaid coverage.

- Consider putting your home into a house preservation trust and other appreciated assets into an irrevocable asset protection trust.

- Check out long-term care insurance policies. You may find one that offers important protection at a price that makes sense.

- Consider making a living will and durable power of attorney for health care.

- Consider transferring your home to children or others but retaining a life estate. That guarantees you the right to live there.

OPTIONS AVAILABLE WHEN ONE ENTERS A NURSING HOME AND LEAVES A SPOUSE AT HOME

Should you have to go into a nursing home, leaving a spouse at home:

- You should, where practical, pay off debts and change money into exempt assets, such as a home, household goods, personal effects, car, property producing income for support, life insurance, and burial plots and expenses. Exempt assets (other than the house) may then be transferred to others.

You may even prepay some upcoming costs.

- You should transfer the house into the name of your spouse-at-home, and at the same time the spouse-at-home should change his or her will so that the house won't revert to you (and then to the nursing home) if he or she dies. Even better, the spouse-at-home should put the house and any other remaining assets into a revocable living trust.

- You may consider making a gift to children or others. First figure out how much the spouse-at-home will be allowed to keep (one-half of the total or $74,820, whichever is less); then transfer about half of the remaining assets. Again, the children may want to consider a family asset protection trust.

- See if you can make any gifts that trigger no ineligibility period, such as to a child living with the parents for two years or more.

- Apply for Medicaid and argue that the spouse-at-home needs the assets to generate enough income to live on.

- Consider shifting assets into the name of the healthy spouse, who may then purchase an annuity. Some of the additional income can be accumulated for heirs.

- Your spouse-at-home may protect both assets and income by getting a divorce. In some states, a support order can protect income for the spouse-at-home without actually going through a divorce.

OPTIONS AVAILABLE WHEN AN UNMARRIED PERSON ENTERS A NURSING HOME

Should you be an unmarried person entering a nursing home, you should:

- Where practical, consider transferring money into exempt assets, particularly a house. However, in many states, the protection for a house disappears soon after an unmarried person enters a nursing home. And the state's estate recovery program may grab the home anyhow.

- Consider making a gift of about half of your assets to children or others. The rest will be spent during the ineligibility period, but after that period has run out, at least the transferred assets should be protected. Your children may consider placing transferred assets into a family asset protection trust.

- Shift assets to a family member who can take advantage of a medical deduction.

- See if you can make any gifts that trigger no ineligibility period, such as to a child who lived with you for at least two years prior to your nursing home admission.

- Pay your children for services provided.

- If your goal is to maximize care for yourself, not to leave assets to heirs, consider a self-care trust.

- Consider selling the home to a family member on a land contract; the mortgage payments will go to the nursing home, but the additional nursing charges will be paid by Medicaid.

- Place assets into a limited liability company and then make discounted gifts.

Sample Medicaid Plans

Following are four sample Medicaid plans illustrating how one's parents might employ the strategies described in this book to protect a portion of their life savings.

Situation 1

Your parents own a home and have additional assets (CDs and stock) totaling $100,000. Some assets are owned jointly with rights of survivorship, others are owned individually. Your parents' income is about $25,000 annually, excluding interest and dividends, an amount sufficient for them to live on.

They have three children—Joe, who lives in town, and two others, who live elsewhere. Your parents have a good relationship with all three children but are closest with Joe because of his proximity. Your parents' wills are simple, leaving everything to each other and then to the children in equal shares.

Now your father has become seriously ill. Although he's mentally competent, he may soon have to enter a nursing home. Here is a possible plan that could benefit your parents in this situation:

Plan 1

1. Each parent should prepare one durable power of attorney naming the other as attorney-in-fact and a second naming Joe as attorney-in-fact. If necessary to maintain family harmony, they could also make durable powers of attorney naming each of their other children. They should give the durable powers of attorney to a third person (like their lawyer) to hold until it becomes necessary to use them.

2. Both parents should consider making living wills and durable powers of attorney for health care.

3. They should transfer the house into your mother's name, and your mother may empty joint accounts and use the money to open accounts in her own name.

4. Assume that the house has a $50,000 mortgage. That could be paid off by selling some stock or cashing in a CD when it becomes due.

5. Your parents could also buy a new refrigerator and stove to replace the ones they've had for fifteen years, and prepay funeral costs.

6. Your mother might consider purchasing an annuity.

7. Your mother may make a tax-free transfer of a portion of the assets to the children. The children, in turn, might choose to create a family asset protection trust.

8. Assets remaining in your mother's name, including the house, should be put into a revocable living trust that does not include your father as a beneficiary.

Situation 2

Your father passed away many years ago and your mother has needed full-time care for the last few years. You moved in with her two years ago and have been helping to dress, bathe, and feed her. But you are now sixty-three and won't be able to manage all of her needs for much longer. You are the only living child.

Besides the house, your mother has about $50,000.

Plan 2

1. Your mother should prepare a durable power of attorney naming you as attorney-in-fact. She also should make a durable power of attorney for health care and a living will.

2. Your mother could invest some or all of her cash in the house, paying off the mortgage, making improvements, and/or purchasing household goods.

3. Your mother could then transfer the house to you. This transfer can be done before she goes into a nursing home without affecting her Medicaid eligibility because you have lived in the house for two years, helping your mother stay out of an institution.

4. Your mother can set aside funds for her funeral expenses and burial plots for herself and you.

5. A portion of any of the $50,000 that remains may be given to you as payment for services rendered. If you can't convince the Medicaid bureaucrats that the payment to you is really a payment for work (since you and your mother had no written contract and payments were not contemporaneous with the work) rather than a gift, at worst the payment would trigger a relatively short period of ineligibility.

Situation 3

Your parents are both in their fifties and doing quite well. They want to plan ahead to avoid impoverishment by nursing-home costs.

They presently own a home, and their remaining assets total about $150,000. They have three children.

Plan 3

1. Your parents should make durable powers of attorney for each other and, probably, for at

least one of the children. They should also make durable powers of attorney for health care and living wills.

2. Your parents should look closely at long-term care insurance policies. At their age the policies may be available at a reasonable premium.

3. They are probably too young to give away most or all of their assets. But they may want to make small look-back gifts every few months.

4. Place assets into a revocable living trust to avoid probate.

Situation 4

Your seventy-five-year-old father has assets of $150,000 and is living off the income from them; he also owns his home. He is currently healthy but is worried about what may happen if he becomes ill. He has three children but is somewhat concerned about giving away his assets to them while he is alive, because if one of them got divorced or died, his assets might end up with the in-law.

Plan 4

1. Your father might consider gifting about half of his assets to the children, creating a twenty-five-month ineligibility period. The children, who understand their father's con-

cerns about his financial security, then create a family asset protection trust.

2. His remaining assets should be put into a revocable living trust designed to avoid probate at his death.

3. The house can be put into a house protection trust to shelter it from the nursing home while maintaining the capital gains tax breaks.

4. Your father should make a durable power of attorney, a health care power of attorney, and a living will.

No problem facing older Americans and their families is more severe than that posed by the catastrophic costs of long-term care, and our government has done little to address the roots of the problem.

If we care about the quality of our lives and the lives of our parents and grandparents, we must all continue to pressure our elected officials to act in the best interests of the elderly. We will all be better off once the politicians finally decide to adopt a system that allows older Americans to obtain long-term care without having to impoverish themselves and their families.

Until that time comes, families are on their own and must protect themselves. With the tips provided in this book, older Americans should be able to avoid the Medicaid trap and protect their savings from catastrophic nursing-home care costs.

Appendix A
Durable Power of Attorney Forms

In chapter 12, I discussed the usage and advantage of a durable power of attorney. The first form that follows was prepared by Barbara Gilder Quint for *Family Circle* magazine (June 1, 1987). She drafted it at the time as a sample form for use in every state except Florida, Missouri, North Carolina, South Carolina, and Wyoming. If you live in Wyoming, a similar preprinted form is available in stationery stores for about a dollar. Subsequently in this appendix are sample durable power of attorney forms applicable to the other states. Also included are forms provided by the state legislatures in New York, California, Colorado, Connecticut, Illinois, Minnesota, Texas, and Wisconsin. While the *Family Circle* form was drafted to be acceptable in these states as well as most others, there are some differences, and third parties who may be asked to rely on the use of a durable power of attorney will probably be more familiar with their own state's version.

Each form is followed by a set of explanations designed to help clarify the form's provisions.

NOTE: These forms and the explanations are intended only to help you understand the benefits and uses of a durable power of attorney. Always see an experienced attorney to help with your planning and to prepare your legal documents, including durable powers of attorney. These documents are too important to try to do on your own; a mistake can be costly.

DURABLE GENERAL POWER OF ATTORNEY

STATE OF _____

COUNTY OF _____

       Know all Men by These Presents, which are intended to constitute a DURABLE GENERAL POWER OF ATTORNEY,

That I _____
                                (Name of principal)

_____
                               (Address of principal)

do hereby appoint _____
                               (Name of agent)

_____
                               (Address of agent)
                                   and

_____
     (Name of agent if more than one agent is designated)

_____
    (Address of agent if more than one agent is designated)

My Attorney(s)-in-Fact TO ACT (jointly) (severally), as my true and lawful Attorney(s)-in-Fact, for me and in my name, place and stead:

       (A) Power with Respect to Accounts and Instruments. To establish or open accounts, certificates of deposit and any other form of account or instrument for me with financial institutions of any kind; to modify, terminate, make deposits to and write checks on and endorse checks for or make withdrawals from all accounts in my name or with respect to which I am an authorized signatory; to negotiate, endorse or transfer any checks or other instruments with respect to any such accounts; to contract for any services rendered by any financial institution; and to add property to any trust agreement created by me.

       (B) Power with Respect to Safe-Deposit Boxes. To contract with any institution for the maintenance of a safe-deposit box in my name; to have access to all safe-deposit boxes in my name or with respect to which I am an authorized signatory; to add to and remove from the contents of any such safe-deposit box and to terminate any and all contracts for such boxes.

       (C) Power to Sell and Buy. To sell and buy personal, intangible or mixed property, upon such terms and conditions as my Attorney(s)-in-Fact deems appropriate; to use any credit card held in my name to make such purchases and to sign such charge slips as may be necessary to use such credit cards; and to repay from any funds belonging to me any money borrowed and to pay for any purchases made or cash advanced using credit cards issued to me.

       (D) Power to Exercise Rights in Securities. To exercise all rights with respect to securities that I now own, or may hereafter acquire; to establish, utilize and terminate brokerage accounts; and to invest and reinvest any of my assets in stocks, common and/or preferred, bonds (including, without limitation, United States Treasury Bonds or other United States government obligations which may be redeemed at par for the purpose of applying the entire amount of principal and accrued interest thereon to the payment of the Federal estate tax, if any, occasioned by my death), notes, debentures, loans, mortgages, common trust funds, or other securities or property, real or personal, upon such terms and conditions as my Attorney(s)-in-Fact deems appropriate.

(E) (Power to Borrow Money (including any Insurance Policy Loans). To borrow money for my account upon such terms and conditions as my Attorney(s)-in-Fact may deem appropriate and to secure such borrowing by the granting of security interests in any property or interest in property which I may now or hereafter own; to borrow money upon any life insurance policies owned by me upon my life for any purpose and to grant a security interest in such policy to secure any such loans; and no insurance company shall be under any obligation whatsoever to determine the need for such loan or the application of the proceeds therefrom.

(F) Power with Respect to Real Property. To purchase real property, to manage, maintain and alter all real property belonging to me, and to lease, sell, mortgage, encumber or otherwise dispose of all interests in real property belonging to me, upon such terms and conditions as my Attorney(s)in-Fact deems appropriate; to renew leases of the same or to execute, acknowledge and deliver leases therefor; to execute deeds of conveyance either with or without covenants of general warranty; to pay and satisfy all mortgages, encumbrances, taxes and assessments that may be a lien or charge upon any of my real property; and to receive rentals from and the proceeds of sale of any of my real property. For purposes of this Durable General Power of Attorney, real property shall include, without limitation, the real property known as _____.

(G) Power to Demand, Compromise and Receive. To demand, arbitrate, settle, sue for, collect, receive, deposit, expand for my benefit, reinvest or make such other appropriate dispositions of, as my Attorney(s)-in-Fact deems appropriate, all cash rights to payments of cash, property (personal, intangible and/or mixed), rights and/or benefits to which I am now or may in the future become entitled, regardless of the identity of the individual or public or private entity involved (and for purposes of receiving Social Security benefits, my Attorney(s)-in-Fact is herewith appointed my "Representative Payee"); to compound, compromise, settle and adjust all claims and demands whatsoever which I may now owe or be liable for; and to utilize all lawful means and methods for such purposes.

(H) Power with Respect to Taxes. To make, prepare, sign and file for me and on my behalf any and all required tax estimates and returns, federal, state or local, as well as any waivers, affidavits, schedules or other forms required or permitted to be filed in connection therewith, and to protest and appeal any assessments or determinations of tax against me which my Attorney(s)-in-Fact deems to have been made without proper warrant.

(I) Power with Respect to Documents. To sign, acknowledge, record and deliver agreements, affidavits, bills of sale, stock powers, deeds, leases, mortgages, notes, receipts, releases, satisfactions, journal entries, certificates and such other documents which may be necessary or convenient in execution of the powers hereinbefore expressly conferred upon my Attorney(s)-in-Fact; to execute and deliver applications for automobile license plates and certificates of title and to endorse for transfer and to deliver certificates of title; and to execute and deliver applications for insurance (including, without limitation, insurance on my life) and to cancel and select the amounts therefor.

(J) Power to Engage Services. To engage the services of and compensate attorneys-at-law, appraisers, accountants, brokers, real estate managers, investment counsel and such other persons as may be proper or convenient to advise and assist in the management, maintenance and disposition of my property.

(K) Power to Incur Obligations. To incur obligations for the maintenance, support, health, care, well-being, comfort and welfare of me and my family and to satisfy such obligations out of my money or property; and to consent on my behalf to medical and surgical procedures.

I further give and grant to my said Attorney(s)-in-Fact full power and authority to do and perform every act necessary to be done in the exercise of any of the foregoing powers as fully as I might or could do if personally present, with full power of substitution and revocation, hereby ratifying and confirming all that my said Attorney(s)-in-Fact shall lawfully do, or cause to be done by virtue hereof.

This instrument may not be changed orally.

This power of attorney is durable and shall not be affected by the subsequent disability or incompetence of the principal or by any lapse of time.

TO INDUCE ANY THIRD PARTY TO ACT HEREUNDER, I HEREBY AGREE THAT ANY THIRD PARTY RECEIVING A DULY EXECUTED COPY OR FACSIMILE OF THIS INSTRUMENT MAY ACT HEREUNDER, AND THAT REVOCATION OR TERMINATION HEREOF SHALL BE INEFFECTIVE AS TO SUCH THIRD PARTLY UNLESS AND UNTIL ACTUAL NOTICE OR KNOWLEDGE OF SUCH REVOCATION OR TERMINATION SHALL HAVE BEEN RECEIVED BY SUCH THIRD PARTY AND I FOR MYSELF AND FOR MY HEIRS, EXECUTORS, LEGAL REPRESENTATIVES AND ASSIGNS, HEREBY AGREE TO INDEMNIFY AND HOLD HARMLESS ANY SUCH THIRD PARTY FROM AND AGAINST ANY AND ALL CLAIMS THAT MAY ARISE AGAINST SUCH THIRD PARTY BY REASON OF SUCH THIRD PARTY HAVING RELIED ON THE PROVISIONS OF THIS INSTRUMENT.

In witness whereof, I have hereunto signed my name this _____ day of _____, 19____

_____
(Signature of Principal)

Specimen Signature of Attorney(s)-in-Fact:

_____

Signed in the presence of:

_____

_____
Witness

_____
Witness

CERTIFICATE OF NOTARY

STATE OF _____)
) SS:
COUNTY OF _____)

On the _____ day of _____, 19___, before me personally came _____, whose identity is well known to me and known to me to be the individual described in and who executed the foregoing instrument, and (he) (she) acknowledged to me that (he) (she) executed the same.

_____
Notary Public

My commission expires:

_____

3

Durable General Power of Attorney

Explanation

As you can see, this Durable General Power of Attorney form is filled with legalese. Don't be scared off by this confusing language. The explanations that follow should provide you with a clear understanding of the terms used.

Introduction: At the top left go the name of your state and county. Below that go your name and address (you are the "principal"—the person making the durable general power of attorney).

The next lines are for the name(s) and address(es) of the person(s) to whom you are giving the durable general power of attorney (called the "agent[s]" or "attorney[s]-in-fact"). Talk to your lawyer about any specific requirements for your state.

If you have decided to name more than one attorney-in-fact, you must decide whether to strike the word *jointly* or *severally*. If you want to require your attorneys-in-fact to act together to use the power of attorney, you would leave the word *jointly* and strike the word *severally*. But if you prefer to allow either of your attorneys-in-fact on his or her own to exercise the powers provided in the power of attorney, you would strike out the word *jointly* and leave the word *severally*.

The following lettered clauses specify broad powers providing your attorney(s)-in-fact with latitude to manage your financial affairs. Powers are separately enumerated to avoid any questions about whether you intended to authorize your attorney(s)-in-fact to undertake specific actions on your behalf.

Clause A: This clause authorizes your attorney(s)-in-fact to open and manage accounts, CDs, and other instruments for you in financial institutions. It also says that your attorney(s)-in-fact may add to any trust agreement you may have created.

Clause B: This clause allows your attorney(s)-in-fact to maintain and gain access to safe-deposit boxes in your name.

Clause C: This clause permits your attorney(s)-in-fact to buy and sell items and to use your credit cards.

Clause D: This clause lets your attorney(s)-in-fact invest in securities on your behalf and manage and handle those securities. This is broad enough to allow your attorney(s)-in-fact to vote at stockholders meetings.

Clause E: This clause authorizes your attorney(s)-in-fact to borrow money in your name.

Clause F: This clause gives your attorney(s)-in-fact broad authority to manage, sell, buy, mortgage, and/or lease real estate, including your home. In the blank you would fill in the address(es) of your residence and any other real estate you own. You don't have to change the durable general power of attorney each time you buy or sell real estate. Note that in the District of Columbia, no deed of conveyance may be executed by an attorney-in-fact. Recording requirements vary greatly from state to state.

Clause G: This clause authorizes your attorney(s)-in-fact to take any necessary action with respect to rights you have or may have in the future to money or property. It also lets your attorney(s)-in-fact handle claims made against you. The term *representative payee* is defined in chapter 12.

Clause H: This clause gives your attorney(s)-in-fact the power to deal with your taxes. Although you might prefer to forget about this, it's important that tax forms be prepared and taxes paid, to avoid possible penalties.

Clause I: This clause spells out the right of your attorney(s)-in-fact to sign and execute all sorts of documents on your behalf. It also allows your attorney(s)-in-fact to handle your applications for license plates, certificates of title, and insurance.

Clause J: This clause allows your attorney(s)-in-fact to hire specialists to assist in handling your financial affairs.

Clause K: This clause generally authorizes your attorney(s)-in-fact to incur and pay bills for your maintenance, support, and care. It also empowers your attorney(s)-in-fact to make certain health care decisions.

Closing Paragraphs: The first paragraph following the lettered clauses is a catchall authorizing your attorney(s)-in-fact to do anything you could do.

The next line is self-explanatory—you can't change the terms of the document orally.

The final sentence before the paragraph in all capital letters is *crucial* to making your power of attorney *durable*, so that it remains valid at the time you will need it most—during your incapacity.

Some banks and insurance companies have traditionally been unwilling to accept or act on any preprinted power of attorney form that they did not prepare themselves. The last full paragraph, printed in all capital letters, attempts to deal with this problem. That paragraph will protect third parties relying on the durable general power of attorney and, it is hoped, encourage them to accept this form. However, since there can be no assurance that this will work, you should contact your bank and insurance company to discuss their forms and procedures.

Finally, the document is signed and dated at the end before two witnesses and a notary. While not every state requires two witnesses and a notary, you won't lose anything by having all three. The attorney(s)-in-fact signs his or her name under yours. The notary then fills in and signs the bottom portion. A notary is authorized by the state or federal government to administer oaths and attest to the authenticity of signatures.

UNIFORM STATUTORY FORM POWER OF ATTORNEY

(California Civil Code Section 2475)

NOTICE: THE POWERS GRANTED BY THIS DOCUMENT ARE BROAD AND SWEEPING. THEY ARE EXPLAINED IN THE UNIFORM STATUTORY FORM POWER OF ATTORNEY ACT (CALIFORNIA CIVIL CODE SECTIONS 2475–2499.5, INCLUSIVE). IF YOU HAVE ANY QUESTIONS ABOUT THESE POWERS, OBTAIN COMPETENT LEGAL ADVICE. THIS DOCUMENT DOES NOT AUTHORIZE ANYONE TO MAKE MEDICAL AND OTHER HEALTH-CARE DECISIONS FOR YOU. YOU MAY REVOKE THIS POWER OF ATTORNEY IF YOU LATER WISH TO DO SO.

I, _____ ,

(your name and address)

appoint _____

(name and address of the person appointed, or of each person appointed if you want to designate more than one)

as my agent (attorney-in-fact) to act for me in any lawful way with respect to the following initialed subjects: **TO GRANT ALL OF THE FOLLOWING POWERS, INITIAL THE LINE IN FRONT OF (N) AND IGNORE THE LINES IN FRONT OF THE OTHER POWERS. TO GRANT ONE OR MORE, BUT FEWER THAN ALL, OF THE FOLLOWING POWERS, INITIAL THE LINE IN FRONT OF EACH POWER YOU ARE GRANTING. TO WITHHOLD A POWER, DO NOT INITIAL THE LINE IN FRONT OF IT. YOU MAY, BUT NEED NOT, CROSS OUT EACH POWER WITHHELD.**

Initial:

_____ (A) Real property transactions.

_____ (B) Tangible personal property transactions.

_____ (C) Stock and bond transactions.

_____ (D) Commodity and option transactions.

_____ (E) Banking and other financial institution transactions.

_____ (F) Business operating transactions.

_____ (G) Insurance and annuity transactions.

_____ (H) Estate, trust, and other beneficiary transactions.

_____ (I) Claims and litigation.

_____ (J) Personal and family maintenance.

_____ (K) Benefits from social security, medicare, medicaid, or other governmental programs, or civil or military service.

_____ (L) Retirement plan transactions.

_____ (M) Tax matters.

_____ (N) **ALL OF THE POWERS LISTED ABOVE.**

YOU NEED NOT INITIAL ANY OTHER LINES IF YOU INITIAL LINE (N).

SPECIAL INSTRUCTIONS:
ON THE FOLLOWING LINES YOU MAY GIVE SPECIAL INSTRUCTIONS LIMITING OR EXTENDING THE POWERS GRANTED TO YOUR AGENT.

_____

_____

_____

_____

_____

_____

_____

UNLESS YOU DIRECT OTHERWISE ABOVE, THIS POWER OF ATTORNEY IS EFFECTIVE IM-MEDIATELY AND WILL CONTINUE UNTIL IT IS REVOKED. This power of attorney will continue to be effective even though I become incapacitated. **STRIKE THE PRECEDING SENTENCE IF YOU DO NOT WANT THIS POWER OF ATTORNEY TO CONTINUE IF YOU BECOME INCAPACI-TATED.**

Exercise of Power of Attorney Where
More than One Agent Designated

If I have designated more than one agent, the agents are to act _____. **IF YOU APPOINT MORE THAN ONE AGENT AND YOU WANT EACH AGENT TO BE ABLE TO ACT ALONE WITHOUT THE OTHER AGENT JOINING, WRITE THE WORD "SEPARATELY" IN THE BLANK SPACE ABOVE. IF YOU DO NOT INSERT ANY WORD IN THE BLANK SPACE, OR IF YOU INSERT THE WORD "JOINTLY", THEN ALL OF YOUR AGENTS MUST ACT OR SIGN TO-GETHER.** I agree that any third party who receives a copy of this document may act under it. Revocation of the power of attorney is not effective as to a third party until the third party has actual knowledge of the revocation. I agree to indemnify the third party for any claims that arise against the third party because of reliance on this power of attorney.

Signed this _____ day of _____, 19_____

_____
(your signature)

_____
(your social security number)

2

State of _____

County of _____

CERTIFICATE OF ACKNOWLEDGEMENT OF
NOTARY PUBLIC

State of California   )

)SS

County of _____)

On _____ before me, _____ (here insert name and title of the officer), personally appeared _____

_____

_____

personally known to me (or proved to me on the basis of satisfactory evidence) to be the person(s) whose name(s) is/are subscribed to the within instrument and acknowledged to me that he/she/they executed the same in his/her/their authorized capacity(ies), and that by his/ her/their signature(s) on the instrument the person(s), or the entity upon behalf of which the person(s) acted, executed the instrument. WITNESS my hand and official seal.

Signature _____ _____ (Seal)

Uniform Statutory Form Power of Attorney
(California)

Explanation

The explanations that follow should provide you with a clear understanding of the terms used in the Uniform Statutory Form Power of Attorney for California.

Notice: The notice confirms what the book has already stated: the powers given to your agent(s) (attorney(s)-in-fact) are broad. Read the notice carefully.

Paragraph 1: The first blank line is for your name and address. On the next lines go the name(s) and address(es) of the person(s) to whom you are giving the power of attorney (called the "agent(s)" or "attorney(s)-in-fact").

Paragraph 2: The following lettered clauses specify broad powers providing your agent(s) with wide latitude to manage your affairs. Powers are separately enumerated to avoid any questions about whether you intended to authorize your agent(s) to undertake specific actions on your behalf. If you choose not to give all of these powers to your agent(s), you would leave blank and draw a line through those powers you want to exclude.

Line A: This line gives your agent(s) broad authority to mortgage, sell, buy, accept, manage, lease, and/or otherwise deal with real estate, including your home.

Line B: This line permits your agent(s) broad authority to buy, sell, manage, receive, mortgage, lease, and/or otherwise handle transactions involving items of personal property.

Line C: This line lets your agent(s) invest in securities on your behalf and manage, receive, sell, mortgage, and/or otherwise handle stocks and bonds for you. This is broad enough to allow your agent(s) to vote at stockholders meetings.

Line D: This line allows your agent(s) to invest in commodities and options on your behalf and to manage, sell, receive, mortgage, and/or otherwise handle commodities and options for you.

Line E: This line authorizes your agent(s) to handle banking transactions, including opening and managing accounts, CDs, and other instruments in financial institutions, signing checks, making withdrawals, and having access to your safe-deposit box.

Line F: This line allows your agent(s) to engage in any business transactions for you.

Line G: This line authorizes your agent(s) to handle any insurance and annuity matters for you, including obtaining, managing, maintaining, or terminating insurance and annuities, paying premiums, and obtaining benefits for you.

Line H: This line permits your agent(s) to act for you with respect to estate, trust, and other beneficiary matters, including establishing trusts, receiving inheritances, and participating in the administration of estates.

Line I: This line gives your agent(s) the right to handle claims and litigation for you, including bringing a lawsuit for you, defending you against claims, and settling disputes for you.

Line J: This line authorizes your agent(s) to handle your personal and family affairs, to take steps to provide for the support and welfare of your family, and to maintain your relationships with family, friends, and organizations.

Line K: This line enables your agent(s) to handle any matters you may have with government benefits and/or programs, including making and receiving proceeds of any claims and maximizing benefits from government programs.

Line L: This line allows your agent(s) to handle retirement plan transactions for you, including selecting payment options, making or changing beneficiary designations, making contributions and rollovers, and borrowing from retirement plans.

Line M: This line gives your agent(s) authority to deal with your taxes. Although you might prefer to forget about this, it's important that tax forms be prepared and taxes paid, to avoid possible problems.

Line N: This line is a catchall authorizing your agent(s) to do all of the tasks listed above.

Special Instructions Paragraph: In the space that follows you could add other provisions or limitations, but if you do this, make sure your additions or changes comply with the law.

Next Paragraph. These lines are *crucial* to making your power of attorney *durable*, so that it remains valid at the time you will need it the most—during your incapacity. Note also that this is not a springing durable power of attorney but is effective and can be used *immediately*.

Next Paragraph: If you have decided to name more than one agent, you would fill in the next blank with either the word *separately* or *jointly*. "Separately" means that either of your agents on his or her own will be able to exercise the powers provided in the power of attorney; "jointly" means that your agents must act together to use your power of attorney.

Some banks and insurance companies have been unwilling to accept or act on any power of 'attorney form that they did not prepare themselves. The next language attempts to deal with this problem. The language should protect third parties relying on the document and, it's hoped, encourage them to accept it.

Finally, you would sign and date the document at the end before a notary. The notary fills in and signs the bottom portion. A notary is authorized by the state or federal government to administer oaths and attest to the authenticity of signatures.

COLORADO STATUTORY POWER OF ATTORNEY FOR PROPERTY

NOTICE: UNLESS YOU LIMIT THE POWER IN THIS DOCUMENT, THIS DOCUMENT GIVES YOUR AGENT THE POWER TO ACT FOR YOU, WITHOUT YOUR CONSENT, IN ANY WAY THAT YOU COULD ACT FOR YOURSELF. THE POWERS GRANTED BY THIS DOCUMENT ARE BROAD AND SWEEPING. THEY ARE EXPLAINED IN THE "UNIFORM STATUTORY FORM POWER OF ATTORNEY ACT," PART 13 OF ARTICLE 1 OF TITLE 15, COLORADO REVISED STATUTES, AND PART 6 OF ARTICLE 14 OF TITLE 15, COLORADO REVISED STATUTES. IF YOU HAVE ANY QUESTIONS ABOUT THESE POWERS, OBTAIN COMPETENT LEGAL ADVICE. THIS DOCUMENT DOES NOT AUTHORIZE ANYONE TO MAKE MEDICAL OR OTHER HEALTH-CARE DECISIONS FOR YOU. YOU MAY REVOKE THIS POWER OF ATTORNEY IF YOU LATER WISH TO DO SO.

THE PURPOSE OF THIS POWER OF ATTORNEY IS TO GIVE THE PERSON YOU DESIGNATE (YOUR "AGENT") BROAD POWERS TO HANDLE YOUR PROPERTY AND AFFAIRS, WHICH MAY INCLUDE POWERS TO PLEDGE, SELL, OR OTHERWISE DISPOSE OF ANY REAL OR PERSONAL PROPERTY WITHOUT ADVANCE NOTICE TO YOU OR APPROVAL BY YOU. THIS FORM DOES NOT IMPOSE A DUTY ON YOUR AGENT TO EXERCISE GRANTED POWERS; BUT WHEN POWERS ARE EXERCISED, YOUR AGENT MUST USE DUE CARE TO ACT FOR YOUR BENEFIT AND IN ACCORDANCE WITH THE PROVISIONS OF THIS FORM AND MUST KEEP A RECORD OF RECEIPTS, DISBURSEMENTS, AND SIGNIFICANT ACTIONS TAKEN AS AGENT. YOU MAY NAME SUCCESSOR AGENTS UNDER THIS FORM BUT NOT CO-AGENTS. UNTIL YOU REVOKE THIS POWER OF ATTORNEY OR A COURT ACTING ON YOUR BEHALF TERMINATES IT, YOUR AGENT MAY EXERCISE THE POWERS GIVEN HERE THROUGHOUT YOUR LIFETIME, EVEN AFTER YOU MAY BECOME DISABLED, UNLESS YOU EXPRESSLY LIMIT THE DURATION OF THIS POWER IN THE MANNER PROVIDED BELOW.

YOU MAY HAVE OTHER RIGHTS OR POWERS UNDER COLORADO LAW NOT SPECIFIED IN THIS FORM.

I, _____ (INSERT YOUR FULL NAME AND ADDRESS), APPOINT _____ (INSERT THE FULL NAME AND ADDRESS OF THE PERSON APPOINTED) AS MY AGENT (ATTORNEY-IN-FACT) TO ACT FOR ME IN ANY LAWFUL WAY WITH RESPECT TO THE FOLLOWING INITIALED SUBJECTS:

TO GRANT ONE OR MORE OF THE FOLLOWING POWERS, INITIAL THE LINE IN FRONT OF EACH POWER YOU ARE GRANTING. TO WITHHOLD A POWER, DO NOT INITIAL THE LINE IN FRONT OF IT. YOU MAY, BUT NEED NOT, CROSS OUT EACH POWER WITHHELD.

INITIAL:

_____ (A) Real property transactions (when property recorded).
_____ (B) Tangible personal property transactions.
_____ (C) Stock and bond transactions.
_____ (D) Commodity and option transactions.
_____ (E) Banking and other financial institution transactions.
_____ (F) Business operating transactions.
_____ (G) Insurance and annuity transactions.

_____ (H) Estate, trust, and other beneficiary transactions.
_____ (I) Claims and litigation.
_____ (J) Personal and family maintenance.
_____ (K) Benefits from social security, medicare, medicaid, or other governmental programs or military service.
_____ (L) Retirement plan transactions.
_____ (M) Tax matters.

UNLESS YOU DIRECT OTHERWISE, THIS POWER OF ATTORNEY IS EFFECTIVE IMMEDIATELY AND WILL CONTINUE UNTIL IT IS REVOKED OR TERMINATED AS SPECIFIED BELOW. STRIKE THROUGH AND WRITE YOUR INITIALS TO THE LEFT OF THE FOLLOWING SENTENCE IF YOU DO NOT WANT THIS POWER OF ATTORNEY TO CONTINUE IF YOU BECOME DISABLED, INCAPACITATED, OR INCOMPETENT.

1. _____ THIS POWER OF ATTORNEY WILL CONTINUE TO BE EFFECTIVE EVEN THOUGH I BECOME DISABLED, INCAPACITATED, OR INCOMPETENT.

YOU MAY INCLUDE ADDITIONS TO AND LIMITATIONS ON THE AGENT'S POWERS IN THIS POWER OF ATTORNEY IF THEY ARE SPECIFICALLY DESCRIBED BELOW.

2. THE POWERS GRANTED ABOVE SHALL NOT INCLUDE THE FOLLOWING POWERS OR SHALL BE MODIFIED OR LIMITED IN THE FOLLOWING MANNER (HERE YOU MAY INCLUDE ANY SPECIFIC LIMITATIONS YOU DEEM APPROPRIATE, SUCH AS A PROHIBITION OF OR CONDITIONS ON THE SALE OF PARTICULAR STOCK OR REAL ESTATE OR SPECIAL RULES REGARDING BORROWING BY THE AGENT):

_____

_____

_____

_____

3. IN ADDITION TO THE POWERS GRANTED ABOVE, I GRANT MY AGENT THE FOLLOWING POWERS (HERE YOU MAY ADD ANY OTHER DELEGABLE POWERS, SUCH AS THE POWER TO MAKE GIFTS, EXERCISE POWERS OF APPOINTMENT, NAME OR CHANGE BENEFICIARIES OR JOINT TENANTS, OR REVOKE OR AMEND ANY TRUST SPECIFICALLY REFERRED TO BELOW):

_____

_____

_____

4. SPECIAL INSTRUCTIONS (ON THE FOLLOWING LINES YOU MAY GIVE SPECIAL INSTRUCTIONS TO YOUR AGENT):

_____

_____

_____

YOUR AGENT WILL BE ENTITLED TO REIMBURSEMENT FOR ALL REASONABLE EXPENSES INCURRED IN ACTING UNDER THIS POWER OF ATTORNEY. STRIKE THROUGH AND INITIAL THE NEXT SENTENCE IF YOU DO NOT WANT YOUR AGENT TO ALSO BE ENTITLED TO REASONABLE COMPENSATION FOR SERVICES AS AGENT.

5. _____ MY AGENT IS ENTITLED TO REASONABLE COMPENSATION FOR SERVICES RENDERED AS AGENT UNDER THIS POWER OF ATTORNEY.

THIS POWER OF ATTORNEY MAY BE AMENDED IN ANY MANNER OR REVOKED BY YOU AT ANY TIME. ABSENT AMENDMENT OR REVOCATION, THE AUTHORITY GRANTED IN THIS POWER OF ATTORNEY IS EFFECTIVE WHEN THIS POWER OF ATTORNEY IS SIGNED AND CONTINUES IN EFFECT UNTIL YOUR DEATH, UNLESS YOU MAKE A LIMITATION ON DURATION BY COMPLETING THE FOLLOWING:

6. THIS POWER OF ATTORNEY TERMINATES ON _____ (INSERT A FUTURE DATE OR EVENT, SUCH AS COURT DETERMINATION OF YOUR DISABILITY, WHEN YOU WANT THIS POWER TO TERMINATE PRIOR TO YOUR DEATH).

BY RETAINING THE FOLLOWING PARAGRAPH, YOU MAY, BUT ARE NOT REQUIRED TO, NAME YOUR AGENT AS GUARDIAN OF YOUR PERSON OR CONSERVATOR OF YOUR PROPERTY, OR BOTH, IF A COURT PROCEEDING IS BEGUN TO APPOINT A GUARDIAN OR CONSERVATOR, OR BOTH, FOR YOU. THE COURT WILL APPOINT YOUR AGENT AS GUARDIAN OR CONSERVATOR, OR BOTH, IF THE COURT FINDS THAT SUCH APPOINTMENT WILL SERVE YOUR BEST INTERESTS AND WELFARE. STRIKE THROUGH AND INITIAL PARAGRAPH 7 IF YOU DO NOT WANT YOUR AGENT TO ACT AS GUARDIAN OR CONSERVATOR, OR BOTH.

7. _____ IF A GUARDIAN OF MY PERSON OR A CONSERVATOR FOR MY PROPERTY, OR BOTH, ARE TO BE APPOINTED, I NOMINATE THE AGENT ACTING UNDER THIS POWER OF ATTORNEY AS SUCH GUARDIAN OR CONSERVATOR, OR BOTH, TO SERVE WITHOUT BOND OR SECURITY.

IF YOU WISH TO NAME SUCCESSOR AGENTS, INSERT THE NAME AND ADDRESS OF ANY SUCCESSOR AGENT IN THE FOLLOWING PARAGRAPH:

8. IF ANY AGENT NAMED BY ME SHALL DIE, BECOME INCAPACITATED, RESIGN, OR REFUSE TO ACCEPT THE OFFICE OF AGENT, I NAME THE FOLLOWING, EACH TO ACT ALONE AND SUCCESSIVELY, IN THE ORDER NAMED, AS SUCCESSOR TO SUCH AGENT:

_____

_____

_____

FOR PURPOSES OF THIS PARAGRAPH 8, A PERSON IS CONSIDERED TO BE INCAPACITATED IF AND WHILE THE PERSON IS A MINOR OR A PERSON ADJUDICATED INCAPACITATED OR IF THE PERSON IS UNABLE TO GIVE PROMPT AND INTELLIGENT CONSIDERATION TO BUSINESS MATTERS, AS CERTIFIED BY A LICENSED PHYSICIAN.

I AGREE THAT ANY THIRD PARTY WHO RECEIVES A COPY OF THIS DOCUMENT MAY ACT UNDER IT. REVOCATION OF THE POWER OF ATTORNEY IS NOT EFFECTIVE AS TO A THIRD PARTY UNTIL THE THIRD PARTY LEARNS OF THE REVOCATION. I AGREE TO INDEMNIFY THE THIRD PARTY FOR ANY CLAIMS THAT ARISE AGAINST THE THIRD PARTY BECAUSE OF RELIANCE ON THIS POWER OF ATTORNEY.

SIGNED ON _____, 19___.

IF THERE IS ANYTHING ABOUT THIS FORM THAT YOU DO NOT UNDERSTAND, IT MAY BE IN YOUR BEST INTEREST TO CONSULT A COLORADO LAWYER RATHER THAN SIGN THIS FORM.

_____
(YOUR SIGNATURE)

_____
(YOUR SOCIAL SECURITY NUMBER)

YOU MAY, BUT ARE NOT REQUESTED TO, REQUEST YOUR AGENT AND SUCCESSOR AGENTS TO PROVIDE SPECIMEN SIGNATURES BELOW. IF YOU INCLUDE SPECIMEN SIGNATURES IN THIS POWER OF ATTORNEY, YOU MUST COMPLETE THE CERTIFICATION OPPOSITE THE SIGNATURES OF THE AGENTS.

NOTICE TO AGENTS: BY EXERCISING POWERS UNDER THIS DOCUMENT, THE AGENT ASSUMES THE FIDUCIARY AND OTHER LEGAL RESPONSIBILITIES OF AN AGENT UNDER COLORADO LAW.

SPECIMEN SIGNATURES OF AGENT

I CERTIFY THAT THE SIGNATURES OF MY AGENT (AND SUCCESSORS) ARE CORRECT.

_____
AGENT

_____
PRINCIPAL

_____
SUCCESSOR AGENT

_____
PRINCIPAL

_____
SUCCESSOR AGENT

_____
PRINCIPAL

STATE OF COLORADO)
) SS
COUNTY OF)

      THIS DOCUMENT WAS ACKNOWLEDGED BEFORE ME ON _____ (DATE) BY _____ (NAME OF PRINCIPAL. (WHO CERTIFIES THE CORRECTNESS OF THE SIGNATURE(S) OF THE AGENT(S).)

                                _____

                                NOTARY PUBLIC

                                MY COMMISSION EXPIRES: _____

                                SEAL

Colorado Statutory Power of Attorney for Property

Explanation

The explanations that follow should provide you with a clear understanding of the terms used in the Colorado Statutory Power of Attorney for Property.

Notice: The notice confirms what the book has already stated: the powers given to your agent(s) (attorney[s]-in-fact) are broad. Read the notice carefully. It also reminds the agent(s) to keep good records.

Paragraph 1: The first blank line is for your name and address. On the next line you would fill in the name and address of the person to whom you are giving the power of attorney (called the "agent" or "attorney-in-fact").

Paragraph 2. The following lettered clauses specify broad powers providing your agent with wide latitude to manage your affairs. Powers are separately enumerated to avoid any questions about whether you intended to authorize your agent to undertake specific actions on your behalf. If you choose not to give all of these powers to your agent(s), you would leave blank and draw a line through the powers you want to exclude.

Line A: This line gives your agent(s) broad authority to mortgage, sell, buy, accept, manage, lease, and/or otherwise deal with real estate, including your home.

Line B: This line permits your agent(s) broad authority to buy, sell, manage, receive, mortgage, lease, and/or otherwise handle transactions involving items of personal property.

Line C: This line lets your agent(s) invest in securities on your behalf and manage, receive, sell, mortgage, and/or otherwise handle stocks and bonds for you. This is broad enough to allow your agent(s) to vote at stockholders meetings.

Line D: This line lets your agent(s) invest in commodities and options on your behalf and/or otherwise handle commodities and options for you.

Line E: This line authorizes your agent(s) to handle banking transactions, including opening and manag-ing accounts, CDs, and other instruments in financial institutions, signing checks, making withdrawals, and having access to your safe-deposit box.

Line F: This line allows your agent(s) to engage in any business transactions for you.

Line G: This line authorizes your agent(s) to handle any insurance and annuity matters for you, including obtaining, managing, maintaining, or terminating insurance and annuities, paying premiums, and obtaining benefits for you.

Line H: This line permits your agent(s) to act for you with respect to estate, trust, and other beneficiary matters, including establishing trusts, receiving inheritances, and participating in the administration of estates.

Line I: This line gives your agent(s) the right to handle claims and litigation for you, including bringing a lawsuit for you, defending you against claims, and settling disputes for you.

Line J: This line authorizes your agent(s) to handle your personal and family affairs, to take steps to provide for the support and welfare of your family, and to maintain your relationships with family, friends, and organizations.

Line K: This line enables your agent(s) to handle any matters you may have with government benefits and/or programs, including making and receiving proceeds of any claims and maximizing benefits from government programs.

Line L: This line allows your agent(s) to handle retirement plan transactions for you, including selecting payment options, making or changing beneficiary designations, making contributions and rollovers, and borrowing from retirement plans.

Line M: This line gives your agent(s) authority to deal with your taxes. Although you might prefer to forget about this, it's important that tax forms be prepared and taxes paid, to avoid possible problems.

This next paragraph is *crucial* to making your power of attorney *durable*, so that it remains valid at the time you will need it the most—during your incapacity. Don't initial and strike unless you want the power of attorney to end at your incapacity. Note that unless you say otherwise, this power of attorney becomes effective and can be used immediately.

In the spaces that follow you would add any other provisions or limitations—but if you do this, make sure your additions or changes comply with the law.

Paragraph 5: Do you wish to pay your agent for the work performed? If you do not, you would initial and strike this statement; if you do, you would leave it. With family members, compensation is usually not necessary.

Paragraph 6 allows you to limit the duration of the power of attorney. Be careful—if you limit its duration and it expires, you might not be able to create a new one (if you've become incompetent).

Paragraph 7 allows you to name your agent to serve as guardian and/or conservator, if a court decides that a guardian or conservator is required. Nominating your own guardian and/or conservator is usually better than leaving the selection to the court.

Paragraph 8 states that if you have decided to name one or more successor agents, you would fill in the next lines with his, her, or their name(s) and address(es).

Finally, you would sign and date the document at the end before two witnesses and a notary. The agent and any successor agents would also sign, and you would sign your name next to each one. The notary fills in and signs the bottom portion. A notary is authorized by the state or federal government to administer oaths and attest to the authenticity of signatures.

STATUTORY SHORT FORM
DURABLE GENERAL POWER OF ATTORNEY
(CONNECTICUT)

NOTICE: The powers granted by this document are broad and sweeping. They are defined in the Connecticut Statutory Short Form Power of Attorney Act, sections 1-42 to 1-56, inclusive, of the general statutes, which expressly permits the use of any other or different form of power of attorney desired by the parties concerning.

Know All Men by These Presents, which are intended to constitute a GENERAL POWER OF ATTORNEY pursuant to Connecticut Statutory Short Form Power of Attorney Act:

That I, _____,
(insert name and address of the principal)

do hereby appoint _____

_____

_____

_____

(insert name and address of the agent, or each agent, if more than one is designated)

my attorney(s)-in-fact TO ACT _____ .

If more than one agent is designated and the principal wishes each agent alone to be able to exercise the power conferred, insert in this blank the word "severally." Failure to make any insertion or the insertion of the word "jointly" will require the agents to act jointly.

First: In my name, place and stead in any way which I myself could do, if I were personally present, with respect to the following matters as each of them is defined in the Connecticut Statutory Short Form Power of Attorney Act to the extent that I am permitted by law to act through an agent:

(Strike out and initial in the opposite box any one or more of the subdivisions as to which the principal does NOT desire to give the agent authority. Such elimination of any one or more of subdivisions (A) to (L), inclusive, shall automatically constitute an elimination also of subdivision (M).)

To strike out any subdivision the principal must draw a line through the text of that subdivision AND write his initials in the box opposite.

(A)	real estate transactions;	( )
(B)	chattel and goods transactions;	( )
(C)	bond, share and commodity transactions;	( )
(D)	banking transactions;	( )
(E)	business operating transactions;	( )
(F)	insurance transactions;	( )
(G)	estate transactions;	( )

(H)	claims and litigation;	( )
(I)	personal relationships and affairs;	( )
(J)	benefits from military service;	( )
(K)	records, reports and statements;	( )
(L)	health care decisions;	( )
(M)	all other matters;	( )

_____

_____

_____

(Special provisions and limitations may be included in the statutory short form power of attorney only if they conform to the requirements of the Connecticut Statutory Short Form Power of Attorney Act.)

        Second: With full and unqualified authority to delegate any or all of the foregoing powers to any person or persons whom my attorney(s)-in-fact shall select;

        Third: Hereby ratifying and confirming all that said attorney(s) or substitute(s) do or cause to be done.

        This power of attorney shall not be affected by the subsequent disability or incompetence of the principal.

        In Witness Whereof, I have hereunto signed my name and affixed my seal this _____ day of _____, 19_____.

_____ (Seal)
(Signature of Principal)

Specimen Signature of Attorney(s)-in-Fact:

_____

_____

_____

Signed in the presence of:

_____
Witness

_____
Witness

CERTIFICATE OF NOTARY

STATE OF CONNECTICUT   )

)   SS

COUNTY OF   _____   )

        On the _____ day of _____, 19_____, before me personally came _____, whose identity is well known to me to be the individual described in and who executed the foregoing instrument, and (he) (she) acknowledged to me that (he) (she) executed the same.

_____
Notary Public

My commission expires:

_____

3

Statutory Short Form
Durable General Power of Attorney
(Connecticut)

Explanation

The explanations that follow should provide you with a clear understanding of the terms used in the Statutory Short Form Durable General Power of Attorney for Connecticut.

Notice: The notice confirms what the book has already stated: the powers given to your attorney(s)-in-fact are broad.

Introduction: On the first blank line you would fill in your name and address (you are the "principal," the person making the durable general power of attorney). On the next lines go the name(s) and address(es) of the person(s) to whom you are giving the durable general power of attorney (called the "agent[s]" or "attorney[s]-in-fact").

If you have decided to name more than one attorney-in-fact, you should fill in the next blank with either the word *severally* or the word *jointly*. "Severally" means that either of your attorneys-in-fact on his or her own will be able to exercise the powers provided in the durable general power of attorney; "jointly" means that you attorneys-in-fact must act together to use your durable general power of attorney.

The following lettered clauses specify broad powers providing your attorney(s)-in-fact with wide latitude to manage your affairs. Powers are separately enumerated to avoid any questions about whether you intended to authorize your attorney(s)-in-fact to undertake specific actions on your behalf. If you choose not to give all of these powers to your attorney(s)-in-fact, you must draw a line through the power(s) you want to exclude *and* initial inside the parentheses after such excluded power(s).

Clause A: This clause gives your attorney(s)-in-fact broad authority to mortgage, sell, buy, accept, manage, lease, and/or otherwise deal with real estate, including your home.

Clause B: This clause permits your attorney(s)-in-fact broad authority to buy, sell, manage, receive, mortgage, lease, and/or otherwise handle transactions involving items of personal property.

Clause C: This clause lets your attorney(s)-in-fact invest in securities on your behalf and manage, receive, sell, mortgage, and/or otherwise handle securities for you. This is broad enough to allow your attorney(s)-in-fact to vote at stockholders meetings.

Clause D: This clause authorizes your attorney(s)-in-fact to handle banking transactions, including opening and managing accounts, CDs, and other instruments in financial institutions, signing checks, making withdrawals, and having access to your safe-deposit box.

Clause E: This clause allows your attorney(s)-in-fact to engage in any business transactions for you.

Clause F: This clause authorizes your attorney(s)-in-fact to handle any insurance matters for you, including obtaining, managing, maintaining, or terminating insurance, paying premiums, and obtaining benefits for you.

Clause G: This clause permits your attorney(s)-in-fact to act for you with respect to estate matters, including receiving inheritances and participating in the administration of estates.

Clause H: This clause gives your attorney(s)-in-fact the right to handle claims and litigation for you, including bringing a lawsuit for you, defending you against claims, and settling disputes for you.

Clause I: This clause authorizes your attorney(s)-in-fact to handle your personal affairs, to take steps to provide for the support and welfare of your family, and to maintain your relationships with family, friends, and organizations.

Clause J: This clause enables your attorney(s)-in-fact to handle any matters you may have with the military, including making and receiving proceeds of any claims and maximizing benefits from military service.

Clause K: This clause empowers your attorney(s)-in-fact to make, execute, file, and store records, reports, and statements, including tax returns, for you.

Clause L: This clause authorizes your attorney(s)-in-fact to consent to, refuse to consent to, or withdraw consent to any medical treatment other than that designed solely for the purpose of maintaining physical comfort, the withdrawal of life support systems, or the withdrawal of nutrition and hydration.

Clause M: This clause is a catchall authorizing your attorney(s)-in-fact to do anything you could do.

On the lines that follow, you would add any other provisions or limitations—but if you do this, make sure your additions or changes comply with the law.

The paragraph beginning with "Second" allows your attorney(s)-in-fact to delegate his or her powers to someone else.

The paragraph beginning with "Third" provides that you ratify and confirm actions taken by your attorney(s)-in-fact under the durable general power of attorney. This lets third parties know they can rely on your attorney(s)-in-fact's use of the document.

The next sentence is *crucial* to making your power of attorney *durable,* so that it remains valid at the time you will need it most—during your incapacity.

Finally, you would sign and date the document at the end before two witnesses and a notary. The attorney(s)-in-fact signs his or her name under yours. The notary fills in and signs the bottom portion. A notary is authorized by the state or federal government to administer oaths and attest to the authenticity of signatures.

DURABLE POWER OF ATTORNEY

STATE OF FLORIDA

COUNTY OF _____

      Know all Men by These Presents, which are intended to constitute a DURABLE POWER OF ATTORNEY,

That I _____
(Name of principal)

_____
(Address of principal)

do hereby appoint _____
(Name of agent)

_____
(Address of agent)
and

_____
(Name of agent if more than one agent is designated)

_____
(Address of agent if more than one agent is designated)

My Attorney(s)-in-Fact TO ACT (jointly) (severally), as my true and lawful Attorney(s)-in-Fact, for me and in my name, place and stead:

      (A) Power with Respect to Accounts and Instruments. To establish or open accounts, certificates of deposit and any other form of account or instrument for me with financial institutions of any kind; to modify, terminate, make deposits to and write checks on and endorse checks for or make withdrawals from all accounts in my name or with respect to which I am an authorized signatory; to negotiate, endorse or transfer any checks or other instruments with respect to any such accounts; to contract for any services rendered by any financial institution; and to add property to any trust agreement created by me.

      (B) Power with Respect to Safe-Deposit Boxes. To contract with any institution for the maintenance of a safe-deposit box in my name; to have access to all safe-deposit boxes in my name or with respect to which I am an authorized signatory; to add to and remove from the contents of any such safe-deposit box and to terminate any and all contracts for such boxes.

      (C) Power to Sell and Buy. To sell and buy personal, intangible or mixed property, upon such terms and conditions as my Attorney(s)-in-Fact deems appropriate; to use any credit card held in my name to make such purchases and to sign such charge slips as may be necessary to use such credit cards; and to repay from any funds belonging to me any money borrowed and to pay for any purchases made or cash advanced using credit cards issued to me.

      (D) Power to Exercise Rights in Securities. To exercise all rights with respect to securities that I now own, or may hereafter acquire; to establish, utilize and terminate brokerage accounts; and to invest and reinvest any of my assets in stocks, common and/or preferred, bonds (including, without limitation, United States Treasury Bonds or other United States government obligations which may be redeemed at par for the purpose of applying the entire amount of principal and accrued interest thereon to the payment of the Federal estate tax, if any, occasioned by my death), notes, debentures, loans, mortgages, common trust funds, or other securities or property, real or personal, upon such terms and conditions as my Attorney(s)-in-Fact deems appropriate.

(E) Power to Borrow Money (including any Insurance Policy Loans). To borrow money for my account upon such terms and conditions as my Attorney(s)-in-Fact may deem appropriate and to secure such borrowing by the granting of security interests in any property or interest in property which I may now or hereafter own; to borrow money upon any life insurance policies owned by me upon my life for any purpose and to grant a security interest in such policy to secure any such loans; and no insurance company shall be under any obligation whatsoever to determine the need for such loan or the application of the proceeds therefrom.

(F) Power with Respect to Real Property. To purchase real property, to manage, maintain and alter all real property belonging to me, and to lease, sell, mortgage, encumber or otherwise dispose of all interests in real property belonging to me, upon such terms and conditions as my Attorney(s)-in-Fact deems appropriate; to renew leases of the same or to execute, acknowledge and deliver leases therefor; to execute deeds of conveyance either with or without covenants of general warranty; to pay and satisfy all mortgages, encumbrances, taxes and assessments that may be a lien or charge upon any of my real property; and to receive rentals from and the proceeds of sale of any of my real property. For purposes of this Durable Power of Attorney, real property shall include, without limitation, property held as tenants by entireties and homestead property, and the real property known as _____.

(G) Power to Demand, Compromise and Receive. To demand, arbitrate, settle, sue for, collect, receive, deposit, expand for my benefit, reinvest or make such other appropriate dispositions of, as my Attorney(s)-in-Fact deems appropriate, all cash rights to payments of cash, property (personal, intangible and/or mixed), rights and/or benefits to which I am now or may in the future become entitled, regardless of the identity of the individual or public or private entity involved (and for purposes of receiving Social Security benefits, my Attorney(s)-in-Fact is herewith appointed my "Representative Payee"); to compound, compromise, settle and adjust all claims and demands whatsoever which I may now owe or be liable for; and to utilize all lawful means and methods for such purposes.

(H) Power with Respect to Taxes. To make, prepare, sign and file for me and on my behalf any and all required tax estimates and returns, federal, state or local, as well as any waivers, affidavits, schedules or other forms required or permitted to be filed in connection therewith, and to protest and appeal any assessments or determinations of tax against me which my Attorney(s)-in-Fact deems to have been made without proper warrant.

(I) Power with Respect to Documents. To sign, acknowledge, record and deliver agreements, affidavits, bills of sale, stock powers, deeds, leases, mortgages, notes, receipts, releases, satisfactions, journal entries, certificates and such other documents which may be necessary or convenient in execution of the powers hereinbefore expressly conferred upon my Attorney(s)-in-Fact; to execute and deliver applications for automobile license plates and certificates of title and to endorse for transfer and to deliver certificates of title; and to execute and deliver applications for insurance (including, without limitation, insurance on my life) and to cancel and select the amounts therefor.

(J) Power to Engage Services. To engage the services of and compensate attorneys-at-law, appraisers, accountants, brokers, real estate managers, investment counsel and such other persons as may be proper or convenient to advise and assist in the management, maintenance and disposition of my property.

(K) Power to Incur Obligations. To incur obligations for the maintenance, support, health, care, well-being, comfort and welfare of me and my family and to satisfy such obligations out of my money or property; and to consent on my behalf to medical and surgical procedures.

I further give and grant to my said Attorney(s)-in-Fact full power and authority to do and perform every act necessary to be done in the exercise of any of the foregoing powers as fully as I might or could do if personally present, with full power of substitution and revocation, hereby ratifying and confirming all that my said Attorney(s)-in-Fact shall lawfully do, or cause to be done by virtue hereof.

Anyone dealing with my Attorney(s)-in-Fact under this Durable Power of Attorney may rely on any signed copy, photocopy or similar copy of a signed copy as though it were the original.

This Durable Power of Attorney shall not be affected by my future disability, if any, or lapse of time, except as provided by statute. The power conferred on said Attorney(s)-in-Fact by this instrument shall be exercisable from the date specified in this instrument, notwithstanding a later disability or incapacity on my part, unless otherwise provided by statutes of the State of Florida.

All acts done by said Attorney(s)-in-Fact pursuant to the power conferred during any period of my disability or incompetence shall have the same effect and inure to the benefit of and bind me or my heirs, devisees, and personal representatives, as if I were competent and not disabled.

This Durable Power of Attorney shall be nondelegable and shall be valid until such time as I shall die, revoke this power, or be adjudged incompetent.

This Durable Power of Attorney shall commence on the date of execution hereof.

In witness whereof, I have hereunto signed my name this _____ day of _____, 19____.

_____
(Signature of Principal)

Specimen Signature of Attorney(s)-in-Fact

_____

Signed in the presence of:

_____

_____
Witness

_____
Witness

CERTIFICATE OF NOTARY

STATE OF _____)
) SS
COUNTY OF _____)

The foregoing Durable Power of Attorney was acknowledged before me on this _____ day of _____, 19____, by _____ whose identity is personally known to me and known to me to be the individual described in and who executed the foregoing instrument, or who has produced _____ as identification.

_____
Notary Public, State of Florida

My commission expires:

_____

Commission No. _____

Durable Power of Attorney (Florida)

Explanation

As you can readily see, this Durable Power of Attorney form adapted for use in Florida is filled with legalese. Don't be scared off by this confusing language. The explanations that follow should provide you with a clear understanding of the terms used.

Introduction: At the top left, below "STATE OF FLORIDA," you would fill in the name of your county. Below that go your name and address (you are the "principal," the person making the durable power of attorney).

On the next lines you would fill in the name(s) and address(es) of the person(s) to whom you are giving the durable power of attorney (called the "agent[s]" or "attorney[s]-in-fact").

If you have decided to name more than one attorney-in-fact, you must decide whether to strike the word *jointly* or *severally*. If you want to require your attorneys-in-fact to act together to use the power of attorney, you would leave the word *jointly* and strike the word *severally*. But if you prefer to allow either of your attorneys-in-fact on his or her own to exercise the powers provided in the power of attorney, you would strike out the word *jointly* and leave the word *severally*.

The following lettered clauses specify broad powers providing your attorney(s)-in-fact with latitude to manage your financial affairs. Powers are separately enumerated to avoid any questions about whether you intended to authorize your attorney(s)-in-fact to undertake specific actions on your behalf.

Clause A: This clause authorizes your attorney(s)-in-fact to open and manage accounts, CDs, and other instruments for you in financial institutions. It also says that your attorney(s)-in-fact may add to any trust agreement you may have created.

Clause B: This clause allows your attorney(s)-in-fact to maintain and gain access to safe-deposit boxes in your name.

Clause C: This clause permits your attorney(s)-in-fact to buy and sell items and to use your credit cards.

Clause D: This clause lets your attorney(s)-in-fact invest in securities on your behalf and to manage and handle those securities. This is broad enough to allow your attorney(s)-in-fact to vote at stockholders meetings.

Clause E: This clause authorizes your attorney(s)-in-fact to borrow money in your name.

Clause F: This clause gives your attorney(s)-in-fact broad authority to manage, sell, buy, mortgage, and/or lease real estate, including your home. In the blank you would fill in the address(es) of your residence and any other real estate you own. Even better, fill in the legal description of the properties. You don't have to change the durable family power of attorney each time you buy or sell real estate. Recording requirements vary greatly from state to state.

Clause G: This clause authorizes your attorney(s)-in-fact to take any necessary action with respect to rights you have or may have in the future to money or property. It also lets your attorney(s)-in-fact handle claims made against you. The term *representative payee* is defined in chapter 12.

Clause H: This clause gives your attorney(s)-in-fact the power to deal with your taxes. Although you might prefer to forget about this, it's important that tax forms be prepared and taxes paid, to avoid possible penalties.

Clause I: This clause spells out the right of your attorney(s)-in-fact to sign and execute all sorts of documents on your behalf. It also allows your attorney(s)-in-fact to handle your applications for license plates, certificates of title, and insurance.

Clause J: This clause allows your attorney(s)-in-fact to hire specialists to assist in handling your financial affairs.

Clause K: This clause generally authorizes your attorney(s)-in-fact to incur and pay bills for your maintenance, support, and care. It also empowers your attorney(s)-in-fact to make certain health care decisions.

Closing Paragraphs: The first paragraph following the lettered clauses is a catchall authorizing your attorney(s)-in-fact to do anything you could do.

The next line contains a blank. Fill in the relationship(s) of your attorney(s)-in-fact to you.

The next paragraph allows a copy of your signed durable power of attorney to be used in place of the original.

The following two paragraphs are *crucial* to making your power of attorney *durable*, so that it remains valid at the time you will need it most—during your incapacity.

The next sentence recognizes that the durable power of attorney will be valid until you die, revoke it, or are determined to be incompetent by a judge in a court proceeding. Your attorney(s)-in-fact cannot delegate the authority provided under the durable power of attorney to others.

The last sentence says that the durable power of attorney begins working the moment you sign it.

Finally, you would sign and date the document at the end before two witnesses and a notary. The attorney(s)-in-fact signs under your name. The notary fills in and signs the bottom portion. A notary is authorized by the state or federal government to administer oaths and attest to the authenticity of signatures.

ILLINOIS STATUTORY SHORT FORM POWER
OF ATTORNEY FOR PROPERTY

(NOTICE: THE PURPOSE OF THIS POWER OF ATTORNEY IS TO GIVE THE PERSON YOU DESIGNATE (YOUR "AGENT") BROAD POWERS TO HANDLE YOUR PROPERTY, WHICH MAY INCLUDE POWERS TO PLEDGE, SELL OR OTHERWISE DISPOSE OF ANY REAL OR PERSONAL PROPERTY WITHOUT ADVANCE NOTICE TO YOU OR APPROVAL BY YOU. THIS FORM DOES NOT IMPOSE A DUTY ON YOUR AGENT TO EXERCISE GRANTED POWERS; BUT WHEN POWERS ARE EXERCISED, YOUR AGENT WILL HAVE TO USE DUE CARE TO ACT FOR YOUR BENEFIT AND IN ACCORDANCE WITH THIS FORM AND KEEP A RECORD OF RECEIPTS, DISBURSEMENTS AND SIGNIFICANT ACTIONS TAKEN AS AGENT. A COURT CAN TAKE AWAY THE POWERS OF YOUR AGENT IF IT FINDS THE AGENT IS NOT ACTING PROPERLY. YOU MAY NAME SUCCESSOR AGENTS UNDER THIS FORM BUT NOT CO-AGENTS. UNLESS YOU EXPRESSLY LIMIT THE DURATION OF THIS POWER IN THE MANNER PROVIDED BELOW, UNTIL YOU REVOKE THIS POWER OR A COURT ACTING ON YOUR BEHALF TERMINATES IT, YOUR AGENT MAY EXERCISE THE POWERS GIVEN HERE THROUGHOUT YOUR LIFETIME, EVEN AFTER YOU BECOME DISABLED. THE POWERS YOU GIVE YOUR AGENT ARE EXPLAINED MORE FULLY IN SECTION 3-4 OF THE ILLINOIS "STATUTORY SHORT FORM POWER OF ATTORNEY FOR PROPERTY LAW" OF WHICH THIS FORM IS A PART. THAT LAW EXPRESSLY PERMITS THE USE OF ANY DIFFERENT FORM OF POWER OF ATTORNEY YOU MAY DESIRE. IF THERE IS ANYTHING ABOUT THIS FORM YOU DO NOT UNDERSTAND, YOU SHOULD ASK A LAWYER TO EXPLAIN IT TO YOU.)

POWER OF ATTORNEY made this _____ day of _____ (month), _____ (year).

1. I, _____ (insert name and address of principal), hereby appoint:

_____
(insert name and address of agent)

as my attorney-in-fact (my "agent") to act for me and in my name (in any way I could act in person) with respect to the following powers, as defined in Section 3-4 of the "Statutory Short Form Power of Attorney for Property Law" (including all amendments), but subject to any limitations on or additions to the specified powers inserted in paragraph 2 or 3 below:

(YOU MUST STRIKE OUT ANY ONE OR MORE OF THE FOLLOWING CATEGORIES OF POWERS YOU DO NOT WANT YOUR AGENT TO HAVE. FAILURE TO STRIKE THE TITLE OF ANY CATEGORY WILL CAUSE THE POWERS DESCRIBED IN THAT CATEGORY TO BE GRANTED TO THE AGENT. TO STRIKE OUT A CATEGORY YOU MUST DRAW A LINE THROUGH THE TITLE OF THAT CATEGORY.)

(a) Real estate transactions.
(b) Financial institution transactions.
(c) Stock and bond transactions.
(d) Tangible personal property transactions.
(e) Safe deposit box transactions.
(f) Insurance and annuity transactions.
(g) Retirement plan transactions.

(h)   Social Security, employment and military service benefits.
(i)   Tax matters.
(j)   Claims and litigation.
(k)   Commodity and option transactions.
(l)   Business operations.
(m) Borrowing transactions.
(n)   Estate transactions.
(o)   All other property powers and transactions.

(LIMITATIONS ON AND ADDITIONS TO THE AGENT'S POWER MAY BE INCLUDED IN THIS POWER OF ATTORNEY IF THEY ARE SPECIFICALLY DESCRIBED BELOW.)

2.   The powers granted above shall not include the following powers or shall be modified or limited in the following particulars (here you may include any specific limitations you deem appropriate, such as a prohibition or conditions on the sale of particular stock or real estate or special rules on borrowing by the agent):

_____

_____

_____

_____

3.   In addition to the powers granted above, I grant my agent the following powers (here you may add any other delegable powers including, without limitation, power to make gifts, exercise powers of appointment, name or change beneficiaries or joint tenants or revoke or amend any trust specifically referred to below):

_____

_____

_____

(YOUR AGENT WILL HAVE AUTHORITY TO EMPLOY OTHER PERSONS AS NECESSARY TO ENABLE THE AGENT TO PROPERLY EXERCISE THE POWERS GRANTED IN THIS FORM, BUT YOUR AGENT WILL HAVE TO MAKE ALL DISCRETIONARY DECISIONS. IF YOU WANT TO GIVE YOUR AGENT THE RIGHT TO DELEGATE DISCRETIONARY DECISION-MAKING POWERS TO OTHERS, YOU SHOULD KEEP THE NEXT SENTENCE, OTHERWISE IT SHOULD BE STRUCK OUT.)

4.   My agent shall have the right by written instrument to delegate any or all of the foregoing powers involving discretionary decision-making to any person or persons whom my agent may select, but such delegation may be amended or revoked by any agent (including any successor) named by me who is acting under this power of attorney at the time of reference.

(YOUR AGENT WILL BE ENTITLED TO REIMBURSEMENT FOR ALL REASONABLE EXPENSES INCURRED IN ACTING UNDER THIS POWER OF ATTORNEY. STRIKE OUT THE NEXT SENTENCE IF YOU DO NOT WANT YOUR AGENT TO ALSO BE ENTITLED TO REASONABLE COMPENSATION FOR SERVICES AS AGENT.)

5.   My agent shall be entitled to reasonable compensation for services rendered as agent under this power of attorney.

(THIS POWER OF ATTORNEY MAY BE AMENDED OR REVOKED BY YOU AT ANY TIME AND IN ANY MANNER. ABSENT AMENDMENT OR REVOCATION, THE AUTHORITY GRANTED IN THIS POWER OF ATTORNEY WILL BECOME EFFECTIVE AT THE TIME THIS POWER IS SIGNED AND WILL CONTINUE UNTIL YOUR DEATH UNLESS A LIMITATION ON THE BEGINNING DATE OR DURATION IS MADE BY INITIALING AND COMPLETING EITHER (OR BOTH) OF THE FOLLOWING:)

6.   (_____) This power of attorney shall become effective on _____

_____

_____

(insert a future date or event during your lifetime, such as court determination of your disability, when you want this power to first take effect)

7.   (_____) This power of attorney shall terminate on _____

_____

_____

(insert a future date or event, such as court determination of your disability, when you want this power to terminate prior to your death)

(IF YOU WISH TO NAME SUCCESSOR AGENTS, INSERT THE NAME(S) AND ADDRESS(ES) OF SUCH SUCCESSOR(S) IN THE FOLLOWING PARAGRAPH.)

8.   If any agent named by me shall die, become incompetent, resign or refuse to accept the office of agent, I name the following (each to act alone and successively, in the order named) as successor(s) to such agent:

_____

_____

For purposes of this paragraph 8, a person shall be considered to be incompetent if and while the person is a minor or an adjudicated incompetent or disabled person or the person is unable to give prompt and intelligent consideration to business matters, as certified by a licensed physician.

(IF YOU WISH TO NAME YOUR AGENT AS GUARDIAN OF YOUR ESTATE, IN THE EVENT A COURT DECIDES THAT ONE SHOULD BE APPOINTED, YOU MAY, BUT ARE NOT REQUIRED TO, DO SO BY RETAINING THE FOLLOWING PARAGRAPH. THE COURT WILL APPOINT YOUR AGENT IF THE COURT FINDS THAT SUCH APPOINTMENT WILL SERVE YOUR BEST INTERESTS AND WELFARE. STRIKE OUT PARAGRAPH 9 IF YOU DO NOT WANT YOUR AGENT TO ACT AS GUARDIAN.)

9. If a guardian of my estate (my property) is to be appointed, I nominate the agent acting under this power of attorney as such guardian, to serve without bond or security.

10. I am fully informed as to all the contents of this form and understand the full import of this grant of powers to my agent.

Signed _____

_____
(principal)

(YOU MAY, BUT ARE NOT REQUIRED TO, REQUEST YOUR AGENT AND SUCCESSOR AGENTS TO PROVIDE SPECIMEN SIGNATURES BELOW. IF YOU INCLUDE SPECIMEN SIGNATURES IN THIS POWER OF ATTORNEY, YOU MUST COMPLETE THE CERTIFICATION OPPOSITE THE SIGNATURES OF THE AGENTS.)

Specimen signatures of agent (and successors)

I certify that the signatures of my agent (and successors) are correct.

_____   _____
                                            (principal)
_____
(agent)

_____   _____
                                            (principal)
_____
(successor agent)

_____   _____
                                            (principal)
_____
(successor agent)

(THIS POWER OF ATTORNEY WILL NOT BE EFFECTIVE UNLESS IT IS NOTARIZED, USING THE FORM BELOW.)

State of _____)
) SS:
County of _____)

      The undersigned, a notary public in and for the above county and state, certifies that _____, known to me to be the same person whose name is subscribed as principal to the foregoing power of attorney, appeared before me in person and acknowledged signing and delivering the instrument as the free and voluntary act of the principal, for the uses and purposes therein set forth (and certified to the correctness of the signature(s) of the agent(s)).

      Dated: _____ (SEAL)

_____
Notary Public

      My commission expires _____

      (THE NAME AND ADDRESS OF THE PERSON PREPARING THIS FORM SHOULD BE INSERTED IF THE AGENT WILL HAVE POWER TO CONVEY ANY INTEREST IN REAL ESTATE.)

      This document was prepared by:

_____

_____

Illinois Statutory Short Form Power of Attorney for Property

Explanation

The explanations that follow should provide you with a clear understanding of the terms used in the Illinois Statutory Short Form Power of Attorney for Property.

Notice: The notice confirms what the book has already stated: the powers given to your attorney-in-fact (agent) are broad. Read the notice carefully; it provides a good description of the power of attorney.

Paragraph 1: On the first blank lines you would fill in the date and your name and address.

The next lines are for the name and address of the person to whom you are giving the power of attorney (called the "agent" or "attorney-in-fact").

The following lettered clauses specify broad powers providing your attorney-in-fact with wide latitude to manage your affairs. Powers are separately enumerated to avoid any questions about whether you intended to authorize your attorney-in-fact to undertake specific actions on your behalf. If you choose not to give all of these powers to your attorney-in-fact, you would draw a line through the powers that you want to exclude.

Line a: This line gives your attorney-in-fact broad authority to mortgage, sell, buy, accept, manage, lease, and/or otherwise deal with real estate, including your home.

Line b: This line authorizes your attorney-in-fact to handle banking transactions, including opening and managing accounts, CDs, and other instruments in financial institutions, signing checks, and making withdrawals.

Line c: This line lets your attorney-in-fact invest in securities on your behalf and manage, receive, sell, mortgage, and/or otherwise handle securities for you. This is broad enough to allow your attorney-in-fact to vote at stockholders meetings.

Line d: This line permits your attorney-in-fact broad authority to buy, sell, manage, receive, mortgage, lease, and/or otherwise handle transactions involving items of personal property.

Line e: This line allows your attorney-in-fact to open, close, or have access to your safe-deposit box.

Line f: This line authorizes your attorney-in-fact to handle any insurance and annuity matters for you, including obtaining, managing, maintaining, or terminating insurance and annuities, paying premiums, and obtaining benefits for you.

Line g: This line allows your attorney-in-fact to handle retirement plan transactions for you, including selecting payment options, making or changing beneficiary designations, making contributions and rollovers, and borrowing from retirement plans.

Line h: This line enables your attorney-in-fact to handle any matters you may have with social security, the military, or other employment matters, including making and receiving proceeds of any claims and maximizing benefits from social security and military service, and to handle other employment benefit matters.

Line i: This line gives your attorney-in-fact authority to deal with your taxes. Although you might prefer to forget about this, it's important that tax forms be prepared and taxes paid, to avoid possible problems.

Line j: This line gives your attorney-in-fact the right to handle claims and litigation for you, including bringing a lawsuit for you, defending you against claims, and settling disputes for you.

Line k: This line gives your attorney-in-fact the power to engage in commodities and option transactions for you.

Line l: This line allows your attorney-in-fact to engage in any business transactions for you.

Line m: This line permits your attorney-in-fact to borrow, mortgage, or pledge, pay notes, and handle all other borrowing matters.

Line n: This line permits your attorney-in-fact to act for you with respect to estate matters, including establishing trusts, receiving inheritances, and participating in the administration of estates.

Line o: This line is a catchall authorizing your attorney-in-fact to do anything you could do.

Paragraphs 2 and 3: In the spaces that follow you would add any other provisions or limitations—but if you do this, make sure your additions or changes comply with the law.

Paragraph 4: This paragraph allows your attorney-in-fact to delegate his or her powers to someone else. If you do not want to allow this, you must strike the paragraph.

Paragraph 5: The next line says that your attorney-in-fact will be paid for his or her services. If you appoint a family member, payment may not be necessary, and you could then strike this.

Paragraphs 6 and 7: The next sections allow you to limit the beginning and duration of the power of at-torney. Be careful—if you limit its duration and it expires, you might not be able to create a new one (if you've become incompetent).

Paragraph 8: Here you can name successor attorney(s)-in-fact in case your first choice is unable to help you. It is usually a good idea to name successors.

Paragraph 9: You can and should nominate someone to act as a guardian of your estate in the event that a court decides one is necessary. As explained in the power of attorney, a guardian is someone who will manage your financial affairs.

Finally, you would sign and date the document at the end before two witnesses and a notary. The attorney-in-fact and any successors also sign. The notary fills in and signs the bottom portion. A notary is authorized by the state or federal government to administer oaths and attest to the authenticity of signatures.

STATUTORY SHORT FORM POWER OF ATTORNEY
(MINNESOTA)

IMPORTANT NOTICE: THE POWERS GRANTED BY THIS DOCUMENT ARE BROAD AND SWEEPING. THEY ARE DEFINED IN MINNESOTA STATUTES SECTION 523.24. IF YOU HAVE ANY QUESTIONS ABOUT THESE POWERS, OBTAIN COMPETENT ADVICE. THIS POWER OF ATTORNEY MAY BE REVOKED BY YOU IF YOU WISH TO DO SO. THIS POWER OF ATTORNEY IS AUTOMATICALLY TERMINATED IF IT IS TO YOUR SPOUSE AND PROCEEDINGS ARE COMMENCED FOR DISSOLUTION, LEGAL SEPARATION, OR ANNULMENT OF YOUR MARRIAGE. THIS POWER OF ATTORNEY AUTHORIZES BUT DOES NOT REQUIRE THE ATTORNEY-IN-FACT TO ACT FOR YOU.

PRINCIPAL (Name and Address of Person Granting the Power)

_____

_____

_____

ATTORNEY(S)-IN-FACT (Name(s) and Address(es))

_____

_____

_____

SUCCESSOR ATTORNEY(S)-IN-FACT (Name(s) and Address(es))
   To act if any named attorney-in-fact dies, resigns, or is otherwise unable to serve

First Successor   _____

_____

_____

Second Successor   _____

_____

_____

NOTICE: If more than one attorney-in-fact is designated, make a check or "x" on the line in front of one of the following statements:

_____ Each attorney-in-fact may independently exercise the powers granted.

_____ All attorneys-in-fact must jointly exercise the powers granted.

Know All by These Presents, which are intended to constitute a STATUTORY SHORT FORM POWER OF ATTORNEY pursuant to Minnesota Statutes,

That I, _____,
               (insert name and address of the principal)
do hereby appoint the above named attorney(s)-in-fact to act as my attorney(s)-in-fact:

First: To act for me, in my name, place and stead in any way which I myself could do, if I were personally present, with respect to the following matters as each of them is defined in Minnesota Statutes, section 523.24:

(To grant to the attorney-in-fact any of the following powers, make a check or "x" in the line in front of each power being granted. To delete any of the following powers, do not make a check or "x" in the line in front of the power. You may, but need not, cross out each power being deleted with a line drawn through it (or in similar fashion). Failure to make a check or "x" in the line in front of the power will have the effect of deleting the power unless the line in front of the power of (N) is checked or x-ed.)

Check or "x":

_____ (A) real property transactions; I choose to limit this power to real property in _____ _____ County, Minnesota, described as follows: (Use legal description. Do not use street address.) (NOTE: A person may not grant powers relating to real property transactions in Minnesota to his or her spouse.)

_____

_____

_____

_____ (B) tangible personal property transactions;
_____ (C) bond, share and commodity transactions;
_____ (D) banking transactions;
_____ (E) business operating transactions;
_____ (F) insurance transactions;
_____ (G) beneficiary transactions;
_____ (H) gift transactions;
_____ (I) fiduciary transactions;
_____ (J) claims and litigation;
_____ (K) family maintenance;
_____ (L) benefits from military service;
_____ (M) records, reports, and statements;
_____ (N) all of the powers listed in (A) through (M) above.

Second: (You must indicate below whether or not this power of attorney will be effective if you become incapacitated or incompetent. Make a check or "x" in the line in front of the statement that expresses your intent.)

_____ This power of attorney shall continue to be effective if I become incapacitated or incompetent. It shall not be affected by my later disability or incompetency.

_____ This power of attorney shall not be effective if I become incapacitated or incompetent.

Third: (You must indicate below whether or not this power of attorney authorizes the attorney-in-fact to transfer your property to the attorney-in-fact. Make a check or "x" in the line in front of the statement that expresses your intent.)

_____ This power of attorney authorizes the attorney-in-fact to transfer my property to the attorney-in-fact.

_____ This power of attorney does not authorize the attorney-in-fact to transfer my property to the attorney-in-fact.

Fourth: (You may indicate below whether or not the attorney-in-fact is required to make an accounting. Make a check or "x" on the line in front of the statement that expresses your intent.)

_____ My attorney-in-fact need not render an accounting unless I request it or the accounting is otherwise required by Minnesota Statutes, section 523.21.

_____ My attorney-in-fact must render _____ (monthly, quarterly, annual) accountings to me or _____ (name and address) during my lifetime, and a final accounting to the personal representative of my estate, if any is appointed, after my death.

In Witness Whereof I have hereunto signed my name this _____ day of _____, 19____.

_____
(Signature of Principal)

Specimen Signature of Attorney(s)-in-Fact:

_____

_____

Signed in the presence of:

_____
Witness

_____
Witness

CERTIFICATE OF NOTARY

STATE OF MINNESOTA _____)

)   SS:

COUNTY OF _____)

         On the _____ day of _____, 19____, before me personally came _____, whose identity is well known to me to be the individual described in and who executed the foregoing instrument, and (he) (she) acknowledged to me that (he) (she) executed the same.

_____
                               Notary Public

My commission expires: _____

This instrument was drafted by:

_____

_____

_____

_____

Statutory Short Form Power of Attorney
(Minnesota)

Explanation

The explanations that follow should provide you with a clear understanding of the terms used in the Statutory Short form Power of Attorney for Minnesota.

Notice: The notice confirms what the book has already stated: the powers given to your attorney(s)-in-fact are broad.

In the spaces for the principal go your name and address. The person(s) who will be receiving the power to act for you, the attorney(s)-in-fact, is listed next, along with successors in case your first choice(s) cannot serve. If you name more than one to act at a time, you may choose to have them act separately or together.

Introduction: On the first blank line you would fill in your name and address (you are the "principal," the person making the power of attorney).

The following lettered clauses specify broad powers providing your attorney(s)-in-fact with wide latitude to manage your affairs. Powers are separately enumerated to avoid any questions about whether you intended to authorize your attorney(s)-in-fact to undertake specific actions on your behalf. For any powers you wish to give to your attorney(s)-in-fact, you would place a check mark or "x" in the line before such power(s). Since you cannot foresee all of the possible problems that could arise, you are usually better off giving your attorney(s)-in-fact the broadest possible powers.

Clause A: This clause gives your attorney(s)-in-fact broad authority to mortgage, sell, buy, accept, manage, lease, and/or otherwise deal with real estate, including your home.

Clause B: This clause permits your attorney(s)-in-fact broad authority to buy, sell, manage, receive, mortgage, lease, and/or otherwise handle transactions involving items of personal property.

Clause C: This clause lets your attorney(s)-in-fact invest in securities on your behalf and to manage, receive, sell, mortgage, and/or otherwise handle securities for you. This is broad enough to allow your attorney(s)-in-fact to vote at stockholders meetings.

Clause D: This clause authorizes your attorney(s)-in-fact to handle banking transactions, including opening and managing accounts, CDs, and other instruments in financial institutions, signing checks, making withdrawals, and having access to your safe-deposit box.

Clause E: This clause allows your attorney(s)-in-fact to engage in any business transactions for you.

Clause F: This clause authorizes your attorney(s)-in-fact to handle insurance matters for you, including obtaining, managing, maintaining, or terminating insurance, paying premiums, and obtaining benefits for you.

Clause G: This clause permits your attorney(s)-in-fact to act for you with respect to any matters in which you are or may be a beneficiary, including with respect to trusts, probate estates, guardianships, conservatorships, or escrows.

Clause H: This clause authorizes your attorney(s)-in-fact to make, complete, or otherwise handle any gift transactions for you.

Clause I: This clause allows your attorney(s)-in-fact to handle fiduciary matters for you, including estate administration, guardianship, and conservatorship activities.

Clause J: This clause gives your attorney(s)-in-fact the right to handle claims and litigation for you, including bringing a lawsuit for you, defending you against claims, and settling disputes for you.

Clause K: This clause authorizes your attorney(s)-in-fact to take steps to provide for the support and welfare of your family and to maintain your relationships with family, friends, and organizations.

Clause L: This clause enables your attorney(s)-in-fact to handle any matters you may have with the military, including making and receiving proceeds of any claims and maximizing benefits from military service.

Clause M: This clause empowers your attorney(s)-in-fact to make, execute, file, and store records, reports, and statements, including tax returns, for you.

Clause N: This clause is a catchall authorizing your attorney(s)-in-fact to do anything you could do.

The next section is *crucial* to making your power of attorney *durable,* so that it remains valid at the time you will need it most—during your incapacity. You would check the first line, stating that the power of attorney will be effective if you become incompetent.

The next paragraph, beginning with "Third," allows you to choose whether or not your attorney(s)-in-fact will be permitted to transfer your property to himself or herself.

The "Fourth" paragraph allows you to choose whether the attorney(s)-in-fact will have to provide you with an accounting periodically. An accounting is a written report on activities using the power of money.

Finally, you would sign and date the document at the end before two witnesses and a notary. The attorney(s)-in-fact signs his or her name under yours. The notary fills in and signs the bottom portion. A notary is authorized by the state or federal government to administer oaths and attest to the authenticity of signatures.

DURABLE GENERAL POWER OF ATTORNEY

STATE OF MISSOURI

COUNTY OF _____

       Know all Men by These Presents, which are intended to constitute a DURABLE GENERAL POWER OF ATTORNEY,

That I _____

(Name of principal)

_____

(Address of principal)

do hereby appoint _____

(Name of agent)

_____

(Address of agent)

and

_____

(Name of agent if more than one agent is designated)

_____

(Address of agent if more than one agent is designated)

My Attorney(s)-in-Fact TO ACT (jointly) (severally), as my true and lawful Attorney(s)-in-Fact, for me and in my name, place and stead:

    (A) Power with Respect to Accounts and Instruments. To establish or open accounts, certificates of deposit and any other form of account or instrument for me with financial institutions of any kind; to modify, terminate, make deposits to and write checks on and endorse checks for or make withdrawals from all accounts in my name or with respect to which I am an authorized signatory; to negotiate, endorse or transfer any checks or other instruments with respect to any such accounts; to contract for any services rendered by any financial institution; and to add property to any trust agreement created by me.

    (B) Power with Respect to Safe-Deposit Boxes. To contract with any institution for the maintenance of a safe-deposit box in my name; to have access to all safe-deposit boxes in my name or with respect to which I am an authorized signatory; to add to and remove from the contents of any such safe-deposit box and to terminate any and all contracts for such boxes.

    (C) Power to Sell and Buy. To sell and buy personal, intangible or mixed property, upon such terms and conditions as my Attorney(s)-in-Fact deems appropriate; to use any credit card held in my name to make such purchases and to sign such charge slips as may be necessary to use such credit cards; and to repay from any funds belonging to me any money borrowed and to pay for any purchases made or cash advanced using credit cards issued to me.

    (D) Power to Exercise Rights in Securities. To exercise all rights with respect to securities that I now own, or may hereafter acquire; to establish, utilize and terminate brokerage accounts; and to invest and reinvest any of my assets in stocks, common and/or preferred, bonds (including, without limitation, United States Treasury Bonds or other United States government obligations which may be redeemed at par for the purpose of applying the entire amount of principal and accrued interest thereon to the payment of the Federal estate tax, if any, occasioned by my death), notes, debentures, loans, mortgages, common trust funds, or other securities or property, real or personal, upon such terms and conditions as my Attorney(s)-in-Fact deems appropriate.

(E) Power to Borrow Money (including any Insurance Policy Loans). To borrow money for my account upon such terms and conditions as my Attorney(s)-in-Fact may deem appropriate and to secure such borrowing by the granting of security interests in any property or interest in property which I may now or hereafter own; to borrow money upon any life insurance policies owned by me upon my life for any purpose and to grant a security interest in such policy to secure any such loans; and no insurance company shall be under any obligation whatsoever to determine the need for such loan or the application of the proceeds therefrom.

(F) Power with Respect to Real Property. To purchase real property, to manage, maintain and alter all real property belonging to me, and to lease, sell, mortgage, encumber or otherwise dispose of all interests in real property belonging to me, upon such terms and conditions as my Attorney(s)-in-Fact deems appropriate; to renew leases of the same or to execute, acknowledge and deliver leases therefor; to execute deeds of conveyance either with or without covenants of general warranty; to pay and satisfy all mortgages, encumbrances, taxes and assessments that may be a lien or charge upon any of my real property; and to receive rentals from and the proceeds of sale of any of my real property. For purposes of this Durable General Power of Attorney, real property shall include, without limitation, the real property known as _____.

(G) Power to Demand, Compromise and Receive. To demand, arbitrate, settle, sue for, collect, receive, deposit, expand for my benefit, reinvest or make such other appropriate dispositions of, as my Attorney(s)-in-Fact deems appropriate, all cash rights to payments of cash, property (personal, intangible and/or mixed), rights and/or benefits to which I am now or may in the future become entitled, regardless of the identity of the individual or public or private entity involved (and for purposes of receiving Social Security benefits, my Attorney(s)-in-Fact is herewith appointed my "Representative Payee"); to compound, compromise, settle and adjust all claims and demands whatsoever which I may now owe or be liable for; and to utilize all lawful means and methods for such purposes.

(H) Power with Respect to Taxes. To make, prepare, sign and file for me and on my behalf any and all required tax estimates and returns, federal, state or local, as well as any waivers, affidavits, schedules or other forms required or permitted to be filed in connection therewith, and to protest and appeal any assessments or determinations of tax against me which my Attorney(s)-in-Fact deems to have been made without proper warrant.

(I) Power with Respect to Documents. To sign, acknowledge, record and deliver agreements, affidavits, bills of sale, stock powers, deeds, leases, mortgages, notes, receipts, releases, satisfactions, journal entries, certificates and such other documents which may be necessary or convenient in execution of the powers hereinbefore expressly conferred upon my Attorney(s)-in-Fact; to execute and deliver applications for automobile license plates and certificates of title and to endorse for transfer and to deliver certificates of title; and to execute and deliver applications for insurance (including, without limitation, insurance on my life) and to cancel and select the amounts therefor.

(J) Power to Engage Services. To engage the services of and compensate attorneys-at-law, appraisers, accountants, brokers, real estate managers, investment counsel and such other persons as may be proper or convenient to advise and assist in the management, maintenance and disposition of my property.

(K) Power to Incur Obligations. To incur obligations for the maintenance, support, health, care, well-being, comfort and welfare of me and my family and to satisfy such obligations out of my money or property; and to consent on my behalf to medical and surgical procedures, and to take other actions pertaining to my health.

I further give and grant to my said Attorney(s)-in-Fact full power and authority to do and perform every act necessary to be done in the exercise of any of the foregoing powers as fully as I might or could do if personally present, with full power of substitution and revocation, hereby ratifying and confirming all that my said Attorney(s)-in-Fact shall lawfully do, or cause to be done by virtue hereof.

This instrument may not be changed orally.

This power of attorney is durable as provided for in 486.550 R.S. Mo. et seq. and shall not be affected by the subsequent disability or incompetence of the principal or by any lapse of time; it shall remain in full force and effect until revoked by me.

TO INDUCE ANY THIRD PARTY TO ACT HEREUNDER, I HEREBY AGREE THAT ANY THIRD PARTY RECEIVING A DULY EXECUTED COPY OR FACSIMILE OF THIS INSTRUMENT MAY ACT HEREUNDER, AND THAT REVOCATION OR TERMINATION HEREOF SHALL BE INEFFECTIVE AS TO SUCH THIRD PARTY UNLESS AND UNTIL ACTUAL NOTICE OR KNOWLEDGE OF SUCH REVOCATION OR TERMINATION SHALL HAVE BEEN RECEIVED BY SUCH THIRD PARTY AND I FOR MYSELF AND FOR MY HEIRS, EXECUTORS, LEGAL REPRESENTATIVES AND ASSIGNS, HEREBY AGREE TO INDEMNIFY AND HOLD HARMLESS ANY SUCH THIRD PARTY FROM AND AGAINST ANY AND ALL CLAIMS THAT MAY ARISE AGAINST SUCH THIRD PARTY BY REASON OF SUCH THIRD PARTY HAVING RELIED ON THE PROVISIONS OF THIS INSTRUMENT.

In witness whereof, I have hereunto signed my hand and seal this _____ day of _____, 19____.

_____
(Signature of Principal)

Specimen Signature of Attorney(s)-in-Fact:

_____

_____

Signed in the presence of:

_____

Witness

_____

Witness

CERTIFICATE OF NOTARY

STATE OF _____)
) SS:
COUNTY OF_____)

On the _____ day of _____, 19____, before me personally came _____, whose identity is well known to me and known to me to be the individual described in and who executed the foregoing instrument, and (he) (she) acknowledged to me that (he) (she) executed the same.

_____
Notary Public

My commission expires:

_____

Durable General Power of Attorney
(Missouri)

Explanation

The explanations that follow should provide you with a clear understanding of the terms used in Missouri's Durable General Power of Attorney form.

Introduction: At the top left, below "STATE OF MISSOURI" goes the name of your county. Below that, you would fill in your name and address (you are the "principal," the person making the durable general power of attorney).

On the next line go the name(s) and address(es) of the person(s) to whom you are giving the durable general power of attorney (called the "agent[s]" or "attorney[s]-in-fact").

If you have decided to name more than one attorney-in-fact, you must decide whether to strike the word *jointly* or *severally*. If you want to require your attorneys-in-fact to act together to use the power of attorney, you should leave the word *jointly* and strike the word *severally*. But if you prefer to allow either of your attorneys-in-fact on his or her own to exercise the powers provided in the power of attorney, you should strike out the word *jointly* and leave the word *severally*.

The following lettered clauses specify broad powers providing your attorney(s)-in-fact with latitude to manage your financial affairs. Powers are separately enumerated to avoid any questions about whether you intended to authorize your attorney(s)-in-fact to undertake specific actions on your behalf.

Clause A: This clause authorizes your attorney(s)-in-fact to open and manage accounts, CDs, and other instruments for you in financial institutions. It also says that your attorney(s)-in-fact may add to any trust agreement you may have created.

Clause B: This clause allows your attorney(s)-in-fact to maintain and gain access to safe-deposit boxes in your name.

Clause C: This clause permits your attorney(s)-in-fact to buy and sell items and to use your credit cards.

Clause D: This clause lets your attorney(s)-in-fact invest in securities on your behalf and to manage and handle those securities. This is broad enough to allow your attorney(s)-in-fact to vote at stockholders meetings.

Clause E: This clause authorizes your attorney(s)-in-fact to borrow money in your name.

Clause F: This clause gives your attorney(s)-in-fact broad authority to manage, sell, buy, mortgage, and/or lease real estate, including your home. In the blank you would fill in the address(es) of your residence and any other real estate you own. You don't have to change the durable general power of attorney each time you buy or sell real estate. Recording requirements vary greatly from state to state.

Clause G: This clause authorizes your attorney(s)-in-fact to take any necessary action with respect to rights you have or may have in the future to money or property. It also lets your attorney(s)-in-fact handle claims made against you. The term *representative payee* is defined in chapter 12.

Clause H: This clause gives your attorney(s)-in-fact the power to deal with your taxes. Although you might prefer to forget about this, it's important that tax forms be prepared and taxes paid, to avoid possible penalties.

Clause I: This clause spells out the right of your attorney(s)-in-fact to sign and execute all sorts of documents on your behalf. It also allows your attorney(s)-in-fact to handle your applications for license plates, certificates of title, and insurance.

Clause J: This clause allows your attorney(s)-in-fact to hire specialists to assist in handling your financial affairs.

Clause K: This clause generally authorizes your attorney(s)-in-fact to incur and pay bills for your maintenance, support, and care. It also empowers your attorney(s)-in-fact to make certain health care decisions.

Closing Paragraphs: The first paragraph following the lettered clauses is a catchall authorizing your attorney(s)-in-fact to do anything you could do.

The next line is self-explanatory—you can't change the terms of the document orally.

The following sentence is *crucial* to making your power of attorney *durable,* so that it remains valid at the time you will need it most—during your incapacity.

Some banks and insurance companies have traditionally been unwilling to accept or act on any preprinted power of attorney form that they did not prepare themselves. The last full paragraph, printed in all capital letters, attempts to deal with this problem. That paragraph will protect third parties relying on the durable general power of attorney and, it is hoped, encourage them to accept this form. However, since there can be no assurance that this will work, you should contact your bank and insurance company to discuss their forms and procedures.

Finally, you would sign and date the document at the end before two witnesses and a notary. The attorney(s)-in-fact signs his or her name under yours. The notary fills in and signs the bottom portion. A notary is authorized by the state or federal government to administer oaths and attest to the authenticity of signatures.

STATUTORY SHORT FORM
DURABLE GENERAL POWER OF ATTORNEY
(NEW YORK)

NOTICE: The powers granted by this document are broad and sweeping. They are defined in New York General Obligations Law, Article 5, Title 15, Sections 5–1502A through 5–1503, which expressly permits the use of any other or different form of power of attorney desired by the parties concerned.

Know All Men by These Presents, which are intended to constitute a GENERAL POWER OF ATTORNEY pursuant to Article 5, Title 15 of the New York General Obligations Law:

That I, _____

_____,

(insert name and address of the principal)

do hereby appoint _____

_____

_____,

(insert name and address of the agent, or
each agent, if more than one is designated)

my attorney(s)-in-fact TO ACT _____

(If more than one agent is designated and the principal wishes each agent alone to be able to exercise the power conferred, insert in this blank the word 'severally'. Failure to make any insertion or the insertion of the word 'jointly' will require the agents to act jointly.)

In my name, place and stead in any way which I myself could do, if I were personally present, with respect to the following matters as each of them is defined in Title 15 of Article 5 of the New York General Obligations Law to the extent that I am permitted by law to act through an agent:

(Strike out and initial in the opposite box any one or more of the subdivisions as to which the principal does NOT desire to give the agent authority. Such elimination of any one or more of subdivisions (A) to (L), inclusive, shall automatically constitute an elimination also of subdivision (M).)

To strike out any subdivision the principal must draw a line through the text of that subdivision AND write his initials in the box opposite.

(A)	real estate transactions;	( )
(B)	chattel and goods transactions;	( )
(C)	bond, share and commodity transactions;	( )
(D)	banking transactions;	( )
(E)	business operating transactions;	( )
(F)	insurance transactions;	( )
(G)	estate transactions;	( )
(H)	claims and litigation;	( )
(I)	personal relationships and affairs;	( )
(J)	benefits from military service;	( )

(K) records, reports and statements;   ( )
(L) full and unqualified authority to my attorney(s)-
     in-fact to delegate any or all of the foregoing
     powers to any person or persons whom my
     attorney(s)-in-fact shall select;   ( )
(M) all other matters;   ( )

_____
_____
_____
_____
_____
_____

(Special provisions and limitations may be included in the statutory short form power of attorney only if they conform to the requirements of section 5–1503 of the New York General Obligations Law.)

This power of attorney shall not be affected by the subsequent disability or incompetence of the principal.

TO INDUCE ANY THIRD PARTY TO ACT HEREUNDER, I HEREBY AGREE THAT ANY THIRD PARTY RECEIVING A DULY EXECUTED COPY OR FACSIMILE OF THIS IN-STRUMENT MAY ACT HEREUNDER, AND THAT REVOCATION OR TERMINATION HEREOF SHALL BE INEFFECTIVE AS TO SUCH THIRD PARTY UNLESS AND UNTIL ACTUAL NOTICE OR KNOWLEDGE OF SUCH REVOCATION OR TERMINATION SHALL HAVE BEEN RECEIVED BY SUCH THIRD PARTY, AND I FOR MYSELF AND FOR MY HEIRS, EXECUTORS, LEGAL REPRESENTATIVES AND ASSIGNS, HEREBY AGREE TO INDEMNIFY AND HOLD HARMLESS ANY SUCH THIRD PARTY FROM AND AGAINST ANY AND ALL CLAIMS THAT MAY ARISE AGAINST SUCH THIRD PARTY BY REASON OF SUCH THIRD PARTY HAVING RELIED ON THE PROVISIONS OF THIS INSTRUMENT.

In Witness Whereof, I have hereunto signed my name and affixed my seal this _____ day of _____, 19____.

_____ (Seal)
(Signature of Principal)

Specimen Signature of Attorney(s)-in-Fact:

_____

_____

_____

signed in the presence of:

_____
Witness

_____
Witness

CERTIFICATE OF NOTARY

STATE OF NEW YORK _____)
) SS:
COUNTY OF _____)

On the _____ day of _____, 19____, before me personally came _____, whose identity is well known to me to be the individual described in and who executed the foregoing instrument, and (he) (she) acknowledged to me that (he) (she) executed the same.

_____
Notary Public

My commission expires:

_____

3

Statutory Short Form
Durable General Power of Attorney
(New York)

Explanation

The explanations that follow should provide you with a clear understanding of the terms used in the Statutory Short Form Durable General Power of Attorney for the State of New York.

Notice: The notice confirms what the book has already stated: the powers given to your attorney(s)-in-fact are broad.

Introduction: On the first blank line you would fill in your name and address (you are the "principal," the person making the durable general power of attorney). On the next line go the name(s) and address(es) of the person(s) to whom you are giving the durable general power of attorney (called the "agent[s]" or "attorney[s]-in-fact").

If you have decided to name more than one attorney-in-fact, you would fill in the next blank with either the word *severally* or the word *jointly*. "Severally" means that either of your attorneys-in-fact on his or her own will be able to exercise the powers provided in the durable general power of attorney; *jointly* means that your attorneys-in-fact must act together to use your durable general power of attorney.

The following lettered clauses specify broad powers providing your attorney(s)-in-fact with wide latitude to manage your affairs. Powers are separately enumerated to avoid any questions about whether you intended to authorize your attorney(s)-in-fact to undertake specific actions on your behalf. For any power(s) you decide not to give your attorney(s)-in-fact, you would draw a line through the power(s) you want to exclude *and* initial inside the parentheses after such excluded power(s).

Clause A: This clause gives your attorney(s)-in-fact broad authority to mortgage, sell, buy, accept, manage, lease, and/or otherwise deal with real estate, including your home.

Clause B: This clause permits your attorney(s)-in-fact broad authority to buy, sell, manage, receive, mortgage, lease, and/or otherwise handle transactions involving items of personal property.

Clause C: This clause lets your attorney(s)-in-fact invest in securities on your behalf and to manage, receive, sell, mortgage, and/or otherwise handle securities for you. This is broad enough to allow your attorney(s)-in-fact to vote at stockholders meetings.

Clause D: This clause authorizes your attorney(s)-in-fact to handle banking transactions, including opening and managing accounts, CDs, and other instruments in financial institutions, signing checks, making withdrawals, and having access to your safe-deposit box.

Clause E: This clause allows your attorney(s)-in-fact to engage in any business transactions for you.

Clause F: This clause authorizes your attorney(s)-in-fact to handle insurance matters for you, including obtaining, managing, maintaining, or terminating insurance, paying premiums, and obtaining benefits for you.

Clause G: This clause permits your attorney(s)-in-fact to act for you with respect to estate matters, including receiving inheritances and participating in the administration of estates.

Clause H: This clause gives your attorney(s)-in-fact the right to handle claims and litigation for you, including bringing a lawsuit for you, defending you against claims, and settling disputes for you.

Clause I: This clause authorizes your attorney(s)-in-fact to handle your personal affairs, to take steps to provide for the support and welfare of your family, and to maintain your relationships with family, friends, and organizations.

Clause J: This clause enables your attorney(s)-in-fact to handle any matters you may have with the military, including making and receiving proceeds of any claims and maximizing benefits from military service.

Clause K: This clause empowers your attorney(s)-in-fact to make, execute, and file, store, and keep records, reports, and statements, including tax returns, for you.

Clause L: This clause allows your attorney(s)-in-fact to delegate his or her powers to someone else.

Clause M: This clause is a catchall authorizing your attorney(s)-in-fact to do anything you could do.

On the lines that follow you would add any other provisions or limitations, but if you do this, make sure your additions or changes comply with the law.

The next sentence is *crucial* to your power of attorney *durable,* so that it remains valid at the time you will need it most—during your incapacity.

Some banks and insurance companies have traditionally been unwilling to accept or act on any preprinted power of attorney form that they did not prepare themselves. The last full paragraph, printed in all capital letters, attempts to deal with this problem. That paragraph will protect third parties relying on the durable general power of attorney and, it is hoped, encourage them to accept this form. However, since there can be no assurance that this will work, you should contact your bank and insurance company to discuss their forms and procedures.

Finally, you would sign and date the document at the end before two witnesses and a notary. The attorney(s)-in-fact signs his or her name under yours. The notary fills in and signs the bottom portion. A notary is authorized by the state or federal government to administer oaths and attest to the authenticity of signatures.

DURABLE GENERAL POWER OF ATTORNEY
(NORTH CAROLINA)

NOTICE: THE POWERS GRANTED BY THIS DOCUMENT ARE BROAD AND SWEEPING. THEY ARE DEFINED IN CHAPTER 32A OF THE NORTH CAROLINA GENERAL STATUTES WHICH EXPRESSLY PERMITS THE USE OF ANY OTHER OR DIFFERENT FORM OF POWER OF ATTORNEY DESIRED BY THE PARTIES CONCERNED.

State Of North Carolina

County Of _____

I, _____, the undersigned, hereby appoint _____ my attorney-in-fact for me and give such person full power to act in my name, place and stead in any way which I myself could do if I were personally present with respect to the following matters as each of them is defined in Chapter 32A of the North Carolina General Statutes to the extent that I am permitted by law to act through an agent. (DIRECTIONS: Initial the line opposite any one or more of the subdivisions as to which the principal desires to give the attorney-in-fact authority.)

(1) Real property transactions: _____
(2) Personal property transactions: _____
(3) Bond, share and commodity transactions: _____
(4) Banking transactions: _____
(5) Safe deposits: _____
(6) Business operating transactions: _____
(7) Insurance transactions: _____
(8) Estate transactions: _____
(9) Personal relationships and affairs: _____
(10) Social security and unemployment: _____
(11) Benefits from military service: _____
(12) Tax: _____
(13) Employment of agents: _____

I also give to such person full power to appoint another to act as my attorney-in-fact and full power to revoke such appointment.

This power of attorney shall not be affected by my subsequent incapacity or mental incompetence.

Dated _____, 19____

_____ (Seal)
Signature

STATE OF _____ COUNTY OF _____

On this _____ day of _____, 19____, personally appeared before me the said named _____ to me known and known to me to be the person described in and who executed the foregoing instrument and he (or she) acknowledged that he (or she) executed the same and being duly sworn by me, made oath that the statements in the foregoing instrument are true.

My Commission Expires _____

_____
(Signature of Notary Public)
Notary Public (Official Seal)

Durable General Power of Attorney
(North Carolina)

Explanation

The explanations that follow should provide you with a clear understanding of the terms used in the Durable General Power of Attorney form for the State of North Carolina.

Introduction: At the top left you would fill in the name of your county. Below that you would fill in your name and address in the first blank. (You are called the "principal".) The second blank is for the name(s) and address(es) of the person(s) to whom you are giving the durable general power of attorney (called the "attorney[s]-in-fact").

Chapter 32A of the North Carolina General Statutes, referred to in the durable general power of attorney, contains the laws governing powers of attorney in North Carolina.

The following numbered lines provide broad powers for your attorney(s)-in-fact to manage your affairs. As the directions in the durable general power of attorney indicate, the lines opposite each power you intend to give to your attorney(s)-in-fact must be initialed. Since you usually can't anticipate every eventuality that might arise, you probably would want to give your attorney(s)-in-fact the widest possible latitude.

The North Carolina laws describe each of the numbered powers as follows:

Line 1. Real Property Transactions: This line gives your attorney(s)-in-fact the authority to lease, purchase, exchange, and acquire, and to agree, bargain, and contract for the lease, purchase, exchange, and acquisition of, and to accept, take, receive, and possess any interest in real property whatsoever, on such terms and conditions, and under such covenants, as your attorney(s)-in-fact shall deem proper; and to maintain, repair, improve, manage, insure, rent, lease, sell, convey, subject to liens, mortgage, subject to deeds of trust, and in any way or manner deal with all or any part of any interest in real property whatsoever, that you own at the time of execution or may thereafter acquire, under such terms and conditions, and under such covenants, as your attorney(s)-in-fact shall deem proper.

Line 2. Personal Property Transactions: This line gives your attorney(s)-in-fact the power to lease, purchase, exchange, and acquire, and to agree, bargain, and contract for the lease, purchase, exchange, and acquisition of, and to accept, take, receive, and possess any personal property whatsoever, tangible or intangible, or interest thereto, on such terms and conditions, and under such covenants, as your attorney(s)-in-fact shall deem proper; and to maintain, repair, improve, manage, insure, rent, lease, sell, convey, subject to liens and mortgages, and hypothecate, and in any way or manner deal with all or any part of any personal property whatsoever, tangible or intangible, or any interest therein, that you own at the time of execution or may thereafter acquire, under such terms and conditions, and under such covenants, as your attorney(s)-in-fact shall deem proper.

Line 3. Bond, Share and Commodity Transactions: This line enables your attorney(s)-in-fact to request, ask, demand, sue for, recover, collect, receive, and hold and possess any bond, share, instrument of similar character, commodity interest, or any instrument with respect thereto together with the interest, dividends, proceeds, or other distributions connected therewith, as now are, or shall hereafter become, owned by, or due, owing payable, or belonging to you at the time of execution or in which you may thereafter acquire interest, to have, use, and take all lawful means and equitable and legal remedies, procedures, and writs in your name for the collection and recovery thereof, and to adjust, sell, compromise, and agree for the same, and to make, execute, and deliver for you all endorsements, acquittances, releases, receipts, or other sufficient discharges for the same.

Line 4. Banking Transactions: This line gives your attorney(s)-in-fact the power to make, receive, sign, endorse, execute, acknowledge, deliver, and possess checks, drafts, bills of exchange, letters of credit, notes, stock certificates, withdrawal receipts, and deposit instruments relating to accounts or deposits in, or certificates of deposit of, banks, savings and loans, or other institutions or associations for you.

Line 5. Safe Deposits: This line authorizes your attorney(s)-in-fact to have free access at any time to any safe-deposit box or vault to which you might have access as lessee or owner.

Line 6. Business Operating Transactions: This line allows your attorney(s)-in-fact to conduct, engage in, and transact any and all lawful business of whatever nature or kind for you.

Line 7. Insurance Transactions: This line provides your attorney(s)-in-fact with authority to exercise or perform any act, power, duty, right, or obligation whatsoever in regard to any contract of life, accident, health, disability, or liability insurance or any combination of such insurance procured by you or on your behalf prior to execution; and to procure new, different, or additional contracts of insurance for you and to designate the beneficiary of any such contract of insurance, provided, however, that the agent himself or herself cannot be such beneficiary unless the agent is your spouse, child, grandchild, parent, brother, or sister.

Line 8. Estate Transactions: This line permits your attorney(s)-in-fact to request, ask, demand, sue for, recover, collect, receive, and hold and possess all legacies, bequests, and devises as are owned by, or due, owing, payable, or belonging to you at the time of execution or in which you may thereafter acquire interest, to have, use, and take all lawful means and equitable and legal remedies, procedures, and writs in your name for the collection and recovery thereof, and to adjust, sell, compromise, and agree for the same, and to make, execute, and deliver for you, all endorsements, acquittances, releases, receipts, or other sufficient discharges for the same.

Line 9. Personal Relationships and Affairs: This line gives your attorney(s)-in-fact the power to do all acts necessary for maintaining the customary standard of living of you and your spouse, children, and other dependents; to provide medical, dental, and surgical care, hospitalization, and custodial care for you and your spouse, children, and other dependents; to continue whatever provision has been made by you for you and your spouse, children, and other dependents, with respect to automobiles or other means of transportation; to continue whatever charge accounts have been operated by you for the convenience of you and your spouse, children, and other dependents, to open such new accounts as your attorney(s)-in-fact shall think to be desirable for the accomplishment of any of the purposes enumerated in this section, and to pay the items charged on such accounts by any person authorized or permitted by you or your attorney(s)-in-fact to make such charges; to continue the discharge of any services or duties assumed by you to any parent, relative, or friend of yours; to continue payments incidental to the membership or affiliation of you in any church, club, society, order, or other organization, or to continue contributions thereto.

Line 10. Social Security and Unemployment: This line authorizes your attorney(s)-in-fact to prepare, execute, and file all Social Security, unemployment insurance, and information returns required by the laws of the United States, of any state or subdivision thereof, or of any foreign government.

Line 11. Benefits from Military Service: This line empowers your attorney(s)-in-fact to execute vouchers in your name for any and all allowances and reimbursements payable by the United States or subdivision thereof to you, arising from or based on military service, and to receive, endorse, and collect the proceeds of any check payable to the order of you drawn on the treasurer or other fiscal officer or depository of the United States or subdivision thereof; to take possession of and to order the removal and shipment of any property of yours from any post, warehouse, depot, dock, or other place of storage or safekeeping, either governmental or private, and to execute and to deliver any release, voucher, receipt, bill of lading, shipping ticket, certificate, or other instrument that the agent shall think to be desirable or necessary for such purpose; to prepare, file, and prosecute your claim to any benefit or assistance, financial or otherwise, to which you are, or you claim to be, entitled under the provisions of any statute or regulation existing at the creation of the agency or thereafter enacted by the United States or by any state or by any subdivision thereof, or by any foreign government, which benefit or assistance arises from or is based on military service performed prior to or after execution of this durable general power of attorney.

Line 12. Tax: This line allows your attorney(s)-in-fact to prepare, execute, verify, and file in your name and on your behalf any and all types of tax returns, amended returns, declaration of estimated tax, report, protest, application for correction of assessed valuation of real or other property, appeal, brief, claim for refund, or petition, including petition to the Tax Court of the United States, in connection with any tax imposed or proposed to be imposed by any government, or claimed, levied, or assessed by any government, and to pay any such tax and to obtain any extension of time for any of the foregoing; to execute waivers or consents agreeing to a later determination and assessment of taxes than is provided by any statute of limitations; to execute waivers of restriction on the assessment and collection of deficiency in any tax; to execute closing agreements and all other documents, instruments, and papers relating to any tax liability of any sort; to institute and carry on through counsel any proceeding in connection with determining or contesting any such tax or to recover any tax paid or to resist any claim for additional tax on any proposed assessment or levy thereof; and to enter into any agreements or stipulations for compromise or other adjustment or disposition of any tax.

Line 13. Employment of Agents: This line grants to your attorney(s)-in-fact the right to employ agents such as legal counsel, accountants, or other professional representation as may be appropriate, and to grant such agents such powers of attorney or other appropriate authorization as may be required in connection with such representation or by the Internal Revenue Service or other governmental authority.

Closing Paragraphs: The first full paragraph following the numbered lines gives your attorney(s)-in-fact the power to appoint someone else to substitute for him or her. This may be especially important if your chosen attorney(s)-in-fact became unable to continue to assist you.

The next line is *crucial* to making your power of attorney *durable*, so that it remains valid at the time you will need it most—during your incapacity.

Finally, you would sign and date the document at the end before a notary. The notary fills in, signs, and seals the last portion. A notary is authorized by the state or federal government to administer oaths and attest to the authenticity of signatures.

STATE OF SOUTH CAROLINA   )
)   **POWER OF ATTORNEY**
COUNTY OF   )

KNOW ALL MEN BY THESE PRESENTS THAT I, _____

_____
(insert name and address of principal) ("Principal"), a resident of the State and County aforesaid, have made, constituted and appointed and by these presents do make, constitute and appoint _____

_____
(insert name and address of the agent) my true and lawful attorney ("Attorney") for the purposes here-inafter set forth.

      Subject to the limitations set forth in this paragraph, I have also made, constituted and ap-pointed and by these presents do make, constitute and appoint as my true and lawful standby attorney ("Standby Attorney") _____
(insert name and address of the agent) for the purposes hereinafter set forth. However, in no event is _____ (Standby Attorney) authorized to act hereunder so long as _____ (Attorney) is living, competent to act and has not resigned nor been removed. A Standby Attorney is subject to removal as provided in Article II, paragraph D, hereof.

ARTICLE I

Empowerment of Attorney

      Attorney is authorized in Attorney's absolute discretion from time to time and at any time with respect to my property, real or personal, at any time owned or held by me and without authorization of any court and in addition to any other rights, powers or authority granted by any other provision of this Power of Attorney or by statute or general rules of law, and regardless of whether I am mentally incom-petent or physically or mentally disabled or incapable of managing my property and income, with full power of substitution, as follows:

§A. Powers in General

      To do and perform all and every act, deed, matter and thing whatsoever in and about my es-tate, property and affairs as fully and effectually to all intents and purposes as I might or could do in my own proper person, if personally present, the specifically enumerated powers described below being in aid and exemplification of the full, complete and general power herein granted and not in limitation or definition thereof.

§B. Powers Relating to Management of Assets

      1. To buy, receive, lease as lessor, accept or otherwise acquire; to sell, convey, mortgage, grant options upon, hypothecate, pledge, transfer, exchange, quitclaim or otherwise encumber or dispose of; or to contract or agree for the acquisition, disposal or encumbrance of any property whatsoever or any custody, possession, interest or right therein, for cash or credit and upon such terms, considerations and conditions as Attorney shall think proper, and no person dealing with Attorney shall be bound to see to the application of any monies paid;

      2. To take, hold, possess, invest or otherwise manage any or all of my property or any in-terest therein; to eject, remove or relieve tenants or other persons from, and recover possession of, such property by all lawful means; and to maintain, protect, preserve, insure, remove, store, transport, repair, build on, raze, rebuild, alter, modify or improve the same or any part thereof and/or to lease any property, real or personal, for me or my benefit, as lessee, with or without option to renew; to collect, receive and receipt for rents, issues and profits of my property;

3. To make, endorse, accept, receive, sign, seal, execute, acknowledge and deliver deeds, assignments, agreements, certificates, endorsements, hypothecations, checks, notes, mortgages, vouchers, receipts, consents, waivers releases, undertakings, satisfactions, acknowledgements and such other documents or instruments in writing of whatever kind and nature as may be necessary convenient or proper in the premises;

4. To subdivide, develop or dedicate real property to public use or to make or obtain the vacation of plats and adjust boundaries, to adjust differences in valuation on exchange or partition by giving or receiving consideration, and to dedicate easements to public use without consideration;

5. To invest and reinvest all or any part of my property in any property and undivided interest in property, wherever located, including bonds, debentures, notes, secured or unsecured, stocks of corporations regardless of class, interest in limited partnerships, real estate or any interest in real estate, whether or not productive at the time of investment, interest in trusts, investment trusts, whether of the open and/or closed fund types and participation in common, collective or pooled trust funds or annuity contracts without being limited by any statute or rule of law concerning investments by fiduciaries;

6. To continue and operate any business owned by me and to do any and all things deemed needful or appropriate by Attorney, including the power to incorporate the business and to put additional capital into the business, for such time as Attorney shall deem advisable, without liability for loss resulting from the continuance or operation of the business except for Attorney's own negligence; and to close out, liquidate or sell the business at such time and upon such terms as Attorney shall deem best;

7. To transfer all of my stock and/or securities to my Attorney, as agent (with the beneficial ownership thereof remaining in me), if necessary or convenient, in order to exercise the powers with respect to such stock and/or securities granted herein;

8. To sell or exercise stock subscription or conversion rights;

9. To refrain from voting or to vote shares of stock owned by me at shareholder's meetings in person or by special, limited or general proxy and in general to exercise all the rights, powers and privileges of an owner in respect to any securities constituting my property;

10. To participate in any plan of reorganization or consolidation or merger involving any company or companies with respect to stock or other securities which I own and to deposit such stock or other securities under any plan or reorganization or with any protective committee and to delegate to such committee discretionary power with relation thereto, to pay a proportionate part of the expenses of such committee and any assessments levied under any such plan, to accept and retain new securities received by Attorney pursuant to any such plan, to exercise all conversion, subscription, voting and other rights, of whatsoever nature pertaining to such property, and to pay any amount or amounts of money that Attorney may deem advisable in connection therewith;

11. To institute, prosecute, defend, abandon, compromise, arbitrate and dispose of legal, equitable or administrative hearings, actions, suits, attachments, arrests, distresses or other proceedings or otherwise engage in litigation involving me, my property or any interest of mine;

12. To deal with Attorney in Attorney's individual or any fiduciary capacity, in buying and selling assets, in lending and borrowing money, and in all other transactions, irrespective of the occupancy by the same person of dual positions;

13. To insure my property against damage or loss and Attorney against liability with respect to third persons.

§C. Powers Relating to Custody of Person

1. In general, and in addition to all the specific acts in this section enumerated, to do any other act or acts, which I can do through an agent, for the welfare of my spouse, children and/or dependents or for the preservation and maintenance of my other personal relationships to parents, relatives friends and organizations;

2. To do all acts necessary for maintaining the customary standard of living of my spouse, children and/or dependents of mine, including by way of illustration and not by way of restriction, power to provide living quarters by purchase, lease or by other contract, or by payment of the operating costs, including interest, amortization payments, repairs and taxes, of premises owned by me and occupied by my family and/or dependents, to provide usual educational facilities, and to provide funds for all the current living costs of my spouse, children and/or dependents of mine, including food and incidentals, and if necessary to make all necessary arrangements, contractual or otherwise, for me at any hospital, nursing home, convalescent home or similar establishment;

3. To continue whatever provision has been made by me, prior to the creation of this power or thereafter, for my spouse, children and/or dependents, with respect to automobiles, or other means of transportation, including by way of illustration but not by way of restriction, power to license, to insure and to replace any automobiles owned by me and customarily used by my spouse, children and/or dependents; to apply for a Certificate of Title upon, and endorse and transfer title thereto, any automobile, truck, van, motorcycle or other motor vehicle and to represent in such transfer assignment that the title to said motor vehicle is free and clear of all liens and encumbrances except those specifically set forth in such transfer assignment;

4. To continue whatever charge accounts have been operated by me prior to the creation of this power or thereafter, for the convenience of my spouse, children and/or dependents, to open such new accounts as Attorney shall think to be desirable for the accomplishment of any of the purposes enumerated in this section, and to pay the items charged on such accounts by any person authorized or permitted by me to make such charges prior to the creation of the power;

5. To continue the discharge of any services or duties assumed by me prior to the creation of this power or thereafter, to any parent, relative or friend of mine;

6. To supervise, compromise, enforce, arbitrate, defend or settle any claim by or against me arising out of property damages or personal injuries suffered by or caused by me, or under such circumstances that the loss resulting therefrom will, or may, fall on me; or to intervene in any action or proceeding relating thereto;

7. To continue payments incidental to my membership or affiliation in any church, club, society, order or other organization or to continue contributions thereto;

8. To demand, to receive, to obtain by action, proceeding or otherwise any money or other thing of value to which I am or may become or may claim to be entitled as salary, wages, commissions or other distributions upon any stock, or as interest or principal upon any indebtedness, or any periodic distribution of profits from any partnership or business in which I have or claim an interest, and to endorse, collect or otherwise realize upon any instrument for the payment so received;

9. To prepare, to execute and to file all joint or separate tax, social security, unemployment insurance and information returns for any years required by the laws of the United States, or of any state or subdivision thereof, or of any foreign government, to prepare, to execute and to file all other papers and instruments which Attorney shall think to be desirable or necessary for safeguarding me against excess or illegal taxation or against penalties imposed for claimed violation of any law or other governmental regulation, and to pay, to compromise, or to contest or to apply for refunds in connection with any taxes or assessments for which I am or may be liable, to consent to any gift for the gift tax purposes and to utilize any gift-splitting provision, or to make any tax election;

10. To execute, to acknowledge, to verify, to seal, to file and to deliver any application, consent, petition, notice release, waiver, agreement or other instrument which Attorney may think useful for the accomplishment of any of the purposes enumerated in this section;

11. To hire, to discharge and to compensate any attorney, accountant, expert witness or other assistant(s) where Attorney shall think such action to be desirable for the proper execution by Attorney of any of the powers described in this section, and for the keeping of needed records thereof;

12. To employ and compensate medical personnel including physicians, surgeons, dentists, medical specialists, nurses and paramedical assistants deemed by Attorney needful for the proper care, custody and control of my person and to do so without liability for any neglect, omission, misconduct or

fault of any such physician or other medical personnel, provided such physician or other medical personnel were selected and retained with reasonable care, and to dismiss any such persons at any time, with or without cause;

13. To authorize any and all kinds of medical procedures and treatment including but not limited to medication, therapy, surgical procedures and dental care, and to consent to all such treatment and medical procedures where such consent is required; to obtain the use of medical equipment, devices or other equipment and devices deemed by Attorney needful for proper care, custody and control of my person and to do so without liability for any neglect, omission, misconduct or fault with respect to such medical treatment or other matters authorized herein;

14. To apply for, elect, receive, deposit and utilize on my behalf all benefits payable by any governmental body or agency, state, federal, county, city or other, and to obtain, make claim upon, collect and dispose of insurance and insurance proceeds for my care, custody and control;

15. To house (or provide for housing), support and maintain any animals which I own and to contract for and pay the expenses of proper veterinary care and treatment for such animals, or if the care and maintenance of such animals shall become unreasonably expensive in Attorney's opinion, to dispose of such animals;

16. To deposit in my name and for my account, with any bank, banker or trust company or any building or savings and loan association or any other banking or similar institution, all monies to which I am entitled or which may come into Attorney's hands as such attorney-in-fact, and all bills of exchange, drafts, checks, promissory notes and other securities for money payable belonging to me, and for that purpose to sign my name and endorse each and every such instrument for deposit or collection; and from time to time, or at any time, to withdraw any or all monies deposited to my credit at any bank, banker or trust company or any building or savings and loan association or any other banking or similar institution having monies belonging to me, and, in connection therewith, to draw checks or to make withdrawals in my name; to make, do, execute, acknowledge and deliver, for and upon my behalf and in my name, all such checks, notes and contracts;

17. To endorse, receive, deposit and/or collect checks payable to my order drawn on the Treasurer or other fiscal officer or depository of the United States, or any sovereign state or authority, or any political subdivision or instrumentality thereof, or any private person, firm, corporation or partnership;

18. To have access at any time or times to any safe deposit box rented by me, wheresoever located, and to remove all or any part of the contents thereof, and to surrender or relinquish said safe deposit box, and any institution in which any such safe deposit box may be located shall not incur any liability to me or my estate as a result of permitting Attorney to exercise this power;

19. To borrow money and to encumber, mortgage or pledge any and all of my property in connection with the exercise of any power vested in Attorney;

20. To purchase for my benefit and in my behalf United States Government bonds redeemable at par in payment of United States estate taxes imposed at my death upon my estate;

21. To make advance arrangements for funeral services, including, but not limited to, purchase of a burial plot and marker and such other and related arrangements for services, flowers, ministerial services, transportation and other necessary, related, convenient or appropriate goods and services as my Attorney shall deem advisable or appropriate under the circumstances.

ARTICLE II

Termination, Amendment, Resignation and Removal

§A. *Power Not Affected by Principal's Incapacity*

This Power of Attorney shall not be affected by physical disability or mental incompetence of the principal which renders the principal incapable of managing his own estate. It is my intent that the

4

authority conferred herein shall be exercisable notwithstanding my physical disability or mental incompetence.

§B. Termination and Amendment

This Power of Attorney shall remain in full force and effect until the earlier of the following events: (i) Attorney has resigned as provided herein; (ii) I have revoked this Power of Attorney by written instrument recorded in the public records of the county aforesaid; or (iii) a committee shall have been appointed for me by a court of competent jurisdiction. This Power of Attorney may be amended by me at any time and from time to time but such amendment shall not be effective as to third persons dealing with Attorney without notice of such amendment unless such amendment shall have been recorded in the public records of the county aforesaid.

§C. Resignation

In the event that Attorney shall become unable or unwilling to serve or continue to serve, then Attorney may resign by delivering to me in writing a copy of his resignation and recording the original in the public records of the county aforesaid. Upon such resignation and recording, Attorney shall thereupon be divested of all authority under this Power of Attorney.

§D. Removal

Any person named herein as Attorney may be removed by written instrument executed by me and recorded in the public records of the county aforesaid.

ARTICLE III
Incidental Powers and Binding Effect

In connection with the exercise of the powers herein described, Attorney is fully authorized and empowered to perform any other acts or things necessary, appropriate, or incidental thereto, with the same validity and effect as if I were personally present, competent and personally exercised the powers myself. All acts lawfully done by Attorney hereunder during any period of my disability or mental incompetence shall have the same effect and inure to the benefit of and bind me and my heirs, devises, legatees and personal representatives as if I were mentally competent and not disabled. The powers herein conferred may be exercised by Attorney alone and the signature or act of Attorney on my behalf may be accepted by third persons as fully authorized by me and with the same force and effect as if done under my hand and seal and as if I were present in person, acting on my own behalf and competent. No person who may act in reliance upon the representations of Attorney for the scope of authority granted to Attorney shall incur any liability to me or to my estate as a result of permitting Attorney to exercise any power, nor shall any person dealing with Attorney be responsible to determine or insure the proper application of funds or property.

ARTICLE IV
Miscellaneous

§A. Exculpation

Attorney, Attorney's heirs, successors and assigns are hereby released and forever discharged from any and all liability upon any claim or demand of any nature whatsoever by me, my heirs or assigns, the beneficiaries under my Will or under any trust which I have created or shall hereafter create or any person whomsoever on account of any failure to act as Attorney pursuant to this Power of Attorney.

§B. Definitions

Whenever the word "Attorney" or "Principal" or any modifying or substituted pronoun therefor is used in this Power of Attorney, such words and respective pronouns shall be held and taken to include both the singular and the plural, the masculine, feminine and neuter gender thereof.

§C. Severability

If any part of any provision of this Power of Attorney shall be invalid or unenforceable under applicable law, said part shall be ineffective to the extent of such invalidity only, without in any way affecting the remaining parts of said provision or the remaining provisions of this Power of Attorney.

§D. Compensation

Attorney shall be entitled to reimbursement for all reasonable costs and expenses actually incurred and paid by Attorney on my behalf pursuant to any provision of this Power of Attorney.

§E. Restrictions

Notwithstanding any provision herein to the contrary, Attorney shall not satisfy the legal obligations of Attorney out of any property subject to this Power of Attorney, nor may Attorney exercise this power in favor of Attorney, Attorney's estate, Attorney's creditors or the creditors of Attorney's estate.

§F. Reservations

Notwithstanding any provision hereto to the contrary, Attorney shall have no power or authority whatsoever with respect to (a) any policy of insurance owned by me on the life of Attorney, and (b) any trust created by Attorney as to which I am a trustee.

IN WITNESS WHEREOF, as Principal, I have executed this Power of Attorney as of this _____ day of _____, 19____, in multiple counter-part originals and I have directed that photographic copies of this Power be made which shall have the same force and effect as an original.

_____ (Seal)
Principal

STATE OF SOUTH CAROLINA   )
)   **ATTESTATION**

COUNTY OF _____)

       The foregoing Power of Attorney was made this _____ day of _____,
19____, signed, sealed, published and declared by the Principal as the Principal's appointment and empowerment of an attorney-in-fact, in the presence of us who at the Principal's request and in the Principal's presence and in the presence of each other, have hereunto subscribed our names as witnesses hereto.

_____ of

_____

_____ of

_____

_____ of

_____

STATE OF SOUTH CAROLINA   )
)   **PROBATE**

COUNTY OF _____)

       Personally appeared deponent and made oath that deponent saw the within named Principal sign, seal and as the Principal's act and deed deliver the within Power of Attorney and that deponent, with the other witnesses whose names are subscribed above, witnessed the execution thereof.

_____

SWORN to before me this _____ day

of _____, 19____.

_____ (Seal)

Notary Public for South Carolina

My Commission Expires: _____

Durable Power of Attorney
(South Carolina)

Explanation

The explanations that follow should provide you with a clear understanding of the terms used in the Durable Power of Attorney form for the State of South Carolina.

Introduction: At the top left, after "STATE OF SOUTH CAROLINA" and "COUNTY OF," goes the name of your county. Below that you would fill in your name and address (you are the "principal," the person making the durable power of attorney).

The next lines are for the name and address of the person to whom you are giving the durable power of attorney (called the "agent" or "attorney").

Article I: The following lettered clauses specify broad powers providing your attorney with wide latitude to manage your financial affairs. Powers are separately enumerated to avoid any questions about whether you intended to authorize your attorney to undertake specific actions on your behalf. In addition, the introductory paragraph to Article I indicates that your durable power of attorney can be used whether you are competent or incompetent.

Article II: Section A is *crucial* to making your power of attorney *durable*, so that it remains valid at the time you will need it most—during your incapacity.

Section B specifies that your durable power of attorney will remain in effect until your attorney resigns, you revoke it in a writing that is properly recorded, or a committee is appointed for you by a court. Amendments also are not effective unless they are properly recorded.

Sections C and D set forth the procedure for withdrawal or removal of your attorney.

Article III: The first sentence is a catchall provision authorizing your attorney to do anything you could do.

Article III also provides assurance to third parties, such as banks and insurance companies, that they may rely on actions taken by your attorney under the durable power of attorney.

Article IV: Section A says that your attorney will not be liable to anyone for failing to act as attorney under the durable power of attorney.

Section B is just a definitional section.

Section C says that if any part of the durable power of attorney is held by a court to be invalid, the rest of the document would remain valid.

Section D provides reimbursement for your attorney's costs.

Section E makes it clear that your attorney is to take action under the durable power of attorney only on your behalf, not on his or her own behalf.

Section F says that your attorney cannot take actions concerning insurance that you own on the life of the attorney or a trust created by the attorney for which you are a trustee.

Finally, you would sign and date the document at the end before three witnesses and a notary, who must sign and date the document too. The witnesses would also provide their addresses.

STATUTORY DURABLE POWER OF ATTORNEY

NOTICE: THE POWERS GRANTED BY THIS DOCUMENT ARE BROAD AND SWEEPING. THEY ARE EXPLAINED IN THE DURABLE POWER OF ATTORNEY ACT, CHAPTER XII, TEXAS PROBATE CODE. IF YOU HAVE ANY QUESTIONS ABOUT THESE POWERS, OBTAIN COMPETENT LEGAL ADVICE. THIS DOCUMENT DOES NOT AUTHORIZE ANYONE TO MAKE MEDICAL AND OTHER HEALTH-CARE DECISIONS FOR YOU. YOU MAY REVOKE THIS POWER OF ATTORNEY IF YOU LATER WISH TO DO SO.

I, _____ (insert your name and address), my social security number being _____ (insert your proper Social Security number), appoint _____ (insert the name and address of the person appointed) as my agent (attorney-in-fact) to act for me in any lawful way with respect to the following initialed subjects:

TO GRANT ALL OF THE FOLLOWING POWERS, INITIAL THE LINE IN FRONT OF (N) AND IGNORE THE LINES IN FRONT OF THE OTHER POWERS.

TO GRANT ONE OR MORE, BUT FEWER THAN ALL, OF THE FOLLOWING POWERS, INITIAL THE LINE IN FRONT OF EACH POWER YOU ARE GRANTING.

TO WITHHOLD A POWER, DO NOT INITIAL THE LINE IN FRONT OF IT. YOU MAY, BUT NEED NOT, CROSS OUT EACH POWER WITHHELD.

INITIAL:

_____ (A) real property transactions;
_____ (B) tangible personal property transactions;
_____ (C) stock and bond transactions;
_____ (D) commodity and option transactions;
_____ (E) banking and other financial institution transactions;
_____ (F) business operating transactions;
_____ (G) insurance and annuity transactions;
_____ (H) estate, trust, and other beneficiary transactions;
_____ (I) claims and litigation;
_____ (J) personal and family maintenance;
_____ (K) benefits from social security, Medicare, Medicaid, or other governmental programs or civil or military service;
_____ (L) retirement plan transactions;
_____ (M) tax matters;
_____ (N) ALL OF THE POWERS LISTED IN (A) THROUGH (M). YOU NEED NOT INITIAL ANY OTHER LINES IF YOU INITIAL LINE (N).

SPECIAL INSTRUCTIONS:

ON THE FOLLOWING LINES YOU MAY GIVE SPECIAL INSTRUCTIONS LIMITING OR EXTENDING THE POWERS GRANTED TO YOUR AGENT.

_____

_____

_____

_____

_____

UNLESS YOU DIRECT OTHERWISE ABOVE, THIS POWER OF ATTORNEY IS EFFECTIVE IMMEDIATELY AND WILL CONTINUE UNTIL IT IS REVOKED.

CHOOSE ONE OF THE FOLLOWING ALTERNATIVES BY CROSSING OUT THE ALTERNATIVE NOT CHOSEN:

(A) This power of attorney is not affected by my subsequent disability or incapacity.
(B) This power of attorney becomes effective upon my disability or incapacity.

YOU SHOULD CHOOSE ALTERNATIVE (A) IF THIS POWER OF ATTORNEY IS TO BECOME EFFECTIVE ON THE DATE IT IS EXECUTED.

IF NEITHER (A) NOR (B) IS CROSSED OUT, IT WILL BE ASSUMED THAT YOU CHOSE ALTERNATIVE (A).

I agree that any third party who receives a copy of this document may act under it. Revocation of the durable power of attorney is not effective as to a third party until the third party receives actual notice of the revocation. I agree to indemnify the third party for any claims that arise against the third party because of reliance on this power of attorney.

If any agent named by me dies, becomes legally disabled, resigns, or refuses to act, I name the following (each to act alone and successively, in the order named) as successor(s) to that agent: _____

_____

Signed this _____ day of _____, 19____.

_____
(your signature)

State of _____)
) SS:
County of _____)

This document was acknowledged before me on _____
(date) by _____ (name of principal).

_____
(signature of notarial officer)
(Seal, if any, of notary)

_____
(printed name of notary)

My commission expires:

_____

THE ATTORNEY IN FACT OR AGENT, BY ACCEPTING OR ACTING UNDER THE APPOINTMENT, ASSUMES THE FIDUCIARY AND OTHER LEGAL RESPONSIBILITIES OF AN AGENT.

Statutory Durable Power of Attorney
(Texas)

Explanation

The explanations that follow should provide you with a clear understanding of the terms used in the Statutory Durable Power of Attorney form for the State of Texas.

Notice: The notice confirms what the book has already stated: the powers given to your agent(s) (attorney[s]-in-fact) are broad. Read the notice carefully.

Paragraph 1: The first blank line is for your name and address, followed by your social security number. The next line is for the name and address of the person to whom you are giving the durable power of attorney (called the "agent" or "attorney-in-fact").

Paragraph 2. The following lettered clauses specify broad powers providing your agent(s) with wide latitude to manage your affairs. Powers are separately enumerated to avoid any questions about whether you intended to authorize your agent(s) to undertake specific actions on your behalf. If you choose not to give all of these powers to your agent(s), you would leave blank and draw a line through the powers that you want to exclude.

Line A: This line gives your agent(s) broad authority to mortgage, sell, buy, accept, manage, lease, and/or otherwise deal with real estate, including your home.

Line B: This line permits your agent(s) broad authority to buy, sell, manage, receive, mortgage, lease, and/or otherwise handle transactions involving items of personal property.

Line C: This line lets your agent(s) invest in securities on your behalf and manage, receive, sell, mortgage, and/or otherwise handle stocks and bonds for you. This is broad enough to allow your agent(s) to vote at stockholders meetings.

Line D: This line lets your agent(s) invest in commodities and options on your behalf and manage, sell, receive, mortgage, and/or otherwise handle commodities and options for you.

Line E: This line authorizes your agent(s) to handle banking transactions, including opening and managing accounts, CDs, and other instruments in financial institutions, signing checks, making withdrawals, and having access to your safe-deposit box.

Line F: This line allows your agent(s) to engage in any business transactions for you.

Line G: This line authorizes your agent(s) to handle any insurance and annuity matters for you, including obtaining, managing, maintaining, or terminating insurance and annuities, paying premiums, and obtaining benefits for you.

Line H: This line permits your agent(s) to act for you with respect to estate, trust, and other beneficiary matters, including establishing trusts, receiving inheritances, and participating in the administration of estates.

Line I: This line gives your agent(s) the right to handle claims and litigation for you, including bringing a lawsuit for you, defending you against claims, and settling disputes for you.

Line J: This line authorizes your agent(s) to handle your personal and family affairs, to take steps to provide for the support and welfare of your family, and to maintain your relationships with family, friends, and organizations.

Line K: This line enables your agent(s) to handle any matters you may have with government benefits and/or programs, including making and receiving proceeds of any claims and maximizing benefits from government programs.

Line L: This line allows your agent(s) to handle retirement plan transactions for you, including selecting payment options, making or changing beneficiary designations, making contributions and rollovers, and borrowing from retirement plans.

Line M: This line gives your agent(s) authority to deal with your taxes. Although you might prefer to forget about this, it's important that tax forms be prepared and taxes paid, to avoid possible problems.

Line N: This line is a catchall authorizing your agent(s) to do all of the tasks listed above.

Special Instructions Paragraph: In the space that follows you would add any other provisions or limitations—but if you do this, make sure your additions or changes comply with the law.

Next Paragraph: These lines are *crucial* to making your power of attorney *durable,* so that it remains valid at the time you will need it the most—during your incapacity. To make it durable, and to make it effective immediately, you would keep line (A) and cross out line (B).

Some banks and insurance companies have been unwilling to accept or act on any power of attorney form that they did not prepare themselves. The next language attempts to deal with this problem. The language should protect third parties relying on the document and, it is hoped, encourage them to accept it.

The next paragraph allows you to name successor agents in case your first choice cannot serve. It is usually a good idea to name one or two successors.

Finally, you would sign and date the document at the end before a notary. The notary fills in and signs the bottom portion. A notary is authorized by the state or federal government to administer oaths and attest to the authenticity of signatures.

STATUTORY POWER OF ATTORNEY

NOTICE: THIS IS AN IMPORTANT DOCUMENT. BEFORE SIGNING THIS DOCUMENT, YOU SHOULD KNOW THESE IMPORTANT FACTS. THE PURPOSE OF THIS POWER OF ATTORNEY IS TO GIVE THE PERSON WHOM YOU DESIGNATE (YOUR "AGENT") BROAD POWERS TO HANDLE YOUR PROPERTY, WHICH MAY INCLUDE POWERS TO PLEDGE, SELL OR OTHERWISE DISPOSE OF ANY REAL OR PERSONAL PROPERTY WITHOUT ADVANCE NOTICE TO YOU OR APPROVAL BY YOU. THE POWERS WILL EXIST EVEN AFTER YOU BECOME DISABLED, INCAPACITATED OR INCOMPETENT UNLESS YOU STRIKE THAT PROVISION. THE POWERS THAT YOU GIVE YOUR AGENT ARE EXPLAINED MORE FULLY IN SECTION 243.10 OF THE WISCONSIN STATUTES. THIS DOCUMENT DOES NOT AUTHORIZE ANYONE TO MAKE MEDICAL OR OTHER HEALTH-CARE DECISIONS FOR YOU. IF THERE IS ANYTHING ABOUT THIS FORM THAT YOU DO NOT UNDERSTAND, YOU SHOULD ASK A LAWYER TO EXPLAIN IT TO YOU.

I, _____ (insert your name and address), appoint _____ (insert the name and address of the person appointed, or of each person appointed, if you want to designate more than one) as my agent to act for me in any lawful way with respect to the powers initialed below. If the person or persons appointed are unable or unwilling to act as my agent, I appoint _____ (insert name and address of alternate person appointed) to act for me in any lawful way with respect to the powers initialed below.

TO GRANT ONE OR MORE OF THE FOLLOWING POWERS, INITIAL THE LINE IN FRONT OF EACH POWER YOU ARE GRANTING.

TO WITHHOLD A POWER, DO NOT INITIAL THE LINE IN FRONT OF IT. YOU MAY, BUT NEED NOT, CROSS OUT EACH POWER WITHHELD.

INITIALS:

_____ 1. Real property transactions.
_____ 2. Tangible personal property transactions.
_____ 3. Stock and bond transactions.
_____ 4. Commodity and option transactions.
_____ 5. Banking and other financial institution transactions.
_____ 6. Business operating transactions.
_____ 7. Insurance and annuity transactions.
_____ 8. Estate, trust, and other beneficiary transactions.
_____ 9. Claims and litigation.
_____ 10. Personal and family maintenance.
_____ 11. Benefits from social security, medicare, medicaid or other governmental programs, or military service.
_____ 12. Retirement plan transactions.
_____ 13. Tax matters.

SPECIAL INSTRUCTIONS:

ON THE FOLLOWING LINES YOU MAY GIVE SPECIAL INSTRUCTIONS LIMITING OR EXTENDING THE POWERS GRANTED TO YOUR AGENT.

_____

_____

_____

This power of attorney will become effective (immediately) (when I become disabled, incapacitated or incompetent). **STRIKE THROUGH ONE.**

I agree that any third party who receives a copy of this document may act under it. Revocation of the power of attorney is not effective as to a third party until the third party learns of the revocation. I agree to reimburse the third party for any loss resulting from claims that arise against the third party because of reliance on this power of attorney.

Signed this _____ day of _____, 19____.

_____
(Your Signature)

_____
(Your Social Security Number)

State of _____)
) SS:
County of _____)

This document was acknowledged before me on _____ (date) by _____ (name of principal).

_____
(Signature of Notarial Officer)
(Seal, if any)

_____
(Title)
My commission expires: _____

BY ACCEPTING OR ACTING UNDER THE APPOINTMENT, THE AGENT ASSUMES THE FIDUCIARY AND OTHER LEGAL RESPONSIBILITIES OF AN AGENT.

Statutory Power of Attorney
(Wisconsin)

Explanation

The explanations that follow should provide you with a clear understanding of the terms used in Wisconsin's Statutory Power of Attorney form.

Notice: The notice confirms what the book has already stated: the powers given to your agent(s) (attorney[s]-in-fact) are broad. Read the notice carefully.

Paragraph 1: On the first blank line go your name and address. The next line is for the name(s) and address(es) of the person(s) to whom you are giving the power of attorney (called the "agent[s]" or "attorney[s]-in-fact"). You may also name one or more successor agent(s) in case your first choice(s) cannot serve.

Paragraph 2: The following numbered clauses specify broad powers providing your agent(s) with wide latitude to manage your affairs. Powers are separately enumerated to avoid any question about whether you intended to authorize your agent(s) to undertake specific actions on your behalf. If you choose not to give all of these powers to your agent(s), you would leave blank and draw a line through the powers you want to exclude.

Line 1: This line gives your agent(s) broad authority to mortgage, sell, buy, accept, manage, lease, and/or otherwise deal with real estate, including your home.

Line 2: This line permits your agent(s) broad authority to buy, sell, manage, receive, mortgage, lease, and/or otherwise handle transactions involving items of personal property.

Line 3: This line lets your agent(s) invest in securities on your behalf and manage, receive, sell, mortgage, and/or otherwise handle stocks and bonds for you. This is broad enough to allow your agent(s) to vote at stockholders meetings.

Line 4: This line lets your agent(s) invest in commodities and options on your behalf and manage, sell, receive, and/or otherwise handle commodities and options for you.

Line 5: This line authorizes your agent(s) to handle banking transactions, including opening and managing accounts, CDs, and other instruments in financial institutions, signing checks, making withdrawals, and having access to your safe-deposit box.

Line 6: This line allows your agent(s) to engage in any business transactions for you.

Line 7: This line authorizes your agent(s) to handle any insurance and annuity matters for you, including obtaining, managing, maintaining, or terminating insurance and annuities, paying premiums, and obtaining benefits for you.

Line 8: This line permits your agent(s) to act for you with respect to estate, trust, and other beneficiary matters, including establishing trusts, receiving inheritances, and participating in the administration of estates.

Line 9: This line give your agent(s) the right to handle claims and litigation for you, including bringing a lawsuit for you, defending you against claims, and settling disputes for you.

Line 10: This line authorizes your agent(s) to handle your personal and family affairs, to take steps to provide for the support and welfare of your family, and to maintain your relationships with family, friends, and organizations.

Line 11: This line enables your agent(s) to handle any matters you may have with government benefits and/or programs, including making and receiving proceeds of any claims and maximizing benefits from government programs.

Line 12: This line allows your agent(s) to handle retirement plan transactions for you, including selecting payment options, making or changing beneficiary designations, making contributions and rollovers, and borrowing from retirement plans.

Line 13: This line gives your agent(s) authority to deal with your taxes. Although you might prefer to forget about this, it's important that tax forms be prepared and taxes paid, to avoid possible problems.

Special Instructions Paragraph: In the space that follows, you would add any other provisions or limitations—but if you do this, make sure your additions or changes comply with the law.

Next Paragraph: The next line makes the durable power of attorney effective either immediately or only after you have become incapacitated (called springing)—see the discussion in the text, pages 89–90, on the pros and cons of each).

Some banks and insurance companies have been unwilling to accept or act on any power of attorney form that they did not prepare themselves. The next language attempts to deal with this problem. The language should protect third parties relying on the document and, it is hoped, encourage them to accept it.

Finally, you would sign and date the document at the end before a notary, and include your social security number. The notary fills in and signs the bottom portion. A notary is authorized by the state or federal government to administer oaths and attest to the authenticity of signatures.

Appendix B
Trusts

This Appendix includes examples of five different types of trusts used in connection with Medicaid planning; each is discussed in the text. The sample trust forms are for:

1. irrevocable asset protection trust
2. irrevocable house preservation trust
3. family asset protection trust (revocable)
4. family asset protection trust (irrevocable)
5. revocable declaration of trust (living trust)

Each of these is presented for illustration purposes only. These should *not* be used without first consulting with an experienced elder law or estate planning attorney. Following each form is an explanation section to help you understand what trusts are all about.

IRREVOCABLE TRUST AGREEMENT

THIS IRREVOCABLE TRUST AGREEMENT is entered into at _____
_____, _____, this _____ day of _____,
19____, by and between _____ of _____,
the Settlor, hereinafter referred to in the first person, and _____,
of _____, the Trustee, hereinafter referred
to sometimes as the "Trustee" and sometimes in the third person impersonal.

ARTICLE I

CREATION OF TRUST

A. Except as provided in Paragraph B of this Article I, this Trust Agreement shall be irrevocable, and I hereby expressly acknowledge that I shall have no right or power, either alone or in conjunction with others, and in any capacity whatsoever, to alter, amend, modify, revoke or terminate this Trust or any of the terms of this Trust Agreement in whole or in part, or otherwise to cause any of the assets of the Trust to revert to me or to my estate.

B. I hereby transfer the property listed in Schedule A of this Trust Agreement to the Trustee. The property and all proceeds, investments and reinvestments thereof and any property hereinafter received by the Trustee from me, my **[wife/husband]**, _____,
or from any other person (such property being hereinafter referred to as the "trust estate") shall be held, administered and distributed in accordance with the terms of the trust herein expressed. I reserve to myself and to others the right to add property to the trust estate by lifetime or testamentary gifts, all of which added property shall be governed by the terms hereof.

ARTICLE II

DISTRIBUTIONS DURING LIFETIME OF SETTLOR

A. NOTWITHSTANDING ANY OTHER PROVISION OF THIS TRUST AGREEMENT, I AND/OR MY **[WIFE/HUSBAND]**, _____, SHALL NOT BE A TRUSTEE OR BENEFICIARY OF THIS TRUST AGREEMENT AND I AND/OR MY **[WIFE/HUSBAND]**, _____, SHALL NOT HAVE ANY LEGAL TITLE OR INTEREST IN THE ASSETS OF THIS TRUST AGREEMENT. THE TRUSTEE IS ABSOLUTELY PROHIBITED FROM MAKING ANY PAYMENTS OF INCOME OR PRINCIPAL TO OR FOR MY BENEFIT OR THE BENEFIT OF MY **[WIFE/HUSBAND]**, _____.

B. The Trust may distribute to or for the benefit of the members of a class composed of my children and issue (living from time to time, of whatever degree and whenever born), out of the net income or principal or both of the trust estate being held hereunder, such amount or amounts (whether the whole or a lesser amount) which shall be necessary to provide for the maintenance, support, health and education of such persons. It is my intention that distributions under this Paragraph B shall be made to or for the benefit of the members of said class in accordance with the maintenance, support, health and educational requirements affecting them individually. It is not my intention to require that the dollar distributions made under this Paragraph B to or for the benefit of each of such members shall be equal, and the Trustee is authorized, in accordance with the provisions of this Paragraph B, to make distributions of

1

principal hereunder to or for the benefit of one of such members to the exclusion of the other without any duty to equalize those distributions. At the end of each taxable year the Trustee shall add any undistributed income to the principal of the trust estate being held hereunder

ARTICLE III

DIVISION OF TRUST ESTATE UPON SETTLOR'S DEATH

Upon my death, the Trustee shall hold, administer and distribute the property held hereunder, as the same shall be constituted after being (a) augmented by property received or to be received by the Trustee as a consequence of my death, including, without limitation, any property received or to be received under the terms of my Last Will and Testament or any Codicil thereto and (b) depleted by any money disbursed by the Trustee pursuant to the provisions of Paragraph C of Article VI hereof (said property as so constituted being hereinafter referred to as "The Family Trust") in accordance with the following provisions of this Trust Agreement.

A. The Family Trust shall be distributed to or held for the benefit of such person or persons out of a class composed of my children and my children's issue (of whatever degree and whenever born), and in such amounts and proportions as I may appoint by my Last Will and Testament or any Codicil thereto; provided, however, anything herein to the contrary notwithstanding, such power of appointment granted under this Paragraph A shall not be exercised in favor of, or to or for the benefit of, me, my **[wife/husband]**, my estate, my **[wife's/husband's]** estate, my creditors, my **[wife's/husband's]** creditors, the creditors of my estate, or the creditors of my **[wife's/husband's]** estate; provided, further, however, that in order for the exercise by me of said power of appointment to be effective, I must exercise such power by specific reference to this Trust Agreement in the provision of my Last Will and Testament or such Codicil. In the event that I fail to exercise such power of appointment, or insofar as any such appointment shall be void or shall not take effect, then the Trustee shall hold, administer and distribute the Family Trust, or any part thereof not effectively appointed by me, pursuant to the provisions of Paragraphs B and C of this Article III.

B. The Trustee shall distribute that part of the Family Trust, if any, that remains after giving effect to the provisions of Paragraph A of this Article III, in equal shares, to my children who survive me, treating as a surviving child of mine for this purpose the collective issue surviving me of any child of mine who shall have predeceased me, the distribution to such issue to be *per stirpes,* the root of the *per stirpes* distribution to be such predeceased child.

C. If, under the provisions of Paragraphs A or B of this Article III, any portion of The Family Trust shall become distributable to any person who is then under the age of twenty-one (21) years, then such portion shall be retained by the Trustee in trust for the benefit of such person. The Trustee shall distribute to or for the benefit of such person out of the net income or principal or both of such portion held for such person, such amount or amounts (whether the whole or a lesser amount) as the Trustee, in its sole discretion, deems necessary or proper suitably to provide for the maintenance, support, health, and education of such person, and shall from time to time add to the principal of such portion the remaining undistributed income, if any, until such person shall attain the age of twenty-one (21) years, whereupon the Trustee shall distribute all of such portion to such person. If such person shall die prior to receiving the complete distribution of the portion held for such person's benefit, such portion shall be distributed free of the trust to such person's estate.

D. If at the time for distribution of The Family Trust or any share or portion of the trust estate being held pursuant to this Article III, there is no person or person's estate entitled under the provisions of this Article III other than this Paragraph D to take such distribution, the Trustee shall divide the trust estate into two (2) equal shares. One such share shall be distributed free of the trust to such person or persons as would be entitled to inherit from me and in the proportions they would so inherit under the laws of the State of _____ as though I had died intestate and domiciled in the State of _____ at the time distribution is so to be made. The other such share shall be distributed free of the trust to such person or persons as would be entitled to inherit from my said **[wife/husband]** and in the proportions they would so inherit under the laws of the State of _____ as though **[she/he]** had died intestate and domiciled in the State of _____ at the time distribution is so to be made.

      E. Notwithstanding any other provisions, in no event shall the Trustee pay any amount to me and/or my **[wife/husband]**. If the Trustee is authorized pursuant to the provision of this Article III to make distributions or payments to or for the benefit of any person (including distributions or payments directed or permitted to be made to a person who is under legal disability or, in the reasonable opinion of the Trustee, is unable properly to administer such distributions or payments), the Trustee may make such distributions or payments in any one or more of the following ways, as the Trustee may deem advisable: (1) directly to such beneficiary; (2) to the legal guardian of such beneficiary; (3) to any custodian then serving for such beneficiary, or to any person designated by the Trustee to serve as a custodian for such beneficiary (any such custodian may be the Trustee); or (4) by the Trustee itself expending such income or principal for the benefit of such beneficiary. The Trustee shall not be required to see to the application of any distribution or payment so made, but the receipt of any of the persons mentioned in Clause (1), (2) or (3) in the immediately preceding sentence shall be a full discharge for the Trustee.

      F. No interest whatsoever in the principal and/or income of any trust estate subject to the provision of Articles II or III shall be alienated, disposed of, or in any manner assigned or encumbered by the person for whom held, voluntarily or involuntarily, while such principal and/or income is in the possession or control of the Trustee. If, by reason of any act of any such person or by operation of law, or by the happening of any event, or for any other reason except by an act of the Trustee specifically authorized hereunder, any such principal and/or income of such trust would but for this Paragraph F cease to be enjoyed by any such person or, by reason of an attempt by any such person to alienate, charge, assign or encumber any of such principal and/or income of such trust, or by reason of the bankruptcy or insolvency of any such person, or by reason of any attachment, garnishment or other proceedings, based upon a valid court judgment, or by reason of any order, finding or judgment of any court either at law or in equity, any of the principal and/or income of such trust would but for this Paragraph F vest in or be enjoyed by some individual, firm or corporation otherwise than as provided herein, then, in any of such events, the trust created for the benefit of such person shall forthwith cease and determine as to such person, who shall thereupon cease to be a beneficiary of such trust **and such person shall be ineligible to serve or to continue to serve as Trustee hereunder.** For purposes of this Paragraph F, the exercise of any power of appointment granted herein or the exercise of any disclaimer by a beneficiary of any rights or benefits under this Trust Agreement shall not cause or result in the provisions of this Paragraph F becoming applicable. Such trust thereafter, subject to all other applicable provisions of this Trust Agreement, shall, during the life of such former beneficiary, be held by the Trustee which, until such former beneficiary's death, may pay to or expend for the benefit of such former beneficiary, out of the principal and/or income of such trust, such sums but such sums only as the Trustee in its absolute discretion may determine, retaining any undistributed principal and/or income until such former beneficiary's death; provided, however, that no payments made under these provisions to or for the benefit of such former beneficiary shall exceed the amounts otherwise payable to such former beneficiary if these provisions had not been invoked. Any undistributed income shall from time to time be added to the principal of such trust. Upon the death of such former beneficiary, such trust as then constituted, including all accrued and undistributed income, shall, subject to all applicable provisions of this Trust Agreement, be distributed to the persons (determined as of the date of death of such former beneficiary) to whom such trust estate would have been so distributable as if such former beneficiary had died prior to the time for any mandatory distribution of the trust estate to such former beneficiary, and as if the provisions of this Paragraph F had never become applicable to the trust of such former beneficiary; provided, however, that for this purpose, if such former beneficiary has a power of appointment over any portion or all of the trust estate, such power of appointment shall be deemed not to have been exercised and the Trustee shall distribute the trust estate in accordance with the provisions of this Trust Agreement notwithstanding any attempted exercise of such power of appointment by said former beneficiary.

G. Any provisions of this Trust Agreement to the contrary notwithstanding, if not already distributed, all accrued and undistributed income and the entire principal of every trust estate then held hereunder shall be paid over and distrusted outright and free of the trust not later than the end of the day immediately preceding the expiration of twenty-one (21) years from and after the death of the last survivor of myself, my said **[wife/husband],** my children and my children's issue living at the date of the execution of this Trust Agreement. Such payment and distribution shall be made to the person or persons for whose benefit the trust estate or estates respectively shall then be held hereunder; provided, however, that if at the time the trust estates are to be distributed pursuant to this Paragraph G, the provisions of the immediately preceding Paragraph F of this Article III shall be in operation as to any such trust, such trust shall be distributed to those persons who would have been entitled to receive such trust as if the former beneficiary for whose benefit such trust was originally created had died immediately preceding the time so provided for such distribution and possessed of said trust estate, such distribution to be outright and free of the trust.

ARTICLE IV

DEFINITIONS

A. The words "issue," "child" and "children," as used herein, shall be deemed to include any legally adopted person as if he or she were the natural child of the adopting parent.

B. Whenever the context so requires, the use of words herein in the singular shall be construed to include the plural, and words in the plural, the singular, and words whether in the masculine, feminine or neuter gender shall be construed to include all of said genders.

C. For purposes of this Trust Agreement, the term "marketable securities" refers to any share of stock in any corporation, certificate of stock or interest in any corporation, note, bond, debenture, or evidence of indebtedness, or any evidence of an interest in or right to subscribe to or purchase any of the foregoing, which are readily tradeable on an established market.

D. For purposes of this Trust Agreement, the word "income" *does* include recognized gains from the sale, exchange or conversion of "marketable securities" but does *not* include any other gains from the sale, exchange or conversion of any other property which are properly allocated to the trust corpus.

E. For purposes of this Trust Agreement, the phrase "net income" refers to "income" as defined above less expenses incurred by the Trustee for management of the trust estate.

F. For purposes of this Trust Agreement, any individual shall be deemed to be unable to continue to serve as Trustee hereunder only when:

1. Such individual's attending physician and at least one other physician licensed in the United States (or, if such individual does not have an attending physician, at least two physicians licensed in the United States) shall have signed and delivered to the Trustee then serving hereunder (or, if such Trustee is the person who is deemed to be unable to continue to serve as Trustee hereunder, then to any fiduciary serving hereunder or to the person who is to succeed such individual as Trustee) their written statements indicating that such individual is incapable in their judgment of attending effectively to such individual's fiduciary duties by reason of mental or physical disability; provided, that the written statements to which reference is made above shall be acknowledged before a notary public and witnessed by two individuals; provided, further, that any person relying on any such written statements by such physicians may presume that the

identity and qualifications of the physicians signing any such statement are in fact who and what they purport to be and such person shall not have any duty to make further inquiry or investigation beyond the review of each written statement itself; provided, further, that no person relying on such written statement shall be liable to any other person or persons for action taken in reliance on such written statement; or

2. Such individual is adjudicated incompetent.

ARTICLE V

POWERS AND DUTIES OF THE TRUSTEE

A. 1. There shall be no duty on the Trustee to pay or see to the payment of any premiums on any policies of life insurance or to take any steps to keep them in force, until such time as the Trustee holds title to any insurance policies hereunder as a part of the corpus of any trust estate. The Trustee furthermore assumes no responsibility with respect to the validity or enforceability of said policies. However, as soon as practicable after receiving notice of the death of the insured under any of such policies, the Trustee shall proceed to collect all amounts payable thereunder. The Trustee shall have full and complete authority to collect and receive any and all such amounts and its receipt therefore shall be a full and complete acquittance to any insurer or payor, who shall be under no obligation to see to the proper application thereof by the Trustee.

2. There shall be no duty on the Trustee to make non-income producing property productive or to convert such property to income producing property.

B. In the administration of the trust created hereunder and in addition to the powers exercised by trustees generally, the Trustee shall have the following powers and authorities without any court order or proceeding, exercisable in the discretion of the Trustee:

1. To purchase as an investment for the trust estate or estates any property, real or personal, belonging to my estate and/or the estate of my **[wife/husband]**, _____;

2. To retain as suitable investments for the trust estate or estates any properties (including, without limitation, securities issued by any corporate Trustee or the holding company of which it is an affiliate) received by it from me, my said **[wife/husband]**, my estate and/or the estate of my said **[wife/husband]**, and whether received by purchase or in any other manner, without regard to any law, statutory or judicial, or any rule or practice of court now or hereafter in force specifying or limiting the permissible investments of trustees, trust companies or fiduciaries generally or requiring the diversification of investments, and without liability to any person whomsoever for loss or depreciation in value thereof;

3. To sell, exchange, convey, mortgage, pledge, lease, control, and manage, and to make contracts concerning, any of the properties, real or personal, comprised in the trust estate or estates, all either publicly or privately and for such considerations and upon such terms as to credit or otherwise as may be reasonable under the circumstances, which leases and contracts may extend beyond the duration of any of the trust created hereunder; to give options therefore; and to execute deeds, transfers, mortgages, leases and other instruments of any kind;

4. To invest and reinvest the properties from time to time comprised in the trust estate or estates in stocks, common and/or preferred, bonds, notes, debentures, loans, mort-

gages, common trust funds, or other securities or property, real or personal, all limitations now or hereafter imposed by law, statutory or judicial, or by any rule or practice of court now or hereafter in force specifying or limiting the permissible investments of trustees, trust companies or fiduciaries generally or requiring the diversification of investments, being hereby expressly waived, it being the intent hereof that the Trustee shall have full power and authority to deal with the trust estate or estates in all respects as though it was the sole owner thereof, without order of court or other authority;

5. To borrow money, from itself or otherwise, with or without security, wherever it deems such action advisable;

6. To exercise voting rights, execute and deliver powers of attorney and proxies and similarly act with reference to shares of stock and other securities comprised in the trust estate or estates in such manner as it deems proper, including, without limitation, the power to participate in or oppose reorganizations, recapitalizations, mergers, consolidations, exchanges, liquidations, arrangements and other corporate actions;

7. To collect all money; in accordance with generally accepted trust accounting principles, to determine whether money or other property coming into its possession shall be treated as principal or income and to charge or apportion expenses, taxes, gains and losses to principal or income;

8. To compromise, adjust and settle claims in favor of or against the trust estate or estates upon such terms and conditions as it may deem best; in the case of any litigation in connection with any part of such trust estate or estates, it may, under advice of its counsel, arbitrate, settle, or adjust any such matter in dispute upon such terms as it may consider just and equitable, and its decision shall be binding upon the beneficiaries;

9. To employ investment counsel, custodians of estate property, brokers, accountants, attorneys, clerical or bookkeeping assistants, and other suitable agents and to pay their reasonable compensation and expenses in addition to any compensation payable to the Trustee, and to execute and deliver powers of attorney; the Trustee shall not be liable for any neglect, omission or wrongdoing of such investment counsel, custodians, brokers, accountants, attorneys, assistants or agents, provided reasonable care shall have been exercised in their selection;

10. To hold title to stock, bonds, or other securities or property, real or personal, in its own name or in the name of its nominee and without indication of any fiduciary capacity or to hold any such bonds or securities in bearer form; the Trustee shall assume full responsibility for the acts of any nominee selected by it;

11. To make all repairs, alterations or improvements of any real property which shall constitute a part of the trust estate or estates; adjust boundaries thereof, and to erect or demolish buildings thereon; and, with respect to such property, to convert for different use, grant easements for adequate consideration, partition, and insure for any or all risks;

12. To pay premiums on any policies of life insurance which may form a part of the trust estate or estates; to cancel, sell, assign, hypothecate, pledge or otherwise dispose of any of said policies; to exercise any right, election, option or privilege granted by any of said policies; to borrow any sums in accordance with the provisions of any of said policies, and to receive all payments, dividends, surrender values, additions, benefits or privileges of any kind which may accrue to any of said policies;

13. To make any allocation, division or distribution required or permitted hereunder in cash or in kind, in real or personal property, or an undivided interest therein, or partly in cash and partly in kind, and to do so without making pro rata allocations, divisions or distributions of specific assets, property allocated, divided or distributed in kind to be taken at its fair market value at the time of such allocation, division or distribution;

14. To receive, in accordance with the provisions of Article I hereof, additional property from me or any other person, the Trustee being authorized and empowered to merge and hold as one any duplicate trusts held for the same beneficiary;

15. To make such expenditures and do such other acts as are reasonably required to manage, improve, protect, preserve, invest or sell any of the trust estates or otherwise properly to administer this Trust.

C. 1. Subject to the limitations set forth in the provisions of the following Subparagraph 2 of this Paragraph C, if the representative of my estate, in such representative's sole discretion, shall determine that appropriate assets of my estate are not available in sufficient amount (or if there are no assets in my estate) to pay the expenses of administration of my estate (but not including my legal debts, my funeral expenses and the expenses of my last illness) and all death taxes chargeable to my estate, including interest and penalties thereon, the Trustee shall, upon the request of the representative of my estate, contribute from the principal of the trust estate the amount of such deficiency; and in connection with any such action the Trustee shall rely upon the written statement of the representative of my estate as to the validity and correctness of the amounts of any such taxes and expenses, and shall furnish funds to such representative so as to enable such representative to discharge the same, or to discharge any part or all thereof itself by making payment directly to the government official or agency or to the person entitled or claiming to be entitled to receive payment thereof. If the Trustee hereunder holds any property that is bequeathed under my Will (other than a residuary bequest), then the Trustee to the extent that such property is held under the Trust Agreement shall distribute such property to the persons entitled to receive such bequest under my Will (other than a residuary bequest) after the deduction, if any, of expenses and taxes to be charged to such bequest pursuant to the provisions of my Will. No consideration need be required by the Trustee from the representative of my estate for any disbursement made by the Trustee pursuant hereto, nor shall there be any obligation upon such representative to repay to the Trustee any of the funds disbursed by it hereunder, and all amounts disbursed by the Trustee pursuant to the authority hereby conferred upon it shall be disbursed without any right in or duty upon the Trustee to seek or obtain contribution or reimbursement from any person or property on account of such payment. The Trustee shall not be responsible for the application of any funds delivered by it to the representative of my estate pursuant to the authority herein granted, nor shall the Trustee be subject to liability to any beneficiary hereunder on account of any payment made by it pursuant to the provisions hereof.

2. Any provisions of this Article V to the contrary notwithstanding, under no circumstances shall the Trustee make any disbursements pursuant to this Paragraph C from (a) assets which are excluded from my gross estate for purposes of the Federal estate tax payable by reason of my death or (b) assets which are not subject to a state inheritance, state estate or other state death tax imposed by reason of my death; provided, however, that assets described in Clause (b) of this sentence (so long as they do not constitute assets described in Clause (a) of this sentence) may be used to the extent that other assets which are included in my gross estate for purposes of Federal estate tax payable by reason of my death and subject to a state inheritance, state estate or other state death tax imposed by reason of my death shall be insufficient to satisfy the Trustee's obligation hereunder.

D. The Trustee shall keep accurate records showing all receipts and disbursements and other transactions involving the trust estate or estates and shall furnish annually to each beneficiary entitled to income (1) a statement of the receipts and disbursements affecting such beneficiary's interest in the trust, and (2) a complete inventory of the trust estate then held for the benefit of such beneficiary.

E. No person, firm or corporation dealing with the Trustee or a nominee of the Trustee or performing any act pursuant to action taken or order given by the Trustee or such nominee shall be obliged to inquire as to the propriety, validity or legality thereof hereunder, nor shall any such person be liable for the application of any money or other consideration paid to the Trustee or such nominee, but, instead, may rely upon any action taken by the Trustee or such nominee pursuant to the powers and authorities conferred upon it under the provisions of this Article V in all respects as if the same were completely unlimited. No transfer agent or registrar of any security held hereunder shall be required to inquire as to the propriety, validity or legality of any transfer made by the Trustee or such nominee.

 F. 1. I and my **[wife/husband]** shall not at any time serve as Trustee hereunder or have any legal title or interest in the trust estate. In the event that said _____ shall be willing or unable to continue to serve as Trustee hereunder, then my _____, _____, of _____, _____, shall serve as successor Trustee hereunder. In the event that both said _____ and said _____ shall be unwilling or unable to serve or continue to serve as Trustee hereunder, then _____, of _____, _____, shall serve as successor Trustee hereunder. Any Trustee shall be entitled to resign as Trustee for any reason whatsoever by giving written notice to the Trustee designated to succeed it, provided that the Trustee designated to succeed it shall first execute a formal written acceptance of the duties and obligations of the Trustee hereunder and file an executed copy of such acceptance with the preceding Trustee. After this is done, and when all sums then due from the trust estate to such predecessor Trustee have been paid, such predecessor Trustee shall transfer the Trust property then in its hands to such successor Trustee and such predecessor Trustee shall thereupon and thereby be discharged of all subsequent duties and obligations under or arising out of its trusteeship.

 2. Any successor Trustee shall have and enjoy all the powers, authorities, duties and immunities hereby vested in and imposed upon the original Trustee and no successor Trustee shall be obliged to inquire into or be in any way accountable for the previous administration of the trust property.

 G. My Trustee is authorized, in its discretion, to sell to, purchase from, borrow funds from, lend funds to, or otherwise deal with, upon such terms and conditions as my Trustee shall deem just and equitable and for full and adequate consideration, the Executor of the Last Will and Testament of myself or my said **[wife/husband]** or the Trustee of any Trust established by me or my said **[wife/husband]** (whether such Trust is a testamentary or inter vivos trust), even though my Trustee may also be serving as Executor under my Will or my said **[wife/husband]**'s Will or as Trustee under any such Trust established by me or by my said **[wife/husband]**.

 H. In determining the amount of any discretionary distributions of income or principal to a beneficiary of a trust created hereunder, the Trustee shall be required to take into account all other means and resources known to or reasonably ascertainable by the Trustee, including Medicaid or any other form of government assistance, which are available to such beneficiary for the purposes for which the Trustee is authorized to make said distributions.

 I. Any Trustee shall be entitled to receive reasonable compensation. Any Trustee shall be entitled to be reimbursed for reasonable expenses it incurs which are necessary to carry out its duties as Trustee hereunder.

 J. No bond shall be required of the Trustee hereunder or any successor Trustee.

 K. The Trustee and any successor Trustee are specifically instructed by the Settlor to maintain the privacy and confidentiality of this instrument and the trust created hereunder, and are in no circumstances to divulge its terms to any probate or other court or other public agency with the exception of a tax authority.

 L. The Trustee and any successor Trustee shall have the authority to merge any trust held hereunder with any other trust, however created, which has similar provisions, the same beneficiaries and the same Trustee.

 M. Notwithstanding any other provision contained herein, an individual Trustee (a) shall have no incident of ownership or power with respect to any policy of insurance upon such Trustee's life, and (b) shall have no power or discretion with respect to the allocation or distribution of assets to the extent that such would discharge such Trustee's legal obligation to support any beneficiary, or directly or indirectly benefit such Trustee, unless necessary to provide for such Trustee's support in reasonable comfort, health care or education at any level, considering such Trustee's other financial resources.

N. No Trustee shall be liable or responsible to any trust beneficiary in any way for failing to make non-income producing property productive or for failing to convert such property to income producing property.

ARTICLE VI

GOVERNING LAW

This Trust Agreement shall be construed under and in accordance with the laws of the State of _____.

IN WITNESS WHEREOF, I have hereunto set my hand, and the Trustee, to evidence its acceptance of the Trust herein expressed, has hereunto set its hand, in duplicate, at _____, _____, _____, on the day and year first above written.

Signed in the presence of:

_____   _____

_____   _____
                                                                        "Settlor"

_____   _____

_____   _____
                                                                        "Trustee"

I, the undersigned legal spouse of the Settlor, hereby waive all community property, dower or courtesy rights which I may have in the hereinabove-described property and give my assent to the provisions of the trust and to the inclusion in it of the said property.

                                        _____

                                        _____

Witness: _____   Witness: _____

STATE OF _____   City
                                    or
COUNTY OF _____   or Town _____

On the _____ day of _____, 19____, personally appeared _____, known to me to be the individual(s) who executed the foregoing instrument, and acknowledged the same to be [his/her] free act and deed, before me.

My commission expires _____   _____
                                          Notary Public

SCHEDULE A

The following is a true and correct Schedule A of the property assigned, delivered and conveyed to _____, Trustee, to be held, treated and disposed of in accordance with the terms of a certain Irrevocable Trust Agreement between _____, the Settlor, and _____, the Trustee, dated _____, 19____, to which Agreement this Schedule A is attached and made a part thereof.

_____

_____

_____

_____

_____

_____

_____

_____

_____

_____

_____

Signed in the presence of:

_____   _____

_____   _____

                                                                            "Settlor"

_____   _____

_____   _____

                                                                            "Trustee"

      I, the undersigned legal spouse of the Settlor, hereby waive all community property, dower or courtesy rights which I may have in the hereinabove-described property and give my assent to the provisions of the trust and to the inclusion in it of the said property.

                                           _____

                                           _____

Witness: _____   Witness: _____

_____   _____

ADDITION OF PROPERTY TO IRREVOCABLE TRUST AGREEMENT

BY _____

DATED _____ _____, 19____

WITH _____, TRUSTEE

_____ (the "Assignor"), pursuant to the terms of the above-described Irrevocable Trust Agreement, does hereby assign, transfer and convey to _____, Trustee, and _____ Trustee, does hereby acknowledge receipt of, the following assets from the Assignor:

_____

_____

_____

_____

_____

_____

_____

_____

_____

_____

_____

_____

_____

_____

_____

_____

_____

_____

The Trustee agrees to hold, manage and administer the above assets as a part of the trust estate created under such Irrevocable Trust Agreement.

At the request of the Trustee, the Assignor shall fully cooperate and execute any and all documents deemed necessary or desirable by it in order to cause the assignment made hereby to be properly recorded.

IN WITNESS WHEREOF, the Assignor and the Trustee have signed their names at _____, _____, on this _____ day of _____, 19____.

Signed in the presence of:

_____   _____

_____   _____, Assignor

_____   _____

_____   _____, Trustee

I, the undersigned legal spouse of the Assignor, hereby waive all community property, dower or courtesy rights which I may have in the hereinabove-described property and give my assent to the inclusion in the trust of the said property.

    _____

    _____

Witness: _____   Witness: _____

STATE OF _____   City
    or
COUNTY OF _____   Town _____

On the _____ day of _____, 19____, personally appeared _____, known to me to be the individual(s) who executed the foregoing instrument, and acknowledged the same to be **[his/her]** free act and deed, before me.

    _____
    Notary Public

My commission expires:

_____

Irrevocable Trust Agreement

Explanation

As you can readily see, this irrevocable asset protection trust agreement is filled with legalese. Don't be scared off by this confusing language. The explanations that follow should provide you with a clear understanding of the terms used.

Introduction: In the first blanks, you would fill in the city and state where you reside and the day, month, and year in which you are executing the agreement. Next go your name and your city and state of residence—"settlor" is your title when you make a trust. Then you would fill in the name and the city and state of residence of the person or institution whom you are naming as trustee.

Remember, neither you nor your spouse can be the trustee. A child or other close relative will probably be your first choice (keeping in mind possible tax consequences where annual distributions of over $10,000 will be made). If no one fits that description, you may have to name an institutional trustee, such as a bank.

Article I(A): This is the section making your trust irrevocable. Once you sign the agreement, you will never be able to change, amend, or revoke it.

Article I(B): This paragraph transfers into the trust all of the items listed on Schedule A at the end of the agreement. You can include on Schedule A just about any item imaginable, including real estate, personal property, savings and checking accounts, boats, cars, and even clothing.

If the property you put into the trust increases in value, the increased value is part of the trust. And if an asset changes form, the new asset still remains in the trust. For example, if the trustee takes $5,000 from a bank account and buys $5,000 worth of stock, that stock remains in the trust.

While you can never remove assets once they are placed into the trust, you can always add to the trust by using the Addition to Trust form following Schedule A.

A testamentary gift, referred to in this paragraph, is a gift given at the time of someone's death, normally contained in a will. For example, you may not put your car into trust immediately, but you may add it to your trust under your will when you die.

IMPORTANT NOTE: In Paragraph I(B) and throughout this trust agreement, you will see references to [**wife/husband**]. If your spouse is a female, you would strike out "husband"; if a male, you would strike out "wife." On the line following [**wife/husband**] you would fill in the name.

Article II: This section specifically provides that you and your spouse cannot get at the income or principal. This is *absolutely crucial* to saving your estate from the grasp of a nursing home if either you or your spouse enters one. With this language, Medicaid cannot require you to spend the principal on the nursing home *because you don't control or even have access to the income or principal.*

Paragraph B gives the trustee the power to give income or principal from the trust to your children and grandchildren if they need funds. Distributions can be made unequally.

Article III: This section describes how your trust principal, less any of your estate taxes, estate administration costs, or funeral expenses will be distributed after you and/or your spouse die.

Paragraph III(A) provides that you may use your will to "appoint" the assets in the trust (state where they should go and in what proportions) at your death. Trust assets cannot be appointed to benefit your creditors.

If not otherwise appointed in your will, the trust principal at your death will be distributed equally to your children. If any of your children has died before your spouse passed away, that child's portion goes to that child's children.

Paragraph III(C) provides that if any person who is to receive a distribution is under age twenty-one, that person's distribution shall be kept in trust until he or she reaches age twenty-one. This provision allows you to make sure that, if you have a young child or grandchild who is to receive a distribution from your trust, that child cannot have control of the funds until he or she is old enough (and, it is hoped, mature enough) to manage those funds. This trust provides for distribution of a child's portion upon reaching age twenty-one, although any age could be chosen and inserted into the trust.

Paragraph III(D) provides for the distribution of the trust if there is no one to receive the principal from your trust under Paragraphs III(A) or (B). If you and your spouse die leaving no living children or grandchildren, Paragraph III(D) takes over. Under III(D), the remaining principal of the trust will be divided into two parts. One part will go to those persons who would inherit from you under the laws of your state as if you had died without a will or a trust. Every state has a law that dictates to whom an estate of someone who dies without a will is to be distributed—usually the closest living relative(s) of the deceased. For example, if you die without children or grandchildren, Paragraph III(D) may mean that your parent or brother collects part of the trust estate.

The other half of the trust estate will be distributed to those persons who would inherit from your deceased spouse under the laws of your state as if he or she had died without a will. The estate is split into two parts so that relatives on both sides of your family are treated equally. For example, rather than having everything go to your cousin, half may go to your cousin and half to your deceased spouse's sister.

The blanks in Paragraph III(D) are for the name of your state.

Part III(E) discusses distributions, after you die, to beneficiaries named in your trust who are under some legal disability or are unable to administer their distributions. Under no circumstances can the trust make distributions to you or to your spouse. If a distribution from your trust is to go to someone who is under a legal disability or unable to manage his or her money, the trustee has four options:

1. Pay the money to the beneficiary.
2. Make the distribution to a legal guardian of the beneficiary.
3. Distribute the beneficiary's portion to a custodian for the beneficiary.
4. Spend the money himself or herself for the benefit of the beneficiary.

If, when you make up your trust, you could predict the ages and physical and mental conditions of all of your beneficiaries at the time of your death, you could spell out which of these four options you would want the trustee to pursue. But since you can't, this trust allows the trustee to choose which option he or she believes is best.

The last sentence of Part III(E) says that once the trustee has made his or her choice and distributed a beneficiary's portion to the beneficiary or to the beneficiary's guardian or custodian, the trustee is off the hook; he or she doesn't have to monitor the use of the distribution after that.

Part III(F), often called a spendthrift clause, provides that nobody but your intended beneficiary can obtain an interest in a distribution under your trust. For example, your child, who will receive a portion of your trust after you're gone, can't sell his or her expected distribution in the future to someone for cash now. And a beneficiary can't put up his or her interest in a distribution as collateral for a loan. After all, you want the person you name in the trust to receive a distribution, not some stranger.

Spendthrift clauses like this are enforced in most, but not all, states. If you have a serious concern that a beneficiary has or may have creditor problems, consult with a local attorney to determine whether this clause will be effective in your state.

Trusts cannot legally tie up assets forever, so Part III(G) is designed to avoid potential problems by limiting the life of the trust.

Article IV: This is the definition section. The most important point here is to recognize that a legally adopted child will be considered a child for purposes of the trust agreement. So by leaving everything to your children equally after you and your spouse die, any adopted child would be treated the same as a natural child.

Article V: This section deals with the powers and duties you are giving to the trustee.

Part V(A) says that after your death, the trustee must collect the money due under any insurance policy on your life. The trustee does not have a duty to pay your life insurance premiums during your lifetime, until and unless the trustee takes title to any insurance policy. In addition, the trustee does not have to change investments to create or maximize income.

Part V(B) is very important, setting forth the powers of the trustee. As you can see, this trust agreement gives the trustee very broad powers to administer the funds and property in the estate, including the power to:

1. Buy real estate or personal property from your or your spouse's estate. Without this power, purchase by your trustee from your estate at death might not be allowed.
2. Keep in the trust anything received from

3. Sell, exchange, mortgage, and do just about anything else with property in the trust.
4. Invest the assets in the trust in just about anything.
5. Borrow money for the trust.
6. Manage stock and other securities.
7. Collect money for the trust.
8. Handle claims and lawsuits for or against the trust.
9. Hire and pay counselors and assistants, like lawyers and accountants, for the trust.
10. Hold property in his or her own name, in the name of a nominee, or in bearer form.
11. Manage real estate in the trust, including repairing, improving, or converting property.
12. Handle life insurance policies in the trust, including paying premiums, canceling or selling policies, cashing in policies, or borrowing against them.
13. Make distributions under the trust in cash or in property.
14. Receive additional property for the trust.
15. Do anything else reasonably required to manage, protect, or preserve the trust assets.

Why put in many specific powers instead of just having item 15, which generally allows the trustee to do anything reasonably necessary? Because with only a general statement, someone with whom the trustee must deal may question his or her power and may refuse to do business with him or her. For example, without specifically giving the trustee the power to sell real estate, buyers, lenders, and escrow agents may be hesitant to deal with him or her, even if your trust agreement generally gives your trustee broad powers. By listing specific powers you can ensure the trustee's ability to manage the trust properly.

Why give the trustee such broad powers anyway? Why not just specify a few actions he or she may take? The reason is simple: you can't predict what the trustee may need to do to manage your estate properly, and if you don't give him or her broad powers, you may hamper him or her and damage your trust estate. For example, if you don't own any stocks, why give the trustee power to manage them? Because at some point it might be in your best interest for your trustee to purchase securities, and you don't want

you, your spouse, or your and your spouse's estates.

your trust agreement to prevent him or her from doing so.

Part V(C) provides for certain payments from your trust upon your death. If the representative of your estate (such as the executor or administrator) decides that the funds left in your estate (not in your trust) are insufficient to pay your estate taxes, expenses of administration, or funeral expenses, he or she can require the trustee to cover those costs. The trustee does not have to get anything in return and your estate representative does not have to repay the money. Once the trustee has paid the representative of your estate, the trustee has no further obligation to monitor the use of these funds.

Part V(D) requires the trustee to keep accurate records showing all transactions in the trust.

Part V(E) is designed to encourage people to deal with the trustee by relieving them of liability in case the trustee takes some action beyond his or her power. For example, if the trustee attempts to sell stock, the buyer can go ahead with the transaction and pay the trustee without worrying about whether the trust really allows the trustee to make that deal.

Part V(F)(1) allows you to name alternative trustees in case your first and/or second choice can't or won't serve when the time comes. In the first blank you would put the name of your first choice for trustee. In the next three blanks you would fill in the relationship to you, the name, and residence of your second choice. In the next two blanks you would fill in the names of your first and second choices for trustee. In the last three blanks you would include the name, city, and state of a third choice for trustee.

Part V(F)(2) gives any successor trustee all of the same powers and duties as the original trustee. It also encourages your chosen successor trustee to accept the job by providing that he or she has no responsibility for anything done by the earlier trustee.

Part V(G) authorizes the trustee to engage in transactions with the executor of your or your spouse's estate or any trustee of any other trust established by you or your spouse. Without this language, a conflict-of-interest issue could arise over these types of dealings.

Part V(H) concerns discretionary distributions by the trustee. Distributions should be made to beneficiaries only after considering their financial status.

In Part V(I) you are providing that the trustee will receive reasonable compensation.

Part V(J) states that the trustee does not have to post a bond. A bond is like an insurance policy; it is designed to protect your trust in case the trustee does something wrong, such as steal assets. Depending on the amount in the trust, a bond could easily cost your trust several hundred dollars. If you've followed the tips in this book and selected the right trustee, you shouldn't need a bond.

Part V(K) instructs the trustee to keep the terms of your trust private to the maximum extent possible. A trust has a great advantage over a will when it comes to passing your assets along after your death. Your estate becomes an open book when it goes through probate; when it passes under a trust, it can be kept from the eyes of nosy neighbors.

Part V(L) allows the trustee to merge trusts that are very similar to avoid duplication of effort and costs.

Part V(M) is a protection for the trustee to avoid the remote possibility of having the trust property included in the trustee's estate, causing adverse tax consequences.

Part V(N) again makes clear that the trustee has no obligation to maximize income.

Article VI: Article VI states that any questions about the trust will be answered by the laws of the state of your primary residence. In the blank space you would fill in the name of your state.

Conclusion: The blanks in the final paragraph are for your city and state. Then you would sign where it says settlor (that's you) and have the trustee sign below that. You and the trustee would each print your name below the signature line. To the left of your and the trustee's signatures, two witnesses to each signature would sign. The witnesses can be the same, but they don't have to be; if they are the same, they must sign twice (once for the settlor and once for the trustee). The witnesses cannot be members of your family.

Your spouse would then sign, with two witnesses signing below. In many states your spouse has a legal interest in your property and must waive his or her rights in writing to the property covered by the trust.

The final section is for a notary public.

Schedule A: Following the end of the trust is Schedule A, on which you would list any items (cash accounts, real estate, personal property, and the like) to be placed under the control of the trustee. Identify each item as best you can, using addresses, registration numbers, account numbers, or other information, wherever possible, to avoid confusion.

On Schedule A you would fill in the name of the trustee in the first blank, your name (the settlor) in the second blank, and the name of the trustee again in the third blank, then date the schedule.

At the bottom, you, the trustee, and your spouse would sign before two independent witnesses.

Addition of Property Form: Finally, included is a form that you can use to add property to the trust later. At the top, you would fill in your name, the date that the trust was originally made, and the name of the trustee. In the first full paragraph you would fill in your name as the assignor, assigning property to the trustee. Then, on the lines that follow, you would list any items to be added to the trust. Again, identify each item as best you can. At the end, you, the trustee, and your spouse would sign before two independent witnesses and a notary.

IRREVOCABLE TRUST AGREEMENT

THIS IRREVOCABLE TRUST AGREEMENT is entered into at
_____, _____, this _____ day of _____, 19____, by and between _____, of _____, the Settlor, hereinafter referred to in the first person, and _____, of _____, the Trustee, hereinafter referred to as the "Trustee" and sometimes in the third person impersonal.

ARTICLE I

CREATION OF TRUST

A. Except as provided in Paragraph B of this Article I, this Trust Agreement shall be irrevocable, and I hereby expressly acknowledge that I shall have no right or power, either alone or in conjunction with others, and in any capacity whatsoever, to alter, amend, modify, revoke or terminate this Trust or any of the terms of this Trust Agreement in whole or in part, or otherwise to cause any of the assets of the Trust to revert to me or to my estate.

B. I hereby transfer the property listed in Schedule A of this Trust Agreement to the Trustee. The property and all proceeds, investments and reinvestments thereof and any property hereinafter received by the Trustee from me, my **[wife/husband]**, _____, or from any other person (such property being hereinafter referred to as the "trust estate") shall be held, administered and distributed in accordance with the terms of the trust herein expressed. I reserve to myself and to others the right to add property to the trust estate by lifetime or testamentary gifts, all of which added property shall be governed by the terms hereof.

ARTICLE II

DISTRIBUTIONS DURING LIFETIME OF SETTLOR

A. NOTWITHSTANDING ANY OTHER PROVISION OF THIS TRUST AGREEMENT, I AND/OR MY **[WIFE/HUSBAND]**, _____, SHALL NOT BE A TRUSTEE OR BENEFICIARY OF THIS TRUST AGREEMENT AND I AND/OR MY **[WIFE/HUSBAND]**, _____, SHALL NOT HAVE ANY LEGAL TITLE OR INTEREST IN THE ASSETS OF THIS TRUST AGREEMENT. THE TRUSTEE IS ABSOLUTELY PROHIBITED FROM MAKING ANY PAYMENTS OF INCOME OR PRINCIPAL TO OR FOR MY BENEFIT OR THE BENEFIT OF MY **[WIFE/HUSBAND]**, _____.

B. While the trust estate holds any interest in any residential real property which is used by me from time to time as a residence, whether permanent or seasonal, including all improvements situated thereupon and all adjoining land used as a part thereof (such interest in any such residential property being hereinafter in this Trust Agreement referred to as the "Real Property"), the Trustee shall accumulate and add to the principal the net income, if any, derived from the trust estate. I and my **[wife/husband]** shall have no legal right to use any real property held by the trust estate as a residence.

C. Unless I shall have previously died, the Trustee shall provide me with written notice of any sale of the Real Property within thirty (30) days after such sale. Upon the sale of the Real Property by

1

the Trustee, the accumulated net income through the date of the sale and the entire net sale proceeds (gross sale proceeds less selling expenses) shall be distributed to or held for the benefit of such person or persons out of a class composed of my children and my children's issue (of whatever degree and whenever born), and in such amounts and proportions as I may appoint by written instrument; provided, however, anything herein to the contrary notwithstanding, such power of appointment granted under this Paragraph C shall not be exercised in favor of, or to or for the benefit of, me, my **[wife/husband]**, my estate, my **[wife's/husband's]** estate, my creditors, my **[wife's/husband's]** creditors, the creditors of my estate, or the creditors of my **[wife's/husband's]** estate; provided, further, however, that in order for the exercise by me of said power of appointment to be effective, I must exercise such power by specific reference to this Trust Agreement in such written instrument. In the event that I fail to exercise such power of appointment, or insofar as any such appointment shall be void or shall not take effect within thirty (30) days after I received written notice from the Trustee of the sale of the Real Property, the Trustee may distribute the accumulated net income through the date of the sale, in equal shares, to my then living children, treating as a then living child of mine for this purpose the then living collective issue of any said child of mine who shall then be deceased, the distribution to such issue to be *per stirpes*, the root of the *per stirpes* distribution to be such deceased child. The Trustee shall add the net sale proceeds to the principal of the trust estate to be held, administered and distributed as provided in Paragraph D of this Article II. See definitions under Article V of this Trust Agreement.

D After the sale of the Real Property, and after the provisions of Paragraph C of this Article II have been provided for, the Trustee may distribute to or for the benefit of the members of a class composed of my children and issue (living from time to time, of whatever degree and whenever born), out of the net income or principal or both of the trust estate being held hereunder, such amount or amounts (whether the whole or a lesser amount) which shall be necessary to provide for the maintenance, support, health and education of such persons. It is my intention that distributions under this Paragraph D shall be made to or for the benefit of the members of said class in accordance with the maintenance, support, health and educational requirements affecting them individually. It is not my intention to require that the dollar distributions made under this Paragraph D to or for the benefit of each of such members shall be equal, and the Trustee is authorized, in accordance with the provisions of this Paragraph D, to make distributions of principal hereunder to or for the benefit of one of such members to the exclusion of the other without any duty to equalize those distributions. At the end of each taxable year the Trustee shall add any undistributed income to the principal of the trust estate being held hereunder.

ARTICLE III

DIVISION OF TRUST ESTATE UPON SETTLOR'S DEATH

Upon my death, the Trustee shall hold, administer and distribute the property held hereunder, as the same shall be constituted after being (a) augmented by property received or to be received by the Trustee as a consequence of my death, including, without limitation, any property received or to be received under the terms of my Last Will and Testament or any Codicil thereto and (b) depleted by any money disbursed by the Trustee pursuant to the provisions of Paragraph C of Article VI hereof (said property as so constituted being hereinafter referred to as "The Family Trust") in accordance with the following provisions of this Trust Agreement.

A. The Family Trust shall be distributed to or held for the benefit of such person or persons out of a class composed of my children and my children's issue (of whatever degree and whenever born), and in such amounts and proportions as I may appoint by my Last Will and Testament or any Codicil thereto; provided, however, anything herein to the contrary notwithstanding, such power of appointment granted under this Paragraph A shall not be exercised in favor of, or to or for the benefit of, me, my **[wife/husband]**, my estate, my **[wife's/husband's]** estate, my creditors, my **[wife's/husband's]** creditors, the creditors of my estate, or the creditors of my **[wife's/husband's]** estate; provided, further, however, that in order for the exercise by me of said power of appointment to be effective, I must exercise such power by specific reference to this Trust Agreement in the provision of my Last Will and Testament or such Codicil. In the event that I fail to exercise such power of appointment, or insofar as any such appointment shall be void or shall not take effect, then the Trustee shall hold, administer and distribute the Family Trust, or any part thereof not effectively appointed by me, pursuant to the provisions of Paragraphs B and C of this Article III.

B. The Trustee shall distribute that part of the Family Trust, if any, that remains after giving effect to the provisions of Paragraph A of this Article III, in equal shares, to my children who survive me, treating as a surviving child of mine for this purpose the collective issue surviving me of any child of mine who shall have predeceased me, the distribution to such issue to be *per stirpes*, the root of the *per stirpes* distribution to be such predeceased child.

C. If, under the provisions of Paragraphs A or B of this Article III, any portion of The Family Trust shall become distributable to any person who is then under the age of twenty-one (21) years, then such portion shall be retained by the Trustee in trust for the benefit of such person. The Trustee shall distribute to or for the benefit of such person out of the net income or principal or both of such portion held for such person, such amount or amounts (whether the whole or a lesser amount) as the Trustee, in its sole discretion, deems necessary or proper suitably to provide for the maintenance, support, health, and education of such person, and shall from time to time add to the principal of such portion the remaining undistributed income, if any, until such person shall attain the age of twenty-one (21) years, whereupon the Trustee shall distribute all of such portion to such person. If such person shall die prior to receiving the complete distribution of the portion held for such person's benefit, such portion shall be distributed free of the trust to such person's estate.

D. If at the time for distribution of The Family Trust or any share or portion of the trust estate being held pursuant to this Article III, there is no person or person's estate entitled under the provisions of this Article III other than this Paragraph D to take such distribution, the Trustee shall divide the trust estate into two (2) equal shares. One such share shall be distributed free of the trust to such person or persons as would be entitled to inherit from me and in the proportions they would so inherit under the laws of the State of _____ as though I had died intestate and domiciled in the State of _____ at the time distribution is so to be made. The other such share shall be distributed free of the trust to such person or persons as would be entitled to inherit from my said **[wife/husband]** and in the proportions they would so inherit under the laws of the State of _____ as though **[he/she]** had died intestate and domiciled in the State of _____ at the time distribution is so to be made.

E. Notwithstanding any other provisions, in no event shall the Trustee pay any amount to me and/or my **[wife/husband]**. If the Trustee is authorized pursuant to the provision of this Article III to make distributions or payments to or for the benefit of any person (including distributions or payments directed or permitted to be made to a person who is under legal disability or, in the reasonable opinion of the Trustee, is unable properly to administer such distributions or payments), the Trustee may make such distributions or payments in any one or more of the following ways, as the Trustee may deem advisable: (I) directly to such beneficiary; (2) to the legal guardian of such beneficiary; (3) to any custodian then serving for such beneficiary, or to any person designated by the Trustee to serve as a custodian for such beneficiary (any such custodian may be the Trustee); or (4) by the Trustee itself expending such income or principal for the benefit of such beneficiary. The Trustee shall not be required to see to the application of any distribution or payment so made, but the receipt of any of the persons mentioned in Clause (1), (2) or (3) in the immediately preceding sentence shall be a full discharge for the Trustee.

F. No interest whatsoever in the principal and/or income of any trust estate subject to the provision of Articles II or III shall be alienated, disposed of, or in any manner assigned or encumbered by the person for whom held, voluntarily or involuntarily, while such principal and/or income is in the possession or control of the Trustee. If, by reason of any act of any such person or by operation of law, or by the happening of any event, or for any other reason except by an act of the Trustee specifically authorized hereunder, any such principal and/or income of such trust would but for this Paragraph F cease to be enjoyed by any such person or, by reason of an attempt by any such person to alienate, charge, assign or encumber any of such principal and/or income of such trust, or by reason of the bankruptcy or insolvency of any such person, or by reason of any attachment, garnishment or other proceedings, based upon a valid court judgment, or by reason of any order, finding or judgment of any court either at law or in equity, any of the principal and/or income of such trust would but for this Paragraph F vest in or be enjoyed by some individual, firm or corporation otherwise than as provided herein, then, in any of such events, the trust created for the benefit of such person shall forthwith cease and determine as to such person, who shall thereupon cease to be a beneficiary of such trust **and such person shall be ineligible to serve or to continue to serve as Trustee hereunder.** For purposes of this Paragraph F, the exercise of any power of appointment granted herein or the exercise of any disclaimer by a beneficiary of any rights or benefits under this Trust Agreement shall not cause or result in the provisions of this Paragraph F becoming applicable. Such trust thereafter, subject to all other applicable provisions of this Trust Agreement, shall, during the life of such former beneficiary, be held by the Trustee which, until such former beneficiary's death, may pay to or expend for the benefit of such former beneficiary, out of the principal and/or income of such trust, such sums but such sums only as the Trustee in its absolute discretion may determine, retaining any undistributed principal and/or income until such former beneficiary's death; provided, however, that no payments made under these provisions to or for the benefit of such former beneficiary shall exceed the amounts otherwise payable to such former beneficiary if these provisions had not been invoked. Any undistributed income shall from time to time be added to the principal of such trust. Upon the death of such former beneficiary, such trust as then constituted, including all accrued and undistributed income, shall, subject to all applicable provisions of this Trust Agreement, be distributed to the persons (determined as of the date of death of such former beneficiary) to whom such trust estate would have been so distributable as if such former beneficiary had died prior to the time for any mandatory distribution of the trust estate to such former beneficiary, and as if the provisions of this Paragraph F had never become applicable to the trust of such former beneficiary; provided, however, that for this purpose, if such former beneficiary has a power of appointment over any portion or all of the trust estate, such power of appointment shall be deemed not to have been exercised and the Trustee shall distribute the trust estate in accordance with the provisions of this Trust Agreement notwithstanding any attempted exercise of such power of appointment by said former beneficiary.

G. Any provisions of this Trust Agreement to the contrary notwithstanding, if not already distributed, all accrued and undistributed income and the entire principal of every trust estate then held hereunder shall be paid over and distrusted outright and free of the trust not later than the end of the day immediately preceding the expiration of twenty-one (21) years from and after the death of the last survivor of myself, my said **[wife/husband]**, my children and my children's issue living at the date of the execution of this Trust Agreement. Such payment and distribution shall be made to the person or persons for whose benefit the trust estate or estates respectively shall then be held hereunder; provided, however, that if at the time the trust estates are to be distributed pursuant to this Paragraph G, the provisions of the immediately preceding Paragraph F of this Article III shall be in operation as to any such trust, such trust shall be distributed to those persons who would have been entitled to receive such trust as if the former beneficiary for whose benefit such trust was originally created had died immediately preceding the time so provided for such distribution and possessed of said trust estate, such distribution to be outright and free of the trust.

ARTICLE IV

DEFINITIONS

A. The words "issue," "child" and "children," as used herein, shall be deemed to include any legally adopted person as if he or she were the natural child of the adopting parent.

B. Whenever the context so requires, the use of words herein in the singular shall be construed to include the plural, and words in the plural, the singular, and words whether in the masculine, feminine or neuter gender shall be construed to include all of said genders.

C. For purposes of this Trust Agreement, the term "marketable securities" refers to any share of stock in any corporation, certificate of stock or interest in any corporation, note, bond, debenture, or evidence of indebtedness, or any evidence of an interest in or right to subscribe to or purchase any of the foregoing, which are readily tradeable on an established market.

D. For purposes of this Trust Agreement, the word "income" *does* include recognized gains from the sale, exchange or conversion of "marketable securities" but does *not* include any other gains from the sale, exchange or conversion of any other property which are properly allocated to the trust corpus.

E. For purposes of this Trust Agreement, the phrase "net income" refers to "income" as defined above less expenses incurred by the Trustee for management of the trust estate.

F. For purposes of this Trust Agreement, any individual shall be deemed to be unable to continue to serve as Trustee hereunder only when:

1. Such individual's attending physician and at least one other physician licensed in the United States (or, if such individual does not have an attending physician, at least two physicians licensed in the United States) shall have signed and delivered to the Trustee then serving hereunder (or, if such Trustee is the person who is deemed to be unable to continue to serve as Trustee hereunder, then to any fiduciary serving hereunder or to the person who is to succeed such individual as Trustee) their written statements indicating that such individual is incapable in their judgment of attending effectively to such individual's fiduciary duties by reason of mental or physical disability; provided, that the written statements to which reference is made above shall be acknowledged before a notary public and witnessed by two individuals; provided, further, that any person relying on any such written statements by such physicians may presume that the identity and qualifications of the physicians signing any such statement are in fact who and what they purport to be and such person shall not have any duty to make further inquiry or investigation beyond the review of each written statement itself; provided, further, that no person relying on such written statement shall be liable to any other person or persons for action taken in reliance on such written statement; or

2. Such individual is adjudicated incompetent.

ARTICLE V

POWERS AND DUTIES OF THE TRUSTEE

A. 1. There shall be no duty on the Trustee to pay or see to the payment of any premiums on any policies of life insurance or to take any steps to keep them in force, until such time as the Trustee holds title to any insurance policies hereunder as a part of the corpus of any trust estate. The Trustee furthermore assumes no responsibility with respect to the validity or enforceability of said policies. However, as soon as practicable after receiving notice of the death of the insured under any of such policies, the Trustee shall proceed to collect all amounts payable thereunder. The Trustee shall have full and complete authority to collect and receive any and all such amounts and its receipt therefore shall be a full and complete acquittance to any insurer or payor, who shall be under no obligation to see to the proper application thereof by the Trustee.

2. There shall be no duty on the Trustee to make non-income producing property productive or to convert such property to income producing property.

B. In the administration of the trust created hereunder and in addition to the powers exercised by trustees generally, the Trustee shall have the following powers and authorities without any court order or proceeding, exercisable in the discretion of the Trustee:

1. To purchase as an investment for the trust estate or estates any property, real or personal, belonging to my estate and/or the estate of my **[wife/husband]**, _____ ;

2. To retain as suitable investments for the trust estate or estates any properties (including, without limitation, securities issued by any corporate Trustee or the holding company of which it is an affiliate) received by it from me, my said **[wife/husband]** my estate and/or the estate of my said **[wife/husband]**, and whether received by purchase or in any other manner, without regard to any law, statutory or judicial, or any rule or practice of court now or hereafter in force specifying or limiting the permissible investments of trustees, trust companies or fiduciaries generally or requiring the diversification of investments, and without liability to any person whomsoever for loss or depreciation in value thereof;

3. To sell, exchange, convey, mortgage, pledge, lease, control, and manage, and to make contracts concerning, any of the properties, real or personal, comprised in the trust estate or estates, all either publicly or privately and for such considerations and upon such terms as to credit or otherwise as may be reasonable under the circumstances, which leases and contracts may extend beyond the duration of any of the trust created hereunder; to give options therefore; and to execute deeds, transfers, mortgages, leases and other instruments of any kind;

4. To invest and reinvest the properties from time to time comprised in the trust estate or estates in stocks, common and/or preferred, bonds, notes, debentures, loans, mortgages, common trust funds, or other securities or property, real or personal, all limitations now or hereafter imposed by law, statutory or judicial, or by any rule or practice of court now or hereafter in force specifying or limiting the permissible investments of trustees, trust companies or fiduciaries generally or requiring the diversification of investments, being hereby expressly waived, it being the intent hereof that the Trustee shall have full power and authority to deal with the trust estate or estates in all respects as though it was the sole owner thereof, without order of court or other authority;

5. To borrow money, from itself or otherwise, with or without security, wherever it deems such action advisable;

6. To exercise voting rights, execute and deliver powers of attorney and proxies and similarly act with reference to shares of stock and other securities comprised in the trust estate or estates in such manner as it deems proper, including, without limitation, the power to participate in or oppose reorganizations, recapitalizations, mergers, consolidations, exchanges, liquidations, arrangements and other corporate actions;

7. To collect all money; in accordance with generally accepted trust accounting principles, to determine whether money or other property coming into its possession shall be treated as principal or income and to charge or apportion expenses, taxes, gains and losses to principal or income;

8. To compromise, adjust and settle claims in favor of or against the trust estate or estates upon such terms and conditions as it may deem best; in the case of any litigation in connection with any part of such trust estate or estates, it may, under advice of its counsel, arbitrate, settle, or adjust any such matter in dispute upon such terms as it may consider just and equitable, and its decision shall be binding upon the beneficiaries;

9. To employ investment counsel, custodians of estate property, brokers, accountants, at-

torneys, clerical or bookkeeping assistants, and other suitable agents and to pay their reasonable compensation and expenses in addition to any compensation payable to the Trustee, and to execute and deliver powers of attorney; the Trustee shall not be liable for any neglect, omission or wrongdoing of such investment counsel, custodians, brokers, accountants, attorneys, assistants or agents, provided reasonable care shall have been exercised in their selection;

10. To hold title to stock, bonds, or other securities or property, real or personal, in its own name or in the name of its nominee and without indication of any fiduciary capacity or to hold any such bonds or securities in bearer form; the Trustee shall assume full responsibility for the acts of any nominee selected by it;

11. To make all repairs, alterations or improvements of any real property which shall constitute a part of the trust estate or estates; adjust boundaries thereof, and to erect or demolish buildings thereon; and, with respect to such property, to convert for different use, grant easements for adequate consideration, partition, and insure for any or all risks;

12. To pay premiums on any policies of life insurance which may form a part of the trust estate or estates; to cancel, sell, assign, hypothecate, pledge or otherwise dispose of any of said policies; to exercise any right, election, option or privilege granted by any of said policies; to borrow any sums in accordance with the provisions of any of said policies, and to receive all payments, dividends, surrender values, additions, benefits or privileges of any kind which may accrue to any of said policies;

13. To make any allocation, division or distribution required or permitted hereunder in cash or in kind, in real or personal property, or an undivided interest therein, or partly in cash and partly in kind, and to do so without making pro rata allocations, divisions or distributions of specific assets, property allocated, divided or distributed in kind to be taken at its fair market value at the time of such allocation, division or distribution;

14. To receive, in accordance with the provisions of Article I hereof, additional property from me or any other person, the Trustee being authorized and empowered to merge and hold as one any duplicate trusts held for the same beneficiary;

15. To make such expenditures and do such other acts as are reasonably required to manage, improve, protect, preserve, invest or sell any of the trust estates or otherwise properly to administer this Trust.

C. 1. Subject to the limitations set forth in the provisions of the following Subparagraph 2 of this Paragraph C, if the representative of my estate, in such representative's sole discretion, shall determine that appropriate assets of my estate are not available in sufficient amount (or if there are no assets in my estate) to pay the expenses of administration of my estate (but not including my legal debts, my funeral expenses and the expenses of my last illness) and all death taxes chargeable to my estate, including interest and penalties thereon, the Trustee shall, upon the request of the representative of my estate, contribute from the principal of the trust estate the amount of such deficiency; and in connection with any such action the Trustee shall rely upon the written statement of the representative of my estate as to the validity and correctness of the amounts of any such taxes and expenses, and shall furnish funds to such representative so as to enable such representative to discharge the same, or to discharge any part or all thereof itself by making payment directly to the government official or agency or to the person entitled or claiming to be entitled to receive payment thereof. If the Trustee hereunder holds any property that is bequeathed under my Will (other than a residuary bequest), then the Trustee to the extent that such property is held under the Trust Agreement shall distribute such property to the persons entitled to receive such bequest under my Will (other than a residuary bequest) after the deduction, if any, of expenses and taxes to be charged to such bequest pursuant to the provisions of my Will. No consideration need be required by the Trustee from the representative of my estate for any disbursement made by the Trustee pursuant hereto, nor shall there be any obligation upon such representative to repay to the Trustee any of the funds disbursed by it hereunder, and all amounts disbursed by the Trustee pursuant to the authority hereby conferred upon it shall be disbursed without any right in or duty upon the Trustee to seek or obtain contribution or reimbursement from any person or property on account of such payment. The Trustee shall not be responsible for the application of any funds delivered by it to the representative of my estate pursuant to the authority herein granted, nor shall the Trustee be subject to liability to any beneficiary hereunder on account of any payment made by it pursuant to the provisions hereof.

2. Any provisions of this Article V to the contrary notwithstanding, under no circumstances shall the Trustee make any disbursements pursuant to this Paragraph C from (a) assets which are excluded from my gross estate for purposes of the Federal estate tax payable by reason of my death or (b) assets which are not subject to a state inheritance, state estate or other state death tax imposed by reason of my death; provided, however, that assets described in Clause (b) of this sentence (so long as they do not constitute assets described in Clause (a) of this sentence) may be used to the extent that other assets which are included in my gross estate for purposes of Federal estate tax payable by reason of my death and subject to a state inheritance, state estate or other state death tax imposed by reason of my death shall be insufficient to satisfy the Trustee's obligation hereunder.

D. The Trustee shall keep accurate records showing all receipts and disbursements and other transactions involving the trust estate or estates and shall furnish annually to each income beneficiary entitled to income (1) a statement of the receipts and disbursements affecting such beneficiary's interest in the trust, and (2) a complete inventory of the trust estate then held for the benefit of such beneficiary.

E. No person, firm or corporation dealing with the Trustee or a nominee of the Trustee or performing any act pursuant to action taken or order given by the Trustee or such nominee shall be obliged to inquire as to the propriety, validity or legality thereof hereunder, nor shall any such person be liable for the application of any money or other consideration paid to the Trustee or such nominee, but, instead, may rely upon any action taken by the Trustee or such nominee pursuant to the powers and authorities conferred upon it under the provisions of this Article V in all respects as if the same were completely unlimited. No transfer agent or registrar of any security held hereunder shall be required to inquire as to the propriety, validity or legality of any transfer made by the Trustee or such nominee.

F. 1. I and my **[wife/husband]** shall not at any time serve as Trustee hereunder or have any legal title or interest in the trust estate. In the event that said _____ shall be unwilling or unable to continue to serve as Trustee hereunder, then my _____, _____, of _____, _____, shall serve as successor Trustee hereunder. In the event that both said _____ and said _____ shall be unwilling or unable to serve or continue to serve as Trustee hereunder, then _____, of _____, _____, shall serve as successor Trustee hereunder. Any Trustee shall be entitled to resign as Trustee for any reason whatsoever by giving written notice to the Trustee designated to succeed it, provided that the Trustee designated to succeed it shall first execute a formal written acceptance of the duties and obligations of the Trustee hereunder and file an executed copy of such acceptance with the preceding Trustee. After this is done, and when all sums then due from the trust estate to such predecessor Trustee have been paid, such predecessor Trustee shall transfer the Trust property then in its hands to such successor Trustee and such predecessor Trustee shall thereupon and thereby be discharged of all subsequent duties and obligations under or arising out of its trusteeship.

2. Any successor Trustee shall have and enjoy all the powers, authorities, duties and immunities hereby vested in and imposed upon the original Trustee and no successor Trustee shall be obliged to inquire into or be in any way accountable for the previous administration of the trust property.

G. My Trustee is authorized, in its discretion, to sell to, purchase from, borrow funds from, lend funds to, or otherwise deal with, upon such terms and conditions as my Trustee shall deem just and equitable and for full and adequate consideration, the Executor of the Last Will and Testament of myself or my said **[wife/husband]** or the Trustee of any Trust established by me or my said **[wife/husband]** (whether such Trust is a testamentary or inter vivos trust), even though my Trustee may also be serving as Executor under my Will or my said **[wife/husband]**'s Will or as Trustee under any such Trust established by me or by my said **[wife/husband]**.

        H. In determining the amount of any discretionary distributions of income or principal to a beneficiary of a trust created hereunder, the Trustee shall be required to take into account all other means and resources known to or reasonably ascertainable by the Trustee, including Medicaid or any other form of government assistance, which are available to such beneficiary for the purposes for which the Trustee is authorized to make said distributions.

        I. Any Trustee shall be entitled to receive reasonable compensation. Any Trustee shall be entitled to be reimbursed for reasonable expenses it incurs which are necessary to carry out its duties as Trustee hereunder.

        J. No bond shall be required of the Trustee hereunder or any successor Trustee.

        K. The Trustee and any successor Trustee are specifically instructed by the Settlor to maintain the privacy and confidentiality of this instrument and the trust created hereunder, and are in no circumstances to divulge its terms to any probate or other court or other public agency with the exception of a tax authority.

        L. The Trustee and any successor Trustee shall have the authority to merge any trust held hereunder with any other trust, however created, which has similar provisions, the same beneficiaries and the same Trustee.

        M. Notwithstanding any other provision contained herein, an individual Trustee (a) shall have no incident of ownership or power with respect to any policy of insurance upon such Trustee's life, and (b) shall have no power or discretion with respect to the allocation or distribution of assets to the extent that such would discharge such Trustee's legal obligation to support any beneficiary, or directly or indirectly benefit such Trustee, unless necessary to provide for such Trustee's support in reasonable comfort, health care or education at any level, considering such Trustee's other financial resources.

        N. No Trustee shall be liable or responsible to any trust beneficiary in any way for failing to make non-income producing property productive or for failing to convert such property to income producing property.

ARTICLE VI

GOVERNING LAW

        This Trust Agreement shall be construed under and in accordance with the laws of the State of _____.

        IN WITNESS WHEREOF, I have hereunto set my hand, and the Trustee, to evidence its acceptance of the Trust herein expressed, has hereunto set its hand, in duplicate, at _____, _____, _____, on the day and year first above written.

Signed in the presence of:

_____   _____

_____   _____

                                                                                  "Settlor"

_____   _____

_____   _____

                                                                                "Trustee"

I, the undersigned legal spouse of the Settlor, hereby waive all community property, dower or courtesy rights which I may have in the hereinabove-described property and give my assent to the provisions of the trust and to the inclusion in it of the said property.

_____

_____

Witness: _____   Witness: _____

STATE OF _____   City
or
COUNTY OF _____   Town _____

On the _____ day of _____, 19___, personally appeared
_____, known to me to be the individual(s) who executed the foregoing instrument, and acknowledged the same to be **[his/her]** free act and deed, before me.

My commission expires _____   _____
Notary Public

SCHEDULE A

The following is a true and correct Schedule A of the property assigned, delivered and conveyed to _____, Trustee, to be held, treated and disposed of in accordance with the terms of a certain Irrevocable Trust Agreement between _____, the Settlor, and _____, the Trustee, dated _____, 19____, to which Agreement this Schedule A is attached and made a part thereof.

_____

_____

_____

_____

_____

_____

_____

_____

_____

_____

_____

_____

_____

_____

_____

_____

_____

_____

_____

_____

Signed in the presence of:

_____   _____

_____   _____

"Settlor"

_____   _____

_____   _____

"Trustee"

      I, the undersigned legal spouse of the Settlor, hereby waive all community property, dower or courtesy rights which I may have in the hereinabove-described property and give my assent to the provisions of the trust and to the inclusion in it of the said property.

_____

_____

Witness: _____   Witness: _____

_____   _____

ADDITION OF PROPERTY TO IRREVOCABLE TRUST AGREEMENT

BY _____

DATED _____ _____, 19____

WITH _____, TRUSTEE

_____ (the "Assignor"), pursuant to the terms of the above-described Irrevocable Trust Agreement, does hereby assign, transfer and convey to _____, Trustee, and _____, Trustee, does hereby acknowledge receipt of, the following assets from the Assignor:

_____

_____

_____

_____

_____

_____

_____

_____

_____

_____

_____

_____

_____

_____

_____

_____

_____

_____

_____

_____

The Trustee agrees to hold, manage and administer the above assets as a part of the trust estate created under such Irrevocable Trust Agreement.

At the request of the Trustee, the Assignor shall fully cooperate and execute any and all documents deemed necessary or desirable by it in order to cause the assignment made hereby to be properly recorded.

IN WITNESS WHEREOF, the Assignor and the Trustee have signed their names at _____, _____, on this _____ day of _____, 19____.

Signed in the presence of:

_____   _____

_____   _____, Assignor

_____   _____

_____   _____, Trustee

I, the undersigned legal spouse of the Assignor, hereby waive all community property, dower or courtesy rights which I may have in the hereinabove-described property and give my assent to the inclusion in the trust of the said property.

_____

_____

Witness: _____   Witness: _____

STATE OF _____   City
                                     or
COUNTY OF _____   Town _____

On the _____ day of _____, 19____, personally appeared _____, known to me to be the individual(s) who executed the foregoing instrument, and acknowledged the same to be **[his/her]** free act and deed, before me.

_____
Notary Public

My commission expires:

_____

Irrevocable Trust Agreement

Explanation

As you can readily see, this irrevocable house preservation trust agreement is filled with legalese. Don't be scared off by this confusing language. The explanations that follow should provide you with a clear understanding of the terms used.

Introduction: In the first blanks you would fill in the city and state where you reside and the day, month, and year in which you are executing the agreement. Next go your name and your city and state of residence—"settlor" is your title when you make a trust. You would then fill in the name, city, and state of the person or institution whom you are naming as trustee.

Remember, neither you nor your spouse can be the trustee. A child or other close relative will probably be your first choice (keeping in mind possible tax consequences where annual distributions of over $10,000 will be made). If no one fits that description, you may have to name an institutional trustee, such as a bank.

Article I(A): This is the section making your trust irrevocable. Once you sign the agreement, you will never be able to change, amend, or revoke it.

Article I(B): This paragraph transfers into the trust all of the items listed on Schedule A at the end of the agreement. You can include on Schedule A just about any item imaginable, including real estate, personal property, savings and checking accounts, boats, cars, and even clothing.

If the property you put into the trust increases in value, the increased value is part of the trust. And if an asset changes form, the new asset still remains in the trust. For example, if the trustee takes $5,000 from a bank account and buys $5,000 worth of stock, that stock remains in the trust.

While you can never remove assets once they are placed into the trust, you can always add to the trust by using the Addition to Trust form following Schedule A.

A testamentary gift, referred to in this paragraph, is a gift given at the time of someone's death, normally contained in a will. For example, you may not put your car into trust immediately, but you may add it to your trust under your will when you die.

IMPORTANT NOTE: In Paragraph I(B) and throughout this trust agreement, you will see references to **[wife/husband]**. If your spouse is a female, you would strike out "husband"; if a male, you would strike out "wife." On the line following **[wife/husband]** you would fill in the name.

Article II: This section specifically provides that you and your spouse cannot get at the income or principal. This is *absolutely crucial* to saving your estate from the grasp of a nursing home if either you or your spouse enters one. With this language, Medicaid cannot require you to spend the principal on the nursing home *because you don't control or even have access to the income or principal.*

Paragraph B provides that if residential real estate is in the trust, income generated (such as rents) will be added to the trust principal. In addition, the trust provides that you and your spouse will have no legal right to live in the home. The trustee may choose to allow you to reside there for free, throw you out, or charge you rent. This is critical to protect your home from nursing-home costs.

Paragraph C says that if the house is sold, you may state that any accumulated income and the sale proceeds shall be paid to some or all of your children and/or grandchildren, in whatever proportions you wish. You, your spouse, and your creditors *cannot* receive the sale proceeds.

Paragraph D gives the trustee the power to distribute house sale proceeds (as well as other trust principal) to some or all of your children and grandchildren for their needs. Again, the proportions do not have to be equal and no distributions need to be made.

Article III: This section describes how your trust principal, less any of your estate taxes, estate administration costs, or funeral expenses, will be distributed after you and/or your spouse die:

Paragraph III(A) provides that you may use your will to "appoint" the assets in the trust (state where they should go and in what proportions) at your death. Trust assets cannot be appointed to benefit your creditors.

If not otherwise appointed in your will, the Trust principal at your death will be distributed equally to your children. If any of your children has died before your spouse passed away, that child's portion goes to that child's children.

Paragraph III(C) provides that if any person who is to receive a distribution is under age twenty-one, that person's distribution shall be kept in trust until he or she reaches age twenty-one. This provision allows you to make sure that if you have a young child or grandchild who is to receive a distribution from your trust, that child cannot have control of the funds until he or she is old enough (and, it is hoped, mature enough) to manage those funds. This trust provides for distribution of a child's portion upon reaching age twenty-one, although any age could be chosen and inserted into the trust.

Paragraph III(D) provides for the distribution of the trust if there is no one to receive the principal from your trust under Paragraphs III(A) or III(B). If you and your spouse die leaving no living children or grandchildren, Paragraph III(D) takes over. Under III(D), the remaining principal of the trust will be divided into two parts. One part will go to those persons who would inherit from you under the laws of your state as if you had died without a will or a trust. Every state has a law that dictates to whom an estate of someone who dies without a will is to be distributed—usually the closest living relative(s) of the deceased. For example, if you die without children or grandchildren, Paragraph III(D) may mean that your parent or brother collects part of the trust estate.

The other half of the trust estate will be distributed to those persons who would inherit from your deceased spouse under the laws of your state as if he or she had died without a will. The estate is split into two parts so that relatives on both sides of your family are treated equally. For example, rather than having everything go to your cousin, half may go to your cousin and half to your deceased spouse's sister.

The blanks in Paragraph III(D) are for the name of your state.

Part III(E) discusses distributions, after you die, to beneficiaries named in your trust who are under some legal disability or are unable to administer their distributions. Under no circumstances can the trust make distributions to you or to your spouse. If a distribution from your trust is to go to someone who is under a legal disability or unable to manage his or her money, the trustee has four options:

1. Pay the money to the beneficiary.
2. Make the distribution to a legal guardian of the beneficiary.
3. Distribute the beneficiary's portion to a custodian for the beneficiary.
4. Spend the money himself or herself for the benefit of the beneficiary.

If, when you make up your trust, you could predict the ages and physical and mental conditions of all of your beneficiaries at the time of your death, you could spell out which of these four options you would want the trustee to pursue. But since you can't, this trust allows the trustee to choose which option he or she believes is best.

The last sentence of Part III(E) says that once the trustee has made his or her choice and distributed a beneficiary's portion to the beneficiary or to the beneficiary's guardian or custodian, the trustee is off the hook; he or she doesn't have to monitor the use of the distribution after that.

Part III(F), often called a spendthrift clause, provides that nobody but your intended beneficiary can obtain an interest in a distribution under your trust. For example, your child, who will receive a portion of your trust after you're gone, can't sell his or her expected distribution in the future to someone for cash now. And a beneficiary can't put up his or her interest in a distribution as collateral for a loan. After all, you want the person you name in the trust to receive a distribution, not some stranger.

Spendthrift clauses like this are enforced in most, but not all, states. If you have a serious concern that a beneficiary has or may have creditor problems, consult with a local attorney to determine whether this clause will be effective in your state.

Trusts cannot legally tie up assets forever, so Part III(G) is designed to avoid potential problems by limiting the life of the trust.

Article IV: This is the definition section. The most important point here is to recognize that a legally adopted child will be considered a child for purposes of the trust agreement. So by leaving everything to your children equally after you and your spouse die, any adopted child would be treated the same as a natural child.

Article V: This section deals with the powers and duties you are giving to the trustee.

Part V(A) says that after your death, the trustee must collect the money due under any insurance policy on your life. The trustee does not have a duty to pay your life insurance premiums during your lifetime, until and unless the trustee takes title to any insurance policy. In addition, the trustee does not have to change investments to create or maximize income.

Part V(B) is very important, setting forth the powers of the trustee. As you can see, this trust agreement gives the trustee very broad powers to administer the funds and property in the estate, including the power to:

1. Buy real estate or personal property from your or your spouse's estate. Without this power, purchase by your trustee from your estate at death might not be allowed.
2. Keep in the trust anything received from you, your spouse, or your and your spouse's estates.
3. Sell, exchange, mortgage, and do just about anything else with property in the trust.
4. Invest the assets in the trust in just about anything.
5. Borrow money for the trust.
6. Manage stock and other securities.
7. Collect money for the trust.
8. Handle claims and lawsuits for or against the trust.
9. Hire and pay counselors and assistants, like lawyers and accountants, for the trust.
10. Hold property in his or her own name, in the name of a nominee, or in bearer form.
11. Manage real estate in the trust, including repairing, improving, or converting property.
12. Handle life insurance policies in the trust, including paying premiums, canceling or selling policies, cashing in policies, or borrowing against them.
13. Make distributions under the trust in cash or in property.
14. Receive additional property for the trust.
15. Do anything else reasonably required to manage, protect, or preserve the trust assets.

Why put in many specific powers instead of just having item 15, which generally allows the trustee to do anything reasonably necessary? Because with only a general statement, someone with whom the trustee must deal may question his or her power and may refuse to do business with him or her. For example, without specifically giving the trustee the power to sell real estate, buyers, lenders, and escrow agents may be hesitant to deal with him or her, even if your trust agreement gives your trustee broad powers. By listing specific powers you can ensure the trustee's ability to manage the trust properly.

Why give the trustee such broad powers anyway? Why not just specify a few actions he or she may take? The reason is simple: you can't predict what the trustee may need to do to manage your estate properly, and if you don't give him or her broad powers, you may hamper him or her and damage your trust estate. For example, if you don't own any stocks, why give the trustee power to manage them? Because at some point it might be in your best interest for your trustee to purchase securities, and you don't want your trust agreement to prevent him or her from doing so.

Part V(C) provides for certain payments from your trust upon your death. If the representative of your estate (such as the executor or administrator) decides that the funds left in your estate (not in your trust) are insufficient to pay your estate taxes, expenses of administration, or funeral expenses, he or she can require the trustee to cover those costs. The trustee does not have to get anything in return and your estate representative does not have to repay the money. Once the trustee has paid the representative of your estate, the trustee has no further obligation to monitor the use of these funds.

Part V(D) requires the trustee to keep accurate records showing all transactions in the trust.

Part V(E) is designed to encourage people to deal with the trustee by relieving them of liability in case the trustee takes some action beyond his or her power. For example, if the trustee attempts to sell stock, the buyer can go ahead with the transaction and pay the trustee without worrying about whether the trust really allows the trustee to make that deal.

Part V(F)(1) allows you to name alternative trustees in case your first and/or second choice can't or won't serve when the time comes. In the first blank you would put the name of your first choice for trustee. In the next three blanks you would fill in the relationship to you, the name, and the residence of your second choice. In the next two blanks you would fill in the names of your first and second choices for trustee. In the last three blanks you would include the name, city, and state of a third choice for trustee.

Part V(F)(2) gives any successor trustee all of the same powers and duties as the original trustee. It also encourages your chosen successor trustee to accept the job by providing that he or she has no responsibility for anything done by the earlier trustee.

Part V(G) authorizes the trustee to engage in transactions with the executor of your or your spouse's estate or any trustee of any other trust established by you or your spouse. Without this language, a conflict-of-interest issue could arise over these types of dealings.

Part V(H) concerns discretionary distributions by the trustee. Distributions should be made to beneficiaries only after considering their financial status.

In Part V(I) you are providing that the trustee will receive reasonable compensation.

Part V(J) states that the trustee does not have to post a bond. A bond is like an insurance policy; it is designed to protect your trust in case the trustee does something wrong, such as steal assets. Depending on the amount in the trust, a bond could easily cost your trust several hundred dollars. If you've followed the tips in this book and selected the right trustee, you shouldn't need a bond.

Part V(K) instructs the trustee to keep the terms of your trust private to the maximum extent possible. A trust has a great advantage over a will when it comes to passing your assets along after your death. Your estate becomes an open book when it goes through probate; when it passes under a trust, it can be kept from the eyes of nosy neighbors.

Part V(L) allows the trustee to merge trusts that are very similar to avoid duplication of effort and costs.

Part V(M) is a protection for the trustee to avoid the remote possibility of having the trust property included in the trustee's estate, causing adverse tax consequences.

Part V(N) again makes clear that the trustee has no obligation to maximize income.

Article VI: Article VI states that any questions about the trust will be answered by the laws of the state of your primary residence. In the blank space you would fill in the name of your state.

Conclusion: The blanks in the final paragraph are for your city and state. Then you would sign where it says settlor (that's you) and have the trustee sign below that. You and the trustee would each print your name below the signature line. To the left of your and the trustee's signatures, two witnesses to each signature would sign. The witnesses can be the same, but they don't have to be; if they are the same, they must sign twice (once for the settlor and once for the trustee). The witnesses cannot be members of your family.

Schedule A: Following the end of the trust is Schedule A, on which you would list any items (cash accounts, real estate, personal property, and the like) to be placed under the control of the trustee. Identify each item as best you can, using addresses, registration numbers, account numbers, or other information, wherever possible, to avoid confusion.

On Schedule A you would fill in the name of the trustee in the first blank, your name (the settlor) in the second blank, and the name of the trustee again in the third blank, then date the schedule.

At the bottom, you, the trustee, and your spouse would each sign before two independent witnesses.

Addition of Property Form: Finally, included is a form that you can use to add property to the trust later. At the top, you would fill in your name, the date that the trust was originally made, and the name of the trustee. In the first full paragraph you would fill in the name of the assignor who is assigning property to the trustee. Then, on the lines that follow, you would list any items to be added to the trust. Again, identify each item as best you can. At the end, you, the trustee, and your spouse would sign before two independent witnesses and a notary.

TRUST AGREEMENT

THIS TRUST AGREEMENT is made at Cleveland, Ohio, this _____ day of _____, 199___, by <u>CHILD ONE</u>, of _____, _____, <u>CHILD TWO</u>, of _____, _____, <u>CHILD THREE</u>, of _____, of _____ and <u>CHILD FOUR</u>, of _____, _____, who, depending upon the context, are hereinafter referred to sometimes as the Settlors (hereinafter referred to in the first person), and sometimes as the Trustees (hereinafter referred to sometimes as the "Trustee" and sometimes in the third person impersonal).

ARTICLE I

CREATION OF TRUST

We hereby deposit with the Trustee the property listed in Schedule A of this Trust Agreement. The Trustee agrees to hold said property, the receipt of which is hereby acknowledged, for the purposes and on the terms and provisions hereinafter set forth, and agrees that it will similarly hold all other property that may be added hereto (a) by any or all of us in our individual capacities (any such property added by any or all of us to be so added only with the consent of the Trustee, which consent shall not be withheld unreasonably), pursuant to the provisions of our Last Wills and Testaments or any Codicils thereto, or by any other manner, and (b) by any other person, by inter vivos transfer (any such property added by any such other person, during his lifetime, to be so added only with the consent of the Trustee, which consent shall not be withheld unreasonably), by last will and testament or codicil thereto, or by any other manner. Any property added by us (or any one of us) during our lifetimes or pursuant to the provisions of our Last Wills and Testaments or any Codicils thereto or by any other manner at or after our deaths, shall be held, administered and distributed in accordance with the applicable provisions of this Trust Agreement unless we shall expressly specify that a particular trust or part thereof hereinafter established shall be the recipient of such property, in which event such property so added by us shall be so held, administered and distributed. Any property added by any such other person shall be held, administered and distributed pursuant to the provisions of Articles III and IV hereof (and the other applicable provisions of this Trust Agreement).

ARTICLE II

RIGHTS RESERVED BY THE SETTLORS

A. We shall have the right, while all of us are living, by written instrument signed by all of us and delivered to the Trustee, (1) to terminate this Trust as to all or any part of the trust estate, (2) to withdraw any assets at any time held hereunder and/or (3) to change the Trustee hereunder. Upon the death of the first of us to die, these rights shall cease.

B. While all of us are living, this Trust Agreement may be amended or modified by an instrument in writing signed by all of us and the Trustee. Upon the death of the first of us to die, this Trust Agreement shall become irrevocable; and, except as provided in Paragraph C of this Article II, none of us shall have any right or power, either alone or in conjunction with others, and in any capacity whatsoever, to alter, amend, modify, revoke or terminate this Trust or any of the terms of this Trust Agreement in whole or in part.

C. Upon the death of any Settlor, such Settlor shall have the power to appoint **[one-fourth]** of The Remaining Trust Estate, as the same is defined in the first sentence of Article IV hereof, pursuant to the provisions of Subparagraphs 1, 2, 3, or 4, as applicable, of Paragraph A of Article IV hereof.

ARTICLE III

DISTRIBUTIONS DURING LIFETIME OF SETTLORS' [**MOTHER/FATHER**],

_____

During the lifetime of our [**mother/father**], _____, the Trustee shall hold, administer and distribute the trust estate held hereunder in accordance with the following provisions.

A. 1. Notwithstanding the provisions of Subparagraph 1 of Paragraph I of Article VI hereof, any one Trustee (whether at such time or times as four (4) Trustees are serving hereunder, at such time or times as three (3) Trustees are serving hereunder, at such time or times as two (2) Trustees are serving hereunder or at such time or times as only one (1) Trustee is serving hereunder) may distribute to or for the benefit of our said [**mother/father**], out of the net income or principal or both of the trust estate being held hereunder, such amount or amounts (whether the whole or a lesser amount), as said Trustee, in its sole and unfettered discretion, deems appropriate for any reason whatsoever; concurrence of more than one Trustee shall not be required. At the end of each taxable year the Trustee shall add any undistributed income to the principal of the trust estate being held hereunder.

2. We do not intend to displace any source of income otherwise available to our said [**mother/father**] for [**his/her**] basic support (such as food and shelter), including any governmental assistance program to which our said [**mother/father**] is or may be entitled. This trust is not intended to be a resource of our said [**mother/father**]. It is not available to [**him/her**]. No part of the corpus or income from the corpus of this trust shall be used to supplant or replace any public assistance benefits which our said [**mother/father**] is to receive from or through any county, state, federal or other governmental agency. Neither the State of _____ nor any Federal, state or local public entity or subdivision, department, or agency thereof may compel the Trustee to pay to it income or principal from the trust estate in reimbursement of costs incurred by such governmental entity in respect of care or services rendered to our said [**mother/father**].

3. The provisions of this Subparagraph 3 shall be applicable only at such time or times as [**four (4)**] Trustees are serving hereunder. Notwithstanding the provisions of Subparagraph 1 of Paragraph I of Article VI hereof, the Trustee may distribute to or for the benefit of the members of a class consisting of said <u>CHILD ONE</u>, said <u>CHILD TWO</u>, said <u>CHILD THREE</u>, and said <u>CHILD FOUR</u>, their children and issue (living from time to time, of whatever degree and whenever born) out of the net income or principal or both of the trust estate being held hereunder, such amount or amounts (whether the whole or a lesser amount), as the Trustee, in its sole discretion, deems appropriate for any reason whatsoever, but only with the concurrence of all four trustees. It is our intention that distributions under this Subparagraph 3 shall be made to or for the benefit of such persons in accordance with the circumstances affecting them individually. It is not our intention to require that the dollar distributions made under this Subparagraph 3 to or for the benefit of such persons shall be equal, and the Trustee is authorized, in accordance with the provisions of this Subparagraph 3, to make distributions of net income or principal or both hereunder to or for the benefit of one of such persons to the exclusion of the other without any duty to equalize those distributions. At the end of each taxable year the Trustee shall add any undistributed income to the principal of the trust estate being held hereunder.

B. The Trustee shall reimburse each Settlor annually, out of the assets of the trust estate, such amount as shall be equal to the excess of (a) all income taxes, Federal, state and local (including interest and penalties thereon) which become payable by such Settlor for the preceding calendar year by reason of the existence of this Trust Agreement during such preceding calendar year over (b) the income taxes, Federal, state and local (including interest and penalties thereon) that would have been payable by such Settlor for the preceding calendar year if this Trust Agreement had not been in existence during such preceding calendar year. The Trustee shall pay this amount at such times as such Settlor may in writing request as funds are needed to pay said income taxes (including interest and penalties thereon).

ARTICLE IV

ADMINISTRATION OF TRUST ESTATE UPON DEATH OF SETTLORS' [**MOTHER/FATHER**], _____

Upon the death of our [**mother/father**], _____, the Trustee shall hold, administer and distribute the assets of the trust estate held hereunder which remain after the provisions of Article III hereof have been provided for (such property being hereinafter referred to as "The Remaining Trust Estate"), in accordance with the following provisions.

A. The Trustee shall divide The Remaining Trust Estate, if any, into [**four (4)**] equal shares to be distributed as follows:

1. The Trustee shall distribute one (1) such equal share of The Remaining Trust Estate to said CHILD ONE, if [**he/she**] is then living. If said CHILD ONE is not then living, the Trustee shall, subject to the following provisos, distribute such equal share of The Remaining Trust Estate to or for the benefit of such person or persons out of the class composed of said PARENT NAME's children and [**his/her**] children's issue (of whatever degree and whenever born), and in such amounts and proportions as said CHILD ONE may appoint by [**his/her**] Last Will and Testament or any Codicil thereto; provided, however, anything herein to the contrary notwithstanding, such power of appointment granted under this Subparagraph 1 shall not be exercised in favor of, or to or for the benefit of, said CHILD ONE, [**his/her**] estate, [**his/her**] creditors, or the creditors of [**his/her**] estate; provided, further, however, that in order for the exercise by said CHILD ONE of said power of appointment to be effective, [**he/she**] must exercise such power by specific reference to this Trust Agreement in the provisions of [**his/her**] Last Will and Testament or such Codicil. If said CHILD ONE fails to exercise such power of appointment, or insofar as any such appointment shall be void or shall not take effect, then the Trustee shall distribute such share of The Remaining Trust Estate, in equal shares, to said CHILD ONE's children who are then living, treating as a then living child of said CHILD ONE for this purpose the then living collective issue of any child of said CHILD ONE who shall then be deceased, the distribution to such issue to be *per stirpes*, the root of the *per stirpes* distribution to be such deceased child.

2. The Trustee shall distribute one (1) such equal share of The Remaining Trust Estate to said CHILD TWO if [**he/she**] is then living. If said CHILD TWO is not then living, the Trustee shall, subject to the following provisos, distribute such equal share of The Remaining Trust Estate to or for the benefit of such person or persons out of the class composed of said PARENT NAME's children and [**his/her**] children's issue (of whatever degree and whenever born), and in such amounts and proportions as said CHILD TWO may appoint by [**his/her**] Last Will and Testament or any Codicil thereto; provided, however, anything herein to the contrary notwithstanding, such power of appointment granted under this Subparagraph 2 shall not be exercised in favor of, or to or for the benefit of, said CHILD TWO, [**his/her**] estate, [**his/her**] creditors, or the creditors of [**his/her**] estate; provided, further, however, that in order for the exercise by said CHILD TWO of said power of appointment to be effective, [**he/she**] must exercise such power by specific reference to this Trust Agreement in the provisions of [**his/her**] Last Will and Testament or such Codicil. If said CHILD TWO fails to exercise such power of appointment, or insofar as any such appointment shall be void or shall not take effect, then the Trustee shall distribute such share of The Remaining Trust Estate, in equal shares, to said CHILD TWO's children who are then living, treating as a then living child of said CHILD TWO for this purpose the then living collective issue of any child of said CHILD TWO who shall then be deceased, the distribution to such issue to be *per stirpes*, the root of the *per stirpes* distribution to be such deceased child.

3. The Trustee shall distribute one (1) such equal share of The Remaining Trust Estate to said CHILD THREE, if [**he/she**] is then living. If said CHILD THREE is not then living, the Trustee shall, subject to the following provisos, distribute such equal share of The Remaining Trust Estate to or for the benefit of such person or persons out of the class composed of said PARENT NAME's children and [**his/her**] children's issue (of whatever degree and whenever born), and in such amounts and pro-portions as said CHILD THREE may appoint by [**his/her**] Last Will and Testament or any Codicil

thereto; provided, however, anything herein to the contrary notwithstanding, such power of appointment granted under this Subparagraph 3 shall not be exercised in favor of, or to or for the benefit of, said CHILD THREE, [his/her] estate, [his/her] creditors, or the creditors of [his/her] estate; provided, further, however, that in order for the exercise by said CHILD THREE of said power of appointment to be effective, [he/she] must exercise such power by specific reference to this Trust Agreement in the provisions of [his/her] Last Will and Testament or such Codicil. If said CHILD THREE fails to exercise such power of appointment, or insofar as any such appointment shall be void or shall not take effect, then the Trustee shall distribute such share of The Remaining Trust Estate, in equal shares, to said CHILD THREE's children who are then living, treating as a then living child of said CHILD THREE for this purpose the then living collective issue of any child of said CHILD THREE who shall then be deceased, the distribution to such issue to be *per stirpes,* the root of the *per stirpes* distribution to be such deceased child.

      4. The Trustee shall distribute one (1) such equal share of The Remaining Trust Estate to said CHILD FOUR, if [he/she] is then living. If said CHILD FOUR is not then living, the Trustee shall, subject to the following provisos, distribute such equal share of The Remaining Trust Estate to or for the benefit of such person or persons out of the class composed of said PARENT NAME's children and [his/her] children's issue (of whatever degree and whenever born), and in such amounts and proportions as said CHILD FOUR may appoint by [his/her] Last Will and Testament or any Codicil thereto; provided, however, anything herein to the contrary notwithstanding, such power of appointment granted under this Subparagraph 4 shall not be exercised in favor of, or to or for the benefit of, said CHILD FOUR, [his/her] estate, [his/her] creditors, or the creditors of [his/her] estate; provided, further, however, that in order for the exercise by said CHILD FOUR of said power of appointment to be effective, [he/she] must exercise such power by specific reference to this Trust Agreement in the provisions of [his/her] Last Will and Testament or such Codicil. If said CHILD FOUR fails to exercise such power of appointment, or insofar as any such appointment shall be void or shall not take effect, then the Trustee shall distribute such share of The Remaining Trust Estate, in equal shares, to said CHILD FOUR's children who are then living, treating as a then living child of said CHILD FOUR for this purpose the then living collective issue of any child of said CHILD FOUR who shall then be deceased, the distribution to such issue to be *per stirpes,* the root of the *per stirpes* distribution to be such deceased child.

      5. In the event that one or more of the distributions provided for in Subparagraphs 1 through 4 of this Paragraph A cannot be made because there is no person then living entitled to take distribution thereunder, then such distribution shall be made to those then living persons entitled to take distribution under said Subparagraphs 1 through 4, in shares proportionate to the shares which such persons are entitled to receive under the provisions of said Subparagraphs 1 through 4.

      B. If, at the time for distribution of any share or portion of the trust estate being held pursuant to this Article IV, there is no person or person's estate entitled under the provisions of this Article IV other than this Paragraph B to take such distribution, the Trustee shall distribute, free of the trust, such share or portion to such person or persons as would be entitled to inherit from said PARENT'S NAME and in the proportions they would so inherit under the laws of the State of _____ as though [he/she] had died intestate, not survived by a spouse and domiciled in the State of _____ at the time distribution is so to be made.

      C. If the Trustee is authorized pursuant to the provisions of this Trust Agreement to make distributions or payments to or for the benefit of any person (including distributions or payments directed or permitted to be made to a person who is under legal disability or, in the reasonable opinion of the Trustee, is unable properly to administer such distributions or payments), the Trustee may make such distributions or payments in any one or more of the following ways, as the Trustee may deem advisable: (1) directly to such beneficiary, (2) to the legal guardian of such beneficiary or (3) to any Custodian then serving for such beneficiary or to any person designated by the Trustee to serve as a Custodian for such person (any such Custodian may be any one of the [four (4)] Trustees serving in their individual capacity). The Trustee shall not be required to see to the application of any distribution or payment so made, but the receipt of any of the persons mentioned in Clause (1), (2), or (3) in the immediately preceding sentence shall be a full discharge for the Trustee.

D. No interest whatsoever in the principal and/or income of any trust estate being administered under the provisions of this Article IV shall be alienated, disposed of, or in any manner assigned or encumbered by the person for whom held, voluntarily or involuntarily, while such principal and/or income is in the possession or control of the Trustee. If, by reason of any act of any such person or by operation of law, or by the happening of any event, or for any other reason except by an act of the Trustee specifically authorized hereunder, any such principal and/or income of The Remaining Trust Estate would but for this Paragraph D cease to be enjoyed by any such person or, by reason of an attempt by any such person to alienate, charge, assign or encumber any of such principal and/or income of The Remaining Trust Estate, or by reason of the bankruptcy or insolvency of any such person, or by reason of any attachment, garnishment or other proceeding, based upon a valid court judgment, or by reason of any order, finding or judgment of any court either at law or in equity, any of the principal and/or income of The Remaining Trust Estate would but for this Paragraph D vest in or be enjoyed by some individual, firm or corporation otherwise than as provided herein, then, in any of such events, the trust hereby created for the benefit of such person shall forthwith cease and determine as to such person, who shall thereupon cease to be a beneficiary under this Article IV, and such person shall be ineligible to serve or to continue to serve as Trustee hereunder. For purposes of this Paragraph D, the exercise of any power of appointment granted herein or the exercise of any disclaimer by a beneficiary of any rights or benefits under this Trust Agreement shall not cause or result in the provisions of this Paragraph D becoming applicable. Such trust thereafter, subject to all other applicable provisions of this Trust Agreement and of the trust of which such person was a beneficiary, shall, during the life of such former beneficiary, be held by the Trustee which, until such former beneficiary's death, may pay to or expend for the benefit of such former beneficiary, out of the principal and/or income of such trust, such sums but such sums only as the Trustee in its absolute discretion may determine, and may also pay to or expend for the benefit of the spouse, child or children of such former beneficiary, out of the principal and/or income of such trust, such sums but such sums only as the Trustee in its absolute discretion may determine, retaining any undistributed principal and/or income until such former beneficiary's death; provided, however, that no payments made under these provisions to or for the benefit of such former beneficiary and any such former beneficiary's spouse, child or children shall exceed the amounts otherwise payable to such former beneficiary if these provisions had not been invoked. Any undistributed income shall from time to time be added to the principal of such trust. Upon the death of such former beneficiary, such trust as then constituted, including all accrued and undistributed income, shall, subject to all applicable provisions of this Trust Agreement and of the trust for the benefit of such former beneficiary, be distributed to the persons (determined as of the date of death of such former beneficiary) to whom such trust estate would have been so distributable as if such former beneficiary had died prior to the time for any mandatory distribution of the trust estate to such former beneficiary (or, if such former beneficiary would not have been entitled to any mandatory distribution of the trust estate during such former beneficiary's lifetime under the provisions of this Trust Agreement, then to the persons who would be entitled to take distribution upon such former beneficiary's death under the provisions of this Trust Agreement), and as if the provisions of this Paragraph D had never become applicable to the trust of such former beneficiary.

E. Any provisions of this Trust Agreement to the contrary notwithstanding, if not already distributed, all accrued and undistributed income and the entire principal of every trust estate then held hereunder shall be paid over and distributed outright and free of the trust not later than the end of the day immediately preceding the expiration of twenty-one (21) years from and after the death of the last to die of said <u>PARENT'S NAME</u>, said <u>CHILD ONE</u>, said <u>CHILD TWO</u>, said <u>CHILD THREE</u>, and said <u>CHILD FOUR</u>, and their children and issue living at the date of death of the first to die of said <u>CHILD ONE</u>, said <u>CHILD TWO</u>, said <u>CHILD THREE</u>, and said <u>CHILD FOUR</u>. Such payment and distribution shall be made to the person or persons for whose benefit the trust estate or estates respectively shall then be held hereunder; provided, however, that if at such time the provisions of the immediately preceding Paragraph D of this Article IV shall be in operation as to any trust, such trust shall be distributed to those persons who would have been entitled to receive such trust as if the former beneficiary for whose benefit such trust was originally created had died immediately preceding the time so provided for such distribution and possessed of said trust estate, such distribution to be outright and free of the trust.

ARTICLE V

DEFINITIONS

A. The words "issue," "child" and "children," as used herein, shall be deemed to include any legally adopted person as if he or she were the natural child of the adopting parent, provided such adopted person was adopted prior to the age of majority.

B. Whenever the context so requires, the use of words herein in the singular shall be construed to include the plural, and the words in the plural, the singular, and words whether in the masculine, feminine or neuter gender shall be construed to include all of said genders.

C. For purposes of this Trust Agreement, any individual shall be deemed to be unable to continue to serve as Trustee hereunder only when:

(1) Such individual's attending physician and at least one other physician licensed in the United States (or, if such individual does not have an attending physician, at least two physicians licensed in the United States) (provided, however, that neither my nor such person's attending physician or any other physician acting hereunder shall be PARENT'S NAME, CHILD ONE, CHILD TWO, CHILD THREE, CHILD FOUR or a child or issue of such individuals) shall have signed and delivered to the Trustee then serving hereunder (or, if such Trustee is the person who is deemed to be unable to continue to serve as Trustee hereunder, then to any fiduciary serving hereunder or to the person who is to succeed such individual as Trustee) their written statements indicating that such individual is incapable in their judgment of attending effectively to such individual's fiduciary duties by reason of mental or physical disability; provided, that the written statements to which reference is made above shall be acknowledged before a notary public and witnessed by two individuals, one of whom may be the notary public; provided, further, that any person relying on any such written statements by such physicians may presume that the identity and qualifications of the physicians signing any such statement are in fact who and what they purport to be, and such person shall not have any duty to make further inquiry or investigation beyond the review of each written statement itself; provided, further, that no person relying on such written statement shall be liable to any other person or persons for action taken in reliance on such written statement; or

(2) Such person is adjudicated incompetent.

ARTICLE VI

POWERS AND DUTIES OF TRUSTEE

A. There shall be no duty on the Trustee to pay or see to the payment of any premiums on any policies of life insurance or to take any steps to keep them in force, until such time as the Trustee holds title to any insurance policies hereunder as a part of the corpus of any trust estate. The Trustee furthermore assumes no responsibility with respect to the validity or enforceability of said policies. However, as soon as practicable after receiving notice of the death of the insured under any of such policies, the Trustee shall proceed to collect all amounts payable thereunder. The Trustee shall have full and complete authority to collect and receive any and all such amounts and its receipt therefor shall be a full and complete acquittance to any insurer or payor, who shall be under no obligation to see to the proper application thereof by the Trustee.

B. In the administration of the trusts created hereunder and in addition to the powers exercised by trustees generally, the Trustee shall have the following powers and authorities without any court order or proceeding, exercisable in the discretion of the Trustee:

1. To purchase as an investment for the trust estate or estates any property, real or personal, belonging to our estates;

2. To retain as suitable investments for the trust estate or estates any properties received by it from us and/or our estates, and whether received by purchase or in any other manner, without regard to any law, statutory or judicial, or any rule or practice of court now or hereafter in force specifying or limiting the permissible investments of trustees, trust companies or fiduciaries generally or requiring the diversification of investments, and without liability to any person whomsoever for loss or depreciation in value thereof;

3. To sell, exchange, convey, mortgage, pledge, lease, control, and manage, and to make contracts concerning, any of the properties, real or personal, comprised in the trust estate or estates, all either publicly or privately and for such considerations and upon such terms as to credit or otherwise as may be reasonable under the circumstances, which leases and contracts may extend beyond the duration of any of the trusts created hereunder; to give options therefor; and to execute deeds, transfers, mortgages, leases and other instruments of any kind;

4. To invest and reinvest the properties from time to time comprised in the trust estate or estates in stocks, common and/or preferred, bonds, notes, debentures, loans, mortgages, common trust funds, or other securities or property, real or personal, all limitations now or hereafter imposed by law, statutory or judicial, or by any rule or practice of court now or hereafter in force specifying or limiting the permissible investments of trustees, trust companies or fiduciaries generally or requiring the diversification of investments, being hereby expressly waived, it being the intent hereof that the Trustee shall have full power and authority to deal with the trust estate or estates in all respects as though it were the sole owner thereof, without order of court or other authority;

5. To borrow money, from itself or otherwise, with or without security, whenever it deems such action advisable;

6. To exercise voting rights, execute and deliver powers of attorney and proxies and similarly act with reference to shares of stock and other securities comprised in the trust estate or estates in such manner as it deems proper, including, without limitation, the power to participate in or oppose reorganizations, recapitalizations, mergers, consolidations, exchanges, liquidations, arrangements and other corporate actions;

7. To collect all money; in accordance with generally accepted trust accounting principles, to determine whether money or other property coming into its possession shall be treated as principal or income and to charge or apportion expenses, taxes, gains and losses to principal or income;

8. To compromise, adjust and settle claims in favor of or against the trust estate or estates upon such terms and conditions as it may deem best; in the case of any litigation in connection with any part of such trust estate or estates, it may, under advice of its counsel, arbitrate, settle, or adjust any such matter in dispute upon such terms as it may consider just and equitable, and its decision shall be binding upon the beneficiaries;

9. To employ investment counsel, custodians of estate property, brokers, accountants, attorneys, clerical or bookkeeping assistants, and other suitable agents and to pay their reasonable compensation and expenses in addition to any compensation payable to the Trustee, and to execute and deliver powers of attorney; to appoint and remove by written instrument, containing such terms and conditions as it may deem appropriate, any natural or legal person or persons as special Trustee to hold all or any part of any real property or other interest in property held in the trust estate or estates and which the Trustee determines, in its sole discretion, it cannot or, because of legal limitations on its powers, it deems inadvisable to hold as Trustee hereunder, and such special Trustee, except as specifically limited by the appointing instrument, shall have the powers, authorities and discretion under this Paragraph B granted to the Trustee with respect to the trust property held by such special Trustee; the Trustee shall not be liable for any neglect, omission or wrongdoing of such investment counsel, custodians, brokers, accountants, attorneys, assistants, agents or special Trustees, provided reasonable care shall have been exercised in their selection;

10. To hold title to stocks, bonds, or other securities or property, real or personal, in its own name or in the name of its nominee and without indication of any fiduciary capacity or to hold any such bonds or securities in bearer form; the Trustee shall assume full responsibility for the acts of any nominee selected by it;

11. To hold as a single fund or unit any part or all of the property comprising any two or more of the separate and distinct shares or portions of The Remaining Trust Estate and to allot undivided interests in such single fund or unit to such separate shares or portions in proportion to the interest of each therein, except that no such holding shall defer the vesting in possession of any estate;

12. To make all repairs, alterations or improvements of any real property which shall constitute a part of the trust estate or estates; adjust boundaries thereof, and to erect or demolish buildings thereon; and, with respect to such property, to convert for different use, grant easements for adequate consideration, partition, and insure for any or all risks;

13. To pay premiums on any policies of life insurance which may form a part of the trust estate or estates; to cancel, sell, assign, hypothecate, pledge or otherwise dispose of any of said policies; to exercise any right, election, option or privilege granted by any of said policies; to borrow any sums in accordance with the provisions of any of said policies, and to receive all payments, dividends, surrender values, additions, benefits or privileges of any kind which may accrue to any of said policies;

14. To make any allocation, division or distribution required or permitted hereunder in cash or in kind, in real or personal property, or an undivided interest therein, or partly in cash and partly in kind and to do so without making pro rata allocations, divisions or distributions of specific assets, property allocated, divided or distributed in kind to be taken at its fair market value at the time of such allocation, division or distribution;

15. To receive, in accordance with the provisions of Article I hereof, additional property from us or any other person, the Trustee being authorized and empowered to merge and hold as one any duplicate trusts held for the same beneficiary; and

16. To make such expenditures and do such other acts as are reasonably required to manage, improve, protect, preserve, invest or sell any of the trust estates or otherwise properly to administer this Trust.

C. The Trustee shall keep accurate records showing all receipts and disbursements and other transactions involving the trust estate or estates and shall furnish annually to each beneficiary currently entitled to income (1) a statement of the receipts and disbursements affecting such beneficiary's interest in the trust and (2) a complete inventory of the trust estate then held for the benefit of such beneficiary.

D. No person, firm or corporation dealing with the Trustee or a nominee of the Trustee or performing any act pursuant to action taken or order given by the Trustee or such nominee shall be obliged to inquire as to the propriety, validity or legality thereof hereunder, nor shall any such person be liable for the application of any money or other consideration paid to the Trustee or such nominee, but, instead, may rely upon any action taken by the Trustee or such nominee pursuant to the powers and authorities conferred upon it under the provisions of this Article VI in all respects as if the same were completely unlimited. No transfer agent or registrar of any security held hereunder shall be required to inquire as to the propriety, validity or legality of any transfer made by the Trustee or such nominee.

E. Any successor Trustee shall have and enjoy all the powers, authorities, duties and immunities hereby vested in and imposed upon the original Trustee and no successor Trustee shall be obliged to inquire into or be in any way accountable for the previous administration of the trust property.

F. In determining the amount of any discretionary distributions of income or principal to a beneficiary of a trust created hereunder, the Trustee may take into account all means and resources known to or reasonably ascertainable by such Trustee which are available to such beneficiary for the purposes for which such Trustee is authorized to make said distributions.

G. The Trustee shall serve without compensation, although the Trustee shall be entitled to be reimbursed for any reasonable expenses it incurs which are necessary to carry out its duties as Trustee hereunder.

H. 1. In the event that any of said <u>CHILD ONE</u>, said <u>CHILD TWO</u>, said <u>CHILD THREE</u> or said <u>CHILD FOUR</u> shall become unwilling or unable to continue to serve as a Trustee hereunder, then such one or ones of said <u>CHILD ONE</u>, said <u>CHILD TWO</u>, said <u>CHILD THREE</u> and said <u>CHILD FOUR</u> who shall be willing and able to continue to serve shall, upon **[their, his, or her]** formal written acceptances or acceptance, serve as Trustees or as sole Trustee hereunder.

2. Any Trustee shall be entitled to resign as Trustee for any reason whatsoever by giving written notice to the Trustee designated to succeed it (or if there is no Trustee then designated to succeed it, to the Trustee who is thereafter designated to succeed it), provided that the Trustee designated to succeed it shall first execute a formal written acceptance of the duties and obligations of the Trustee hereunder and file an executed copy of such acceptance with the preceding Trustee. After this is done, and when all sums then due from the trust estate to such predecessor Trustee have been paid, such predecessor Trustee shall transfer the Trust property then in its hands to such successor Trustee and such predecessor Trustee shall thereupon and thereby be discharged of all subsequent duties and obligations under or arising out of its Trusteeship.

I. The provisions of this Paragraph I shall not apply to the provisions of Subparagraph 1 of Paragraph A of Article III hereof or to the provisions of Subparagraph 3 of Paragraph A of Article III hereof. The provisions of this Paragraph I shall apply for purposes of all other provisions of this Trust Agreement.

1. When only one (1) Trustee is serving, such Trustee shall act alone. When two (2) Trustees are serving, no decision shall be made or proposed action taken by my Trustees except upon the concurrence of both of them. When more than two (2) Trustees are serving, no decision shall be made or proposed action taken by them except upon a majority of all of those serving. Any one (1) Trustee acting alone shall be authorized to take any action authorized hereunder and agreed to by my Trustees in accordance with the immediately preceding two (2) sentences.

2. Each co-Trustee hereunder shall be responsible solely for **[his or her]** own decisions and not for those of **[his or her]** co-Trustee or co-Trustees.

J. No bond shall be required of the Trustee hereunder or any successor Trustee.

ARTICLE VII

GOVERNING LAW

       This Trust Agreement shall be construed under and in accordance with the laws of the State of _____.

       IN WITNESS WHEREOF, we, as Settlors and as Trustees, have executed this Trust Agreement, in quintuplicate, at _____, _____, on the day and year first above written.

Signed in the presence of:

_____   _____

                                                                        "Settlor"

_____   _____

                                                                          "Settlor"

_____   _____

                                                                          "Settlor"

_____   _____

                                                                          "Settlor"

_____   _____

                                                                         "Trustee"

_____   _____

                                                                          "Trustee"

_____   _____

_____   _____
                                                    "Trustee"

_____   _____
                                                    "Trustee"

_____   _____

      We, the undersigned legal spouses of the Settlors, hereby waive all community property, dower or courtesy rights which we may have in the hereinabove-described property and give our assent to the provisions of the trust and to the inclusion in it of the said property.

                                                                       _____

                                                                       _____

Witness: _____   Witness: _____

                                                                        _____

                                                                        _____

Witness: _____   Witness: _____

                                                                        _____

                                                                        _____

Witness: _____   Witness: _____

11

STATE OF _____   City
                                      or
COUNTY OF _____   Town _____

On the _____ day of _____, 19____ personally
appeared _____, known to me to be the
individual(s) who executed the foregoing instrument, and acknowledged the same to be **[his/her]** free act
and deed, before me.

My commission expires: _____   _____
                                             Notary Public

SCHEDULE A

The following is a true and correct Schedule A of the property assigned, delivered and conveyed to _____, Trustee, to be held, treated and disposed of in accordance with the terms of a certain Trust Agreement between _____ _____, the Settlors, and _____, the Trustees, dated _____, 19____, to which Agreement this Schedule A is attached and made a part thereof.

_____

_____

_____

_____

_____

_____

_____

_____

_____

_____

_____

_____

_____

_____

_____

Signed in the presence of:

_____   _____
                                                   "Settlor"

_____   _____
                                                   "Settlor"

_____   _____
                                                   "Settlor"

_____   _____
                                                   "Settlor"

13

_____

_____

"Trustee"

_____

_____

"Trustee"

_____

_____

"Trustee"

_____

_____

"Trustee"

We, the undersigned legal spouses of the Settlors, hereby waive all community property, dower or courtesy rights which we may have in the hereinabove-described property and give our assent to the provisions of the trust and to the inclusion in it of the said property.

_____

_____

Witness: _____   Witness: _____

_____

Witness: _____   Witness: _____

_____

Witness: _____   Witness: _____

_____

Witness: _____   Witness: _____

14

ADDITION OF PROPERTY TO TRUST AGREEMENT

BY _____

DATED _____, 19____

WITH _____, TRUSTEES

_____ (the "Assignor"), pursuant to the terms of the above-described Trust Agreement, does hereby assign, transfer and convey to _____ _____, Trustee and _____, Trustee, does hereby acknowledge receipt of, the following assets from the Assignor:

_____

_____

_____

_____

_____

_____

_____

_____

_____

_____

_____

_____

_____

_____

_____

_____

_____

_____

The Trustee agrees to hold, manage and administer the above assets as a part of the trust estate created under such Trust Agreement.

At the request of the Trustee, the Assignor shall fully cooperate and execute any and all documents deemed necessary or desirable by it in order to cause the assignment made hereby to be properly recorded.

IN WITNESS WHEREOF, the Assignor and the Trustee have signed their names at _____, _____, on this _____ day of _____, 19____.

Signed in the presence of:

_____

_____   _____, Assignor

_____

_____   _____, Trustee

_____   _____, Trustee

_____   _____, Trustee

_____   _____, Trustee

_____

       I, the undersigned legal spouse of the Assignor, hereby waive all community property, dower or courtesy rights which I may have in the hereinabove-described property and give my assent to the inclusion in the trust of the said property.

_____

_____

Witness: _____   Witness: _____

STATE OF _____   City
or
COUNTY OF _____   Town _____

       On the _____ day of _____, 19____, personally appeared _____, known to me to be the individual(s) who executed the foregoing instrument, and acknowledged the same to be **[his/her]** free act and deed, before me.

_____
Notary Public

My commission expires:

_____

Trust Agreement

Explanation

As you can see, this revocable family asset protection trust agreement, to be created by the children of a Medicaid recipient or a potential future Medicaid recipient, is filled with legalese. Don't be scared off by this confusing language. The explanations that follow should provide you with a clear understanding of the terms.

Introduction: In the first blanks you would fill in the day, month, and year in which the agreement is to be executed and the name, city, and state of residence for each person who will be serving as trustee. Remember, neither the Medicaid recipient nor his or her spouse can be the trustee. Children or other close relatives will probably be the first choice.

Article I: This paragraph transfers into the trust all of the items listed on Schedule A at the end of the agreement. You can include on Schedule A just about any item imaginable, including real estate, personal property, savings and checking accounts, boats, cars, and even clothing.

If the property you put into the trust increases in value, the increased value is part of the trust. And if an asset changes form, the new asset remains in the trust. For example, if the trustee takes $5,000 from a bank account and buys $5,000 worth of stock, that stock remains in the trust. You can always add to the trust by using the Addition to Trust form following Schedule A.

Article II: This section provides that all of the settlors, acting together, may revoke or change the trust or withdraw assets at any time, as long as all agree. When one dies then these rights end and the trust becomes irrevocable.

Article III: This section provides that as long as your father or mother is alive, any one of the trustees may use income or assets from the trust for your parent. For this purpose, and *only* this purpose, one trustee may act alone. Before distributions are made, the financial circumstances of your parent must be considered. They do not have any legal right to require distributions from the trust, because if they did, then the trust assets would count against their Medicaid eligibility.

While any one trustee can distribute trust funds to your mother or father, all trustees must agree before any other distributions can be made. Distributions can be made to the children (you and your siblings) and grandchildren from trust income and/or principal, for any reason and in any proportions or amounts whatsoever, but only if all of the trustees agree.

You and your siblings will have to pay income tax on the income—interest and dividends—generated by the trust principal. Even if the income stays in the trust and is not distributed to you and your siblings, you must still pay income tax. But Article III(B) provides that the additional tax on trust income shall be paid from the trust. Note also that distributions of trust income or principal to your father or mother are gifts from the children, and if over $10,000 per child in any year, gift tax returns would have to be filed by the children.

Article IV: This section describes how your trust principal will be distributed after your parent dies.

Paragraph IV(A) provides that each child gets an equal share of the remaining trust principal. If a child had died, his or her will may "appoint" his or her share (state where the share should go and in what proportions), except that trust assets cannot be appointed to a creditor. If a child died before appointing his or her share under a will, then his or her share would go to his or her children; if the deceased child has no children, then his or her share would go to the deceased child's siblings.

Paragraph IV(B) provides for the distribution of the trust in the unlikely event that there's no one to receive the principal from your trust under the earlier provisions. In that case, the assets pass to your parent's next of kin under state law.

Paragraph IV(C) discusses distributions to beneficiaries named in your trust who are under some legal disability or are unable to administer their distributions.

If a distribution from your trust is to go to someone who is under a legal disability or unable to manage his or her money, the trustee has three options:

1. Pay the money to the beneficiary.
2. Make the distribution to a legal guardian of the beneficiary.

3. Distribute the beneficiary's portion to a custodian for the beneficiary.

If, when you make up your trust, you could predict the ages and physical and mental conditions of all of your beneficiaries at the time of your death, you could spell out which of these options you would want the trustee to pursue. But since you can't, this trust allows the trustee to choose which option he or she believes is best.

The last sentence of Part IV(C) says that once the trustee has made his or her choice and distributed a beneficiary's portion to the beneficiary or to the beneficiary's guardian or custodian, the trustee is off the hook; he or she doesn't have to monitor the use of the distribution after that.

Part IV(D), often called a spendthrift clause, provides that nobody but your intended beneficiary can obtain an interest in a distribution under your trust. For example, your child, who may be entitled to receive a portion of your trust, can't sell his or her expected distribution in the future to someone for cash now. And a beneficiary can't put up his or her interest in a distribution as collateral for a loan. After all, you want the person you name in the trust to receive a distribution, not some stranger.

Spendthrift clauses like this are enforced in most, but not all, states. If you have a serious concern that a beneficiary has or may have creditor problems, consult with a local attorney to determine whether this clause will be effective in your state.

Trusts cannot legally tie up assets forever, so Part IV(E) is designed to avoid potential problems by limiting the life of the trust.

Article V: This is the definition section. The most important point here is to recognize that a legally adopted child will be considered a child for purposes of the trust agreement. So by leaving your share to your children, any adopted child would be treated the same as a natural child.

Article VI: This section deals with the powers and duties you are giving to the trustee.

Part VI(A) says that after your death, the trustee must collect the money due under any insurance policy. The trustee does not have a duty to pay your life insurance premiums, however, until and unless the trustee takes title to any insurance policy.

Part VI(B) is very important, setting forth the powers of the trustee. As you can see, this trust agreement gives the trustee very broad powers to administer the funds and property in the estate, including the power to:

1. Buy real estate or personal property from your estates. Without this power, purchases by the trustees from their estates might not be allowed.
2. Keep in the trust anything received from you or your estates.
3. Sell, exchange, mortgage, and do just about anything else with property in the trust.
4. Invest the assets in the trust in just about anything.
5. Borrow money for the trust.
6. Manage stock and other securities.
7. Collect money for the trust.
8. Handle claims and lawsuits for or against the trust.
9. Hire and pay counselors and assistants, like lawyers and accountants, for the trust.
10. Hold property in his or her own name, in the name of a nominee, or in bearer form.
11. Maintain one fund for different trust shares.
12. Manage real estate in the trust, including repairing, improving, or converting property.
13. Handle life insurance policies in the trust, including paying premiums, canceling or selling policies, cashing in policies, or borrowing against them.
14. Make distributions under the trust in cash or in property.
15. Receive additional property for the trust.
16. Do anything else reasonably required to manage, protect, or preserve the trust assets.

Why put in many specific powers instead of just having item 16, which generally allows the trustee to do anything reasonably necessary? Because with only a general statement, someone with whom the trustee must deal may question his or her power and may refuse to do business with the trustee. For example, without specifically giving the trustee the power to sell real estate, buyers, lenders, and escrow agents may be hesitant to deal with him or her if your trust agreement only generally gives the trustee broad powers. By listing specific powers, you can ensure the trustee's ability to manage the trust properly.

Why give the trustee such broad powers anyway? Why not just specify a few actions the trustee may take? The reason is simple: you can't predict what the trustee may need to do to manage the trust properly, and if you don't give him or her broad powers, you may hamper and damage your trust estate. For example, if you don't own any stocks, why give the trustee power to manage them? Because at some point it might be in your best interest for your trustee to purchase securities, and you don't want your trust agreement to prevent him or her from doing so.

Part VI(C) requires the trustee to keep accurate records showing all transactions involving the trust.

Part VI(D) is designed to encourage people to deal with the trustee by relieving them of liability in case the trustee takes some action beyond his or her power. For example, if the trustee attempts to sell stock, the buyer can go ahead with the transaction and pay the trustee without worrying about whether the trust really allows the trustee to make that deal.

Part VI(E) gives any successor trustee all of the same powers and duties as the original trustee. It also encourages your chosen successor trustee to accept the job by providing that he or she has no responsibility for anything done by the earlier trustee.

Part VI(F) concerns discretionary distributions by the trustee. Trustees may consider the financial status of any potential beneficiary.

Part VI(G) provides that the trustee will serve without compensation. Since the trustee will be family, that should be no problem.

Part VI(H) provides that if one of the children cannot or will not serve as trustee, the other(s) shall serve alone. For example, if you and your two siblings are serving as trustee and one sibling resigns, you and your one remaining sibling may continue to serve.

Part VI(I) discusses how the trustee may manage the trust. If a time comes when only one trustee is serving, that trustee may act alone. That trustee may not make distributions to anyone except your father or mother but may carry out the other terms of the trust. If two trustees are serving, decisions must be made together. If more than two are serving, decisions may be made by a majority. This does not mean that all trustees must sign every check. The trustees may authorize one person to administer the trust on a day-to-day basis.

Part VI(J) states that the trustee does not have to post a bond. A bond is like an insurance policy; it is designed to protect your trust in case the trustee does something wrong, such as steal assets. Depend-

ing on the amount in the trust, a bond could easily cost your trust several hundred dollars.

Article VII: Article VII states that any questions about the trust will be answered by the laws of the state of your primary residence. In the blank space you would fill in the name of your state.

Conclusion: The blanks in the final paragraphs are for your city and state. Then each child who is creating the trust would sign where it says "Settlor" and each child who is serving as trustee would sign below that. Each person should print his or her name below the signature line. To the left of each signature, two witnesses to each signature must sign. The witnesses can be the same, but they don't have to be; if they are the same, they must sign twice, once for each settlor and once for each trustee. The witnesses cannot be members of your family.

Then each spouse would also sign, with two witnesses signing below. In many states, spouses have a legal interest in your property and must waive their rights in writing to the property covered by the trust.

The final section is for a notary public.

Schedule A: Following the end of the trust is Schedule A, on which you would list any items (cash accounts, real estate, personal property, and the like) to be placed under the control of the trustee. Identify each item as best you can, using addresses, registration numbers, account numbers, and other information wherever possible, to avoid confusion.

On Schedule A you would fill in the name of all of the trustees in the first blank, all of the settlors in the second blank, and all of the trustees again in the third blank. Then you would date the schedule.

At the bottom, each of the settlors, trustees, and spouses would sign before two independent witnesses.

Addition of Property Form: Finally, included is a form that can be used to add property to the trust later. At the top, you would fill in the names of the settlors, the date that the trust was originally made, and the names of the trustees. In the first full paragraph you would fill in the name of the assignor who is assigning property to the trustee. Then, on the lines that follow, you would list any items to be added to the trust. Again, identify each item as best you can. At the end, each of the settlors, trustees, and spouses would sign before two independent witnesses and a notary.

IRREVOCABLE TRUST AGREEMENT

THIS TRUST AGREEMENT is made at _____, _____, this _____ day of _____, 199___, by <u>CHILD ONE</u>, of _____, _____, <u>CHILD TWO</u>, of _____, _____, <u>CHILD THREE</u>, of _____, _____ and <u>CHILD FOUR</u>, of _____, _____, who, depending upon the context, are hereinafter referred to sometimes as the Settlors (hereinafter referred to in the first person), and sometimes as the Trustees (hereinafter referred to sometimes as the "Trustee" and sometimes in the third person impersonal).

ARTICLE I

CREATION OF TRUST

We hereby deposit with the Trustee the property listed in Schedule A of this Trust Agreement. The Trustee agrees to hold said property, the receipt of which is hereby acknowledged, for the purposes and on the terms and provisions hereinafter set forth, and agrees that it will similarly hold all other property that may be added hereto (a) by any or all of us in our individual capacities (any such property added by any or all of us to be so added only with the consent of the Trustee, which consent shall not be withheld unreasonably), pursuant to the provisions of our Last Wills and Testaments or any Codicils thereto, or by any other manner, and (b) by any other person, by inter vivos transfer (any such property added by any such other person, during his lifetime, to be so added only with the consent of the Trustee, which consent shall not be withheld unreasonably), by last will and testament or codicil thereto, or by any other manner. Any property added by us (or any one of us) during our lifetimes or pursuant to the provisions of our Last Wills and Testaments or any Codicils thereto or by any other manner at or after our deaths, shall be held, administered and distributed in accordance with the applicable provisions of this Trust Agreement unless we shall expressly specify that a particular trust or part thereof hereinafter established shall be the recipient of such property, in which event such property so added by us shall be so held, administered and distributed. Any property added by any such other person shall be held, administered and distributed pursuant to the provisions of Articles III and IV hereof (and the other applicable provisions of this Trust Agreement).

ARTICLE II

TRUST IS IRREVOCABLE

A. Except as provided in Paragraphs B and C of this Article II, this Trust Agreement shall be irrevocable, and we hereby expressly acknowledge that we shall have no right or power, either alone, together or in conjunction with others, and in any capacity whatsoever, to alter, amend, modify, revoke or terminate this Trust or any of the terms of this Trust Agreement in whole or in part.

B. We reserve to ourselves the right to add property to the trust estate by lifetime or testamentary gifts, in accordance with the provisions of Article I hereof, all of which added property shall be governed by the terms hereof.

C. Upon the death of any Settlor, such Settlor shall have the power to appoint **[one-fourth]** of The Remaining Trust Estate, as the same is defined in the first sentence of Article IV hereof, pursuant to the provisions of Subparagraphs 1, 2, 3, or 4, as applicable, of Paragraph A of Article IV hereof.

1

ARTICLE III

DISTRIBUTIONS DURING LIFETIME OF SETTLORS' [**MOTHER/FATHER**],

_____

During the lifetime of our [**mother/ father**], _____, the Trustee shall hold, administer and distribute the trust estate held hereunder in accordance with the following provisions.

A. 1. Notwithstanding the provisions of Subparagraph 1 of Paragraph I of Article VI hereof, any one Trustee (whether at such time or times as four (4) Trustees are serving hereunder, at such time or times as three (3) Trustees are serving hereunder, at such time or times as two (2) Trustees are serving hereunder or at such time or times as only one (1) Trustee is serving hereunder) may distribute to or for the benefit of our said [**mother/father**], out of the net income or principal or both of the trust estate being held hereunder, such amount or amounts (whether the whole or a lesser amount), as said Trustee, in its sole and unfettered discretion, deems appropriate for any reason whatsoever; concurrence of more than one Trustee shall not be required. At the end of each taxable year the Trustee shall add any undistributed income to the principal of the trust estate being held hereunder.

2. We do not intend to displace any source of income otherwise available to our said [**mother/father**] for [**his/her**] basic support (such as food and shelter), including any governmental assistance program to which our said [**mother/father**] is or may be entitled. This trust is not intended to be a resource of our said [**mother/father**]. It is not available to [**him/her**]. No part of the corpus or income from the corpus of this trust shall be used to supplant or replace any public assistance benefits which our said [**mother/father**] is to receive from or through any county, state, federal or other governmental agency. Neither the State of _____ nor any Federal, state or local public entity or subdivision, department, or agency thereof may compel the Trustee to pay to it income or principal from the trust estate in reimbursement of costs incurred by such governmental entity in respect of care or services rendered to our said [**mother/father**].

B. The Trustee shall reimburse each Settlor annually, out of the assets of the trust estate, such amount as shall be equal to the excess of (a) all Federal, state and local income taxes (including interest and penalties thereon) which become payable by such Settlor for the preceding calendar year over (b) the Federal, state and local income taxes (including interest and penalties thereon) that would have been payable by such Settlor for the preceding calendar year if income from this Trust Agreement had not been included in the income of such Settlor during such preceding calendar year. The Trustee shall pay this amount at such times as such Settlor may in writing request as funds are needed to pay said income taxes (including interest and penalties thereon).

ARTICLE IV

ADMINISTRATION OF TRUST ESTATE UPON DEATH

OF SETTLORS' [**MOTHER/FATHER**], _____

Upon the death of our [**mother/father**], _____, the Trustee shall hold, administer and distribute the assets of the trust estate held hereunder which remain after the provisions of Article III hereof have been provided for (such property being hereinafter referred to as "The Remaining Trust Estate"), in accordance with the following provisions.

A. The Trustee shall divide The Remaining Trust Estate, if any, into [**four (4)**] equal shares to be distributed as follows:

1. The Trustee shall distribute one (1) such equal share of The Remaining Trust Estate to said <u>CHILD ONE</u>, if [**he/she**] is then living. If said <u>CHILD ONE</u> is not then living, the Trustee shall, subject to the following provisos, distribute such equal share of The Remaining Trust Estate to or for

the benefit of such person or persons out of the class composed of said <u>PARENT NAME</u>'s children and **[his/her]** children's issue (of whatever degree and whenever born), and in such amounts and proportions as said <u>CHILD ONE</u> may appoint by **[his/her]** Last Will and Testament or any Codicil thereto; provided, however, anything herein to the contrary notwithstanding, such power of appointment granted under this Subparagraph 1 shall not be exercised in favor of, or to or for the benefit of, said <u>CHILD ONE</u>, **[his/her]** estate, **[his/her]** creditors, or the creditors of **[his/her]** estate; provided, further, however, that in order for the exercise by said <u>CHILD ONE</u> of said power of appointment to be effective, **[he/she]** must exercise such power by specific reference to this Trust Agreement in the provisions of **[his/her]** Last Will and Testament or such Codicil. If said <u>CHILD ONE</u> fails to exercise such power of appointment, or insofar as any such appointment shall be void or shall not take effect, then the Trustee shall distribute such share of The Remaining Trust Estate, in equal shares, to said <u>CHILD ONE</u>'s children who are then living, treating as a then living child of said <u>CHILD ONE</u> for this purpose the then living collective issue of any child of said <u>CHILD ONE</u> who shall then be deceased, the distribution to such issue to be *per stirpes,* the root of the *per stirpes* distribution to be such deceased child.

    2. The Trustee shall distribute one (1) such equal share of The Remaining Trust Estate to said <u>CHILD TWO</u>, if **[he/she]** is then living. If said <u>CHILD TWO</u> is not then living, the Trustee shall, subject to the following provisos, distribute such equal share of The Remaining Trust Estate to or for the benefit of such person or persons out of the class composed of said <u>PARENT NAME</u>'s children and **[his/her]** children's issue (of whatever degree and whenever born), and in such amounts and proportions as said <u>CHILD TWO</u> may appoint by **[his/her]** Last Will and Testament or any Codicil thereto; provided, however, anything herein to the contrary notwithstanding, such power of appointment granted under this Subparagraph 2 shall not be exercised in favor of, or to or for the benefit of, said <u>CHILD TWO</u>, **[his/her]** estate, **[his/her]** creditors, or the creditors of **[his/her]** estate; provided, further, however, that in order for the exercise by said <u>CHILD TWO</u>, of said power of appointment to be effective, **[he/she]** must exercise such power by specific reference to this Trust Agreement in the provisions of **[his/her]** Last Will and Testament or such Codicil. If said <u>CHILD TWO</u> fails to exercise such power of appointment, or insofar as any such appointment shall be void or shall not take effect, then the Trustee shall distribute such share of The Remaining Trust Estate, in equal shares, to said <u>CHILD TWO</u>'s children who are then living, treating as a then living child of said <u>CHILD TWO</u> for this purpose the then living collective issue of any child of said <u>CHILD TWO</u> who shall then be deceased, the distribution to such issue to be *per stirpes,* the root of the *per stirpes* distribution to be such deceased child.

    3. The Trustee shall distribute one (1) such equal share of The Remaining Trust Estate to said <u>CHILD THREE</u>, if **[he/she]** is then living. If said <u>CHILD THREE</u> is not then living, the Trustee shall, subject to the following provisos, distribute such equal share of The Remaining Trust Estate to or for the benefit of such person or persons out of the class composed of said <u>PARENT NAME</u>'s children and **[his/her]** children's issue (of whatever degree and whenever born), and in such amounts and proportions as said <u>CHILD THREE</u> may appoint by **[his/her]** Last Will and Testament or any Codicil thereto; provided, however, anything herein to the contrary notwithstanding, such power of appointment granted under this Subparagraph 3 shall not be exercised in favor of, or to or for the benefit of, said <u>CHILD THREE</u>, **[his/her]** estate, **[his/her]** creditors, or the creditors of **[his/her]** estate; provided, further, however, that in order for the exercise by said <u>CHILD THREE</u> of said power of appointment to be effective, **[he/she]** must exercise such power by specific reference to this Trust Agreement in the provisions of **[his/her]** Last Will and Testament or such Codicil. If said <u>CHILD THREE</u> fails to exercise such power of appointment, or insofar as any such appointment shall be void or shall not take effect, then the Trustee shall distribute such share of The Remaining Trust Estate, in equal shares, to said <u>CHILD THREE</u>'s children who are then living, treating as a then living child of said <u>CHILD THREE</u> for this purpose the then living collective issue of any child of said <u>CHILD THREE</u> who shall then be deceased, the distribution to such issue to be *per stirpes,* the root of the *per stirpes* distribution to be such deceased child.

4. The Trustee shall distribute one (1) such equal share of The Remaining Trust Estate to said <u>CHILD FOUR</u>: if **[he/she]** is then living. If said <u>CHILD FOUR</u> is not then living, the Trustee shall, subject to the following provisos, distribute such equal share of The Remaining Trust Estate to or for the benefit of such person or persons out of the class composed of said <u>PARENT NAME</u>'s children and **[his/her]** children's issue (of whatever degree and whenever born), and in such amounts and proportions as said <u>CHILD FOUR</u> may appoint by **[his/her]** Last Will and Testament or any Codicil thereto; provided, however, anything herein to the contrary notwithstanding, such power of appointment granted under this Subparagraph 4 shall not be exercised in favor of, or to or for the benefit of, said <u>CHILD FOUR</u>, **[his/her]** estate, **[his/her]** creditors, or the creditors of **[his/her]** estate; provided, further, however, that in order for the exercise by said <u>CHILD FOUR</u> of said power of appointment to be effective, **[he/she]** must exercise such power by specific reference to this Trust Agreement in the provisions of **[his/her]** Last Will and Testament or such Codicil. If said <u>CHILD FOUR</u> fails to exercise such power of appointment, or insofar as any such appointment shall be void or shall not take effect, then the Trustee shall distribute such share of The Remaining Trust Estate, in equal shares, to said <u>CHILD FOUR</u>'s children who are then living, treating as a then living child of said <u>CHILD FOUR</u> for this purpose the then living collective issue of any child of said <u>CHILD FOUR</u> who shall then be deceased, the distribution to such issue to be *per stirpes,* the root of the *per stirpes* distribution to be such deceased child.

5. In the event that one or more of the distributions provided for in Subparagraphs 1 through 4 of this Paragraph A cannot be made because there is no person then living entitled to take distribution thereunder, then such distribution shall be made to those then living persons entitled to take distribution under said Subparagraphs 1 through 4, in shares proportionate to the shares which such persons are entitled to receive under the provisions of said Subparagraphs 1 through 4.

B. If, at the time for distribution of any share or portion of the trust estate being held pursuant to this Article IV, there is no person or person's estate entitled under the provisions of this Article IV other than this Paragraph B to take such distribution, the Trustee shall distribute, free of the trust, such share or portion to such person or persons as would be entitled to inherit from said <u>PARENT'S NAME</u> and in the proportions they would so inherit under the laws of the State of _____ as though **[he/she]** had died intestate, not survived by a spouse and domiciled in the State of _____ at the time distribution is so to be made.

C. If the Trustee is authorized pursuant to the provisions of this Trust Agreement to make distributions or payments to or for the benefit of any person (including distributions or payments directed or permitted to be made to a person who is under legal disability or, in the reasonable opinion of the Trustee, is unable properly to administer such distributions or payments), the Trustee may make such distributions or payments in any one or more of the following ways, as the Trustee may deem advisable: (1) directly to such beneficiary, (2) to the legal guardian of such beneficiary or (3) to any Custodian then serving for such beneficiary or to any person designated by the Trustee to serve as a Custodian for such person (any such Custodian may be any one of the **[four (4)]** Trustees serving in their individual capacity). The Trustee shall not be required to see to the application of any distribution or payment so made, but the receipt of any of the persons mentioned in Clause (1), (2), or (3) in the immediately preceding sentence shall be a full discharge for the Trustee.

D. No interest whatsoever in the principal and/or income of any trust estate being administered under the provisions of this Article IV shall be alienated, disposed of, or in any manner assigned or encumbered by the person for whom held, voluntarily or involuntarily, while such principal and/or income is in the possession or control of the Trustee. If, by reason of any act of any such person or by operation of law, or by the happening of any event, or for any other reason except by an act of the Trustee specifically authorized hereunder, any such principal and/or income of The Remaining Trust Estate would but for this Paragraph D cease to be enjoyed by any such person or, by reason of an attempt by any such person to alienate, charge, assign or encumber any of such principal and/or income of The Remaining Trust Estate, or by reason of the bankruptcy or insolvency of any such person, or by reason of any attachment, garnishment or other proceeding, based upon a valid court judgment, or by reason of any order, finding or judgment of any court either at law or in equity, any of the principal and/or income of The Remaining Trust Estate would but for this Paragraph D vest in or be enjoyed by some individual, firm or corporation otherwise than as provided herein, then, in any of such events, the trust hereby created for the benefit of such person shall forthwith cease and determine as to such person, who shall thereupon cease to be a beneficiary under this Article IV, and such person shall be ineligible to serve or to continue to serve as Trustee hereunder. For purposes of this Paragraph D, the exercise of any power of appointment granted herein or the exercise of any disclaimer by a beneficiary of any rights or benefits under this Trust Agreement shall not cause or result in the provisions of this Paragraph D becoming applicable. Such trust thereafter, subject to all other applicable provisions of this Trust Agreement and of the trust of which such person was a beneficiary, shall during the life of such former beneficiary, be held by the Trustee which, until such former beneficiary's death, may pay to or expend for the benefit of such former beneficiary, out of the principal and/or income of such trust, such sums but such sums only as the Trustee in its absolute discretion may determine, and may also pay to or expend for the benefit of the spouse, child or children of such former beneficiary, out of the principal and/or income of such trust, such sums but such sums only as the Trustee in its absolute discretion may determine, retaining any undistributed principal and/or income until such former beneficiary's death; provided, however, that no payments made under these provisions to or for the benefit of such former beneficiary and any such former beneficiary's spouse, child or children shall exceed the amounts otherwise payable to such former beneficiary if these provisions had not been invoked. Any undistributed income shall from time to time be added to the principal of such trust. Upon the death of such former beneficiary, such trust as then constituted, including all accrued and undistributed income, shall, subject to all applicable provisions of this Trust Agreement and of the trust for the benefit of such former beneficiary, be distributed to the persons (determined as of the date of death of such former beneficiary) to whom such trust estate would have been so distributable as if such former beneficiary had died prior to the time for any mandatory distribution of the trust estate to such former beneficiary (or, if such former beneficiary would not have been entitled to any mandatory distribution of the trust estate during such former beneficiary's lifetime under the provisions of this Trust Agreement, then to the persons who would be entitled to take distribution upon such former beneficiary's death under the provisions of this Trust Agreement), and as if the provisions of this Paragraph D had never become applicable to the trust of such former beneficiary.

E. Any provisions of this Trust Agreement to the contrary notwithstanding, if not already distributed, all accrued and undistributed income and the entire principal of every trust estate then held hereunder shall be paid over and distributed outright and free of the trust not later than the end of the day immediately preceding the expiration of twenty-one (21) years from and after the death of the last to die of said PARENT'S NAME, said CHILD ONE, said CHILD TWO, said CHILD THREE, and said CHILD FOUR and their children and issue living at the date of death of the signing of this Trust Agreement. Such payment and distribution shall be made to the person or persons for whose benefit the trust estate or estates respectively shall then be held hereunder; provided, however, that if at such time the provisions of the immediately preceding Paragraph D of this Article IV shall be in operation as to any trust, such trust shall be distributed to those persons who would have been entitled to receive such trust as if the former beneficiary for whose benefit such trust was originally created had died immediately preceding the time so provided for such distribution and possessed of said trust estate, such distribution to be outright and free of the trust.

ARTICLE V

DEFINITIONS

A. The words "issue," "child" and "children," as used herein, shall be deemed to include any legally adopted person as if he or she were the natural child of the adopting parent, provided such adopted person was adopted prior to the age of majority.

B. Whenever the context so requires, the use of words herein in the singular shall be construed to include the plural, and the words in the plural, the singular, and words whether in the masculine, feminine or neuter gender shall be construed to include all of said genders.

C. For purposes of this Trust Agreement, any individual shall be deemed to be unable to continue to serve as Trustee hereunder only when:

(1) Such individual's attending physician and at least one other physician licensed in the United States (or, if such individual does not have an attending physician, at least two physicians licensed in the United States) (provided, however, that neither my nor such person's attending physician or any other physician acting hereunder shall be <u>PARENT'S NAME</u>, <u>CHILD ONE</u>, <u>CHILD TWO</u>, <u>CHILD THREE</u>, <u>CHILD FOUR</u> or a child, issue or spouse of such individuals) shall have signed and delivered to the Trustee then serving hereunder (or, if such Trustee is the person who is deemed to be unable to continue to serve as Trustee hereunder, then to any fiduciary serving hereunder or to the person who is to succeed such individual as Trustee) their written statements indicating that such individual is incapable in their judgment of attending effectively to such individual's fiduciary duties by reason of mental or physical disability; provided, that the written statements to which reference is made above shall be acknowledged before a notary public and witnessed by two individuals, one of whom may be the notary public; provided, further, that any person relying on any such written statements by such physicians may presume that the identity and qualifications of the physicians signing any such statement are in fact who and what they purport to be, and such person shall not have any duty to make further inquiry or investigation beyond the review of each written statement itself; provided, further, that no person relying on such written statement shall be liable to any other person or persons for action taken in reliance on such written statement; or

(2) Such person is adjudicated incompetent.

ARTICLE VI

POWERS AND DUTIES OF TRUSTEE

A. There shall be no duty on the Trustee to pay or see to the payment of any premiums on any policies of life insurance or to take any steps to keep them in force, until such time as the Trustee holds title to any insurance policies hereunder as a part of the corpus of any trust estate. The Trustee furthermore assumes no responsibility with respect to the validity or enforceability of said policies. However, as soon as practicable after receiving notice of the death of the insured under any of such policies, the Trustee shall proceed to collect all amounts payable thereunder. The Trustee shall have full and complete authority to collect and receive any and all such amounts and its receipt therefor shall be a full and complete acquittance to any insurer or payor, who shall be under no obligation to see to the proper application thereof by the Trustee.

B. In the administration of the trusts created hereunder and in addition to the powers exercised by trustees generally, the Trustee shall have the following powers and authorities without any court order or proceeding, exercisable in the discretion of the Trustee:

1. To purchase as an investment for the trust estate or estates any property, real or personal, belonging to our estates;

2. To retain as suitable investments for the trust estate or estates any properties received

by it from us and/or our estates, and whether received by purchase or in any other manner, without regard to any law, statutory or judicial, or any rule or practice of court now or hereafter in force specifying or limiting the permissible investments of trustees, trust companies or fiduciaries generally or requiring the diversification of investments, and without liability to any person whomsoever for loss or depreciation in value thereof;

3. To sell, exchange, convey, mortgage, pledge, lease, control, and manage, and to make contracts concerning, any of the properties, real or personal, comprised in the trust estate or estates, all either publicly or privately and for such considerations and upon such terms as to credit or otherwise as may be reasonable under the circumstances, which leases and contracts may extend beyond the duration of any of the trusts created hereunder; to give options therefor; and to execute deeds, transfers, mortgages, leases and other instruments of any kind;

4. To invest and reinvest the properties from time to time comprised in the trust estate or estates in stocks, common and/or preferred, bonds, notes, debentures, loans, mortgages, common trust funds, or other securities or property, real or personal, all limitations now or hereafter imposed by law, statutory or judicial, or by any rule or practice of court now or hereafter in force specifying or limiting the permissible investments of trustees, trust companies or fiduciaries generally or requiring the diversification of investments, being hereby expressly waived, it being the intent hereof that the Trustee shall have full power and authority to deal with the trust estate or estates in all respects as though it were the sole owner thereof, without order of court or other authority;

5. To borrow money, from itself or otherwise, with or without security, whenever it deems such action advisable;

6. To exercise voting rights, execute and deliver powers of attorney and proxies and similarly act with reference to shares of stock and other securities comprised in the trust estate or estates in such manner as it deems proper, including, without limitation, the power to participate in or oppose reorganizations, recapitalizations, mergers, consolidations, exchanges, liquidations, arrangements and other corporate actions;

7. To collect all money; in accordance with generally accepted trust accounting principles, to determine whether money or other property coming into its possession shall be treated as principal or income and to charge or apportion expenses, taxes, gains and losses to principal or income;

8. To compromise, adjust and settle claims in favor of or against the trust estate or estates upon such terms and conditions as it may deem best; in the case of any litigation in connection with any part of such trust estate or estates, it may, under advice of its counsel, arbitrate, settle, or adjust any such matter in dispute upon such terms as it may consider just and equitable, and its decision shall be binding upon the beneficiaries;

9. To employ investment counsel, custodians of estate property, brokers, accountants, attorneys, clerical or bookkeeping assistants, and other suitable agents and to pay their reasonable compensation and expenses in addition to any compensation payable to the Trustee, and to execute and deliver powers of attorney; to appoint and remove by written instrument, containing such terms and conditions as it may deem appropriate, any natural or legal person or persons as special Trustee to hold all or any part of any real property or other interest in property held in the trust estate or estates and which the Trustee determines, in its sole discretion, it cannot or, because of legal limitations on its powers, it deems inadvisable to hold as Trustee hereunder, and such special Trustee, except as specifically limited by the appointing instrument, shall have the powers, author-

ities and discretion under this Paragraph B granted to the Trustee with respect to the trust property held by such special Trustee; the Trustee shall not be liable for any neglect, omission or wrongdoing of such investment counsel, custodians, brokers, accountants, attorneys, assistants, agents or special Trustees, provided reasonable care shall have been exercised in their selection;

10. To hold title to stocks, bonds, or other securities or property, real or personal, in its own name or in the name of its nominee and without indication of any fiduciary capacity or to hold any such bonds or securities in bearer form; the Trustee shall assume full responsibility for the acts of any nominee selected by it;

11. To hold as a single fund or unit any part or all of the property comprising any two or more of the separate and distinct shares or portions of The Remaining Trust Estate and to allot undivided interests in such single fund or unit to such separate shares or portions in proportion to the interest of each therein, except that no such holding shall defer the vesting in possession of any estate;

12. To make all repairs, alterations or improvements of any real property which shall constitute a part of the trust estate or estates; adjust boundaries thereof, and to erect or demolish buildings thereon; and, with respect to such property, to convert for different use, grant easements for adequate consideration, partition, and insure for any or all risks;

13. To pay premiums on any policies of life insurance which may form a part of the trust estate or estates; to cancel, sell, assign, hypothecate, pledge or otherwise dispose of any of said policies; to exercise any right, election, option or privilege granted by any of said policies; to borrow any sums in accordance with the provisions of any of said policies, and to receive all payments, dividends, surrender values, additions, benefits or privileges of any kind which may accrue to any of said policies;

14. To make any allocation, division or distribution required or permitted hereunder in cash or in kind, in real or personal property, or an undivided interest therein, or partly in cash and partly in kind, and to do so without making pro rata allocations, divisions or distributions of specific assets, property allocated, divided or distributed in kind to be taken at its fair market value at the time of such allocation, division or distribution;

15. To receive, in accordance with the provisions of Article I hereof, additional property from us or any other person, the Trustee being authorized and empowered to merge and hold as one any duplicate trusts held for the same beneficiary; and

16. To make such expenditures and do such other acts as are reasonably required to manage, improve, protect, preserve, invest or sell any of the trust estates or otherwise properly to administer this Trust.

C. The Trustee shall keep accurate records showing all receipts and disbursements and other transactions involving the trust estate or estates and shall furnish annually to each beneficiary currently entitled to income (1) a statement of the receipts and disbursements affecting such beneficiary's interest in the trust and (2) a complete inventory of the trust estate then held for the benefit of such beneficiary.

D. No person, firm or corporation dealing with the Trustee or a nominee of the Trustee or performing any act pursuant to action taken or order given by the Trustee or such nominee shall be obliged to inquire as to the propriety, validity or legality thereof hereunder, nor shall any such person be liable for the application of any money or other consideration paid to the Trustee or such nominee, but, instead, may rely upon any action taken by the Trustee or such nominee pursuant to the powers and authorities conferred upon it under the provisions of this Article VI in all respects as if the same were completely unlimited. No transfer agent or registrar of any security held hereunder shall be required to inquire as to the propriety, validity or legality of any transfer made by the Trustee or such nominee.

E. Any successor Trustee shall have and enjoy all the powers, authorities, duties and immunities hereby vested in and imposed upon the original Trustee and no successor Trustee shall be obliged to inquire into or be in any way accountable for the previous administration of the trust property.

F. In determining the amount of any discretionary distributions of income or principal to a beneficiary of a trust created hereunder, the Trustee may take into account all means and resources known to or reasonably ascertainable by such Trustee which are available to such beneficiary for the purposes for which such Trustee is authorized to make said distributions.

G. The Trustee shall serve without compensation, although the Trustee shall be entitled to be reimbursed for any reasonable expenses it incurs which are necessary to carry out its duties as Trustee hereunder.

H. 1. In the event that any of said <u>CHILD ONE</u>, said <u>CHILD TWO</u>, said <u>CHILD THREE</u> or said <u>CHILD FOUR</u> shall become unwilling or unable to continue to serve as a Trustee hereunder, then such one or ones of said <u>CHILD ONE</u> said <u>CHILD TWO</u>, said <u>CHILD THREE</u> and said <u>CHILD FOUR</u> who shall be willing and able to continue to serve shall, upon **[their, his, or her]** formal written acceptances or acceptance, serve as Trustees or as sole Trustee hereunder.

2. Any Trustee shall be entitled to resign as Trustee for any reason whatsoever by giving written notice to the Trustee designated to succeed it (or if there is no Trustee then designated to succeed it, to the Trustee who is thereafter designated to succeed it), provided that the Trustee designated to succeed it shall first execute a formal written acceptance of the duties and obligations of the Trustee hereunder and file an executed copy of such acceptance with the preceding Trustee. After this is done, and when all sums then due from the trust estate to such predecessor Trustee have been paid, such predecessor Trustee shall transfer the Trust property then in its hands to such successor Trustee and such predecessor Trustee shall thereupon and thereby be discharged of all subsequent duties and obligations under or arising out of its Trusteeship.

I. The provisions of this Paragraph I shall not apply to the provisions of Subparagraph 1 of Paragraph A of Article III hereof. The provisions of this Paragraph I shall apply for purposes of all other provisions of this Trust Agreement.

1. When only one (1) Trustee is serving, such Trustee shall act alone. When two (2) Trustees are serving, no decision shall be made or proposed action taken by my Trustees except upon the concurrence of both of them. When more than two (2) Trustees are serving, no decision shall be made or proposed action taken by them except upon the concurrence of a majority of those serving. Any one (1) Trustee acting alone shall be authorized to take any action authorized hereunder and agreed to by my Trustees in accordance with the immediately preceding two (2) sentences.

2. Each co-Trustee hereunder shall be responsible solely for **[his or her]** own decisions and not for those of **[his or her]** co-Trustee or co-Trustees.

J. No bond shall be required of the Trustee hereunder or any successor Trustee.

ARTICLE VII

GOVERNING LAW

This Trust Agreement shall be construed under and in accordance with the laws of the State of _____.

IN WITNESS WHEREOF, we, as Settlors and as Trustees, have executed this Trust Agreement, in quintuplicate, at _____, _____, on the day and year first above written.

Signed in the presence of:

"Settlor"

"Settlor"

"Settlor"

"Settlor"

"Trustee"

"Trustee"

"Trustee"

"Trustee"

We, the undersigned legal spouses of the Settlors, hereby waive all community property, dower or courtesy rights which we may have in the hereinabove-described property and give our assent to the provisions of the trust and to the inclusion in it of the said property.

Witness: _____   Witness: _____

Witness: _____   Witness: _____

Witness: _____   Witness: _____

Witness: _____   Witness: _____

STATE OF _____   City
or
COUNTY OF _____   Town _____

     On the _____ day of _____, 19____, personally appeared _____, known to me to be the individual(s) who executed the foregoing instrument, and acknowledged the same to be **[his/her]** free act and deed, before me.

My commission expires: _____   _____
                                            Notary Public

SCHEDULE A

The following is a true and correct Schedule A of the property assigned, delivered and conveyed to _____, Trustee, to be held, treated and disposed of in accordance with the terms of a certain Irrevocable Trust Agreement between _____, as Settlors, and _____, the Trustees, dated _____ _____, 19____, to which Agreement this Schedule A is attached and made a part thereof.

_____
_____
_____
_____
_____
_____
_____
_____
_____
_____
_____
_____
_____
_____
_____
_____
_____
_____

Signed in the presence of:

_____   _____

_____   _____
                                          "Settlor"

_____   _____
                                          "Settlor"

_____   _____
                                          "Settlor"

_____   _____
                                          "Settlor"

_____   _____

_____   _____
                                            "Trustee"

_____   _____

_____   _____
                                            "Trustee"

_____   _____

_____   _____
                                            "Trustee"

_____   _____
                                            "Trustee"

        We, the undersigned legal spouses of the Settlors, hereby waive all community property, dower or courtesy rights which we may have in the hereinabove-described property and give our assent to the provisions of the trust and to the inclusion in it of the said property.

                                            _____

                                            _____

Witness: _____   Witness: _____

                                            _____

                                            _____

Witness: _____   Witness: _____

                                            _____

                                            _____

Witness: _____   Witness: _____

                                            _____

Witness: _____   Witness: _____

13

ADDITION OF PROPERTY TO DECLARATION OF TRUST

BY _____

    DATED _____ _____, 19____

WITH _____, TRUSTEES

_____ (the "Assignor"), pursuant to the terms of the above-described Declaration of Trust, does hereby assign, transfer and convey to _____, Trustee, and _____, Trustee, does hereby acknowledge receipt of, the following assets from the Assignor:

_____

_____

_____

_____

_____

_____

_____

_____

_____

_____

_____

_____

_____

_____

_____

_____

_____

_____

_____

_____

_____

_____

    The Trustee agrees to hold, manage and administer the above assets as a part of the trust estate created under such Declaration of Trust.

    At the request of the Trustee, the Assignor shall fully cooperate and execute any and all documents deemed necessary or desirable by it in order to cause the assignment made hereby to be properly recorded.

IN WITNESS WHEREOF, the Assignor and the Trustee have signed their names at
_____, _____, on this _____ day of _____, 19____.

Signed in the presence of:

_____   _____

_____   _____, Assignor

_____   _____

_____   _____, Trustee

_____   _____

_____   _____, Trustee

_____   _____

_____   _____, Trustee

_____   _____

_____   _____, Trustee

I, the undersigned legal spouse of the Assignor, hereby waive all community property, dower or courtesy rights which I may have in the hereinabove-described property and give my assent to the inclusion in the trust of said property.

_____

_____

Witness: _____   Witness: _____

STATE OF _____   City
                                          or
COUNTY OF _____   Town _____

On the _____ day of _____, 19____, personally
appeared _____, known to me to be the individual(s) who
executed the foregoing instrument, and acknowledged the same to be [**his/her**] free act and deed, before me.

_____
Notary Public

My commission expires:

_____

15

Irrevocable Trust Agreement

Explanation

As you can see, this irrevocable family asset protection trust agreement to be created by children of a Medicaid recipient or a potential future Medicaid recipient, is filled with legalese. Don't be scared off by this confusing language. The explanations that follow should provide you with a clear understanding of the terms.

Introduction: In the first blanks you would fill in the city and state of your residence, the day, month, and year in which the trust is to be executed, and the name, city, and state of each person who will be serving as trustee. Remember, neither the Medicaid recipient nor his or her spouse can be the trustee. Children or other close relatives will probably be the first choice for trustees.

Article I: This paragraph transfers into the trust all of the items listed on Schedule A at the end of the agreement. You can include on Schedule A just about any item imaginable, including real estate, personal property, savings and checking accounts, boats, cars, and even clothing.

If the property you put into the trust increases in value, the increased value is part of the trust. And if an asset changes form, the new asset remains in the trust. For example, if the trustee takes $5,000 from a bank account and buys $5,000 worth of stock, that stock remains in the trust. You and your spouse can always add to the trust by using the Addition to Trust form following Schedule A.

Article II: This section is very important. It provides that you may revoke or change the trust or withdraw assets at any time.

Article III: This section provides that as long as your father or mother is alive, any one of the trustees may use income or assets from the trust for your parent. For this purpose, and *only* this purpose, one trustee may act alone. Before distributions are made, the financial circumstances of your parent must be considered. They do not have any legal right to require distributions from the trust, because if they did, then the trust assets would count against their Medicaid eligibility.

Article IV: This section describes how your trust principal will be distributed after your parent dies.

Paragraph IV(A) provides that each child gets an equal share of the remaining trust principal. If a child has died, his or her will may "appoint" his or her share (state where the share should go and in what proportions), except that trust assets cannot be appointed to a creditor. If a child died before appointing his or her share under a will, then his or her share would go to his or her children; if the deceased child has no children, then his or her share would go to the deceased child's siblings.

Paragraph IV(B) provides for the distribution of the trust in the unlikely event that there's no one to receive the principal from your trust under the earlier provisions. In that case, the assets pass to your parent's next of kin under state law.

Part IV (C) discusses distributions to beneficiaries named in your trust who are under some legal disability or are unable to administer their distributions. If a distribution from your trust is to go to someone who is under a legal disability or unable to manage his or her money, the trustee has three options:

1. Pay the money to the beneficiary.
2. Make the distribution to a legal guardian of the beneficiary.
3. Distribute the beneficiary's portion to a custodian for the beneficiary.

If, when you make up your trust, you could predict the ages and physical and mental conditions of all of your beneficiaries at the time of your death, you could spell out which of these options you would want the trustee to pursue. But since you can't, this trust allows the trustee to choose which option he or she believes is best.

The last sentence of Part IV(C) says that once the trustee has made his or her choice and distributed a beneficiary's portion to the beneficiary or to the beneficiary's guardian or custodian, the trustee is off the hook; he or she doesn't have to monitor the use of the distribution after that.

Part IV (D), often called a spendthrift clause, provides that nobody but your intended beneficiary can obtain an interest in a distribution under your trust. For example, your child, who will receive a portion of your trust, can't sell his or her expected distribution in the future to someone for cash now. And a beneficiary can't put up his or her interest in a distribution as collateral for a loan. After all, you want the person you name in the trust to receive a distribution, not some stranger.

Spendthrift clauses like this are enforced in most, but not all, states. If you have a serious concern that a beneficiary has or may have creditor problems, consult with a local attorney to determine whether this clause will be effective in your state.

Trusts cannot legally tie up assets forever, so Part IV(E) is designed to avoid potential problems by limiting the life of the trust.

Article V: This is the definition section. The most important point here is to recognize that a legally adopted child will be considered a child for purposes of the trust agreement. So by leaving everything to your children, any adopted child would be treated the same as a natural child.

Article VI: This section deals with the powers and duties you are giving to the trustee.

Part VI(A) says that after your death, the trustee must collect the money due under any insurance policy. The trustee does not have a duty to pay your life insurance premiums until and unless the trustee takes title to any insurance policy.

Part VI(B) is very important, setting forth the powers of the trustee. As you can see, this trust agreement gives the trustee very broad powers to administer the funds and property in the estate, including the power to:

1. Buy real estate or personal property from your or your spouse's estate. Without this power, purchases by your trustee from your estate or your spouse's estate at death might not be allowed.
2. Keep in your trust anything received from you or your estate or your spouse or your spouse's estate.
3. Sell, exchange, mortgage, and do just about anything else with property in the trust.
4. Invest the assets in the trust in just about anything.
5. Borrow money for the trust.
6. Manage stock and other securities.
7. Collect money for the trust.

8. Handle claims and lawsuits for or against the trust.
9. Hire and pay counselors and assistants, like lawyers and accountants, for the trust.
10. Hold property in his or her own name, in the name of a nominee, or in bearer form.
11. Maintain one fund for different trust shares.
12. Manage real estate in the trust, including repairing, improving, or converting property.
13. Handle life insurance policies in the trust, including paying premiums, canceling or selling policies, cashing in policies, or borrowing against them.
14. Make distributions under the trust in cash or in property.
15. Receive additional property for the trust.
16. Do anything else reasonably required to manage, protect, or preserve the trust assets.

Why put in many specific powers instead of just having item 16, which generally allows the trustee to do anything reasonably necessary? Because with only a general statement, someone with whom the trustee must deal may question his or her power and may refuse to do business with him or her. For example, without specifically giving the trustee the power to sell real estate, buyers, lenders, and escrow agents may be hesitant to deal with him or her, even if your trust agreement generally gives him or her broad powers. By listing specific powers, you can ensure the trustee's ability to manage the trust properly.

Why give the trustee such broad powers anyway? Why not just specify a few actions he or she may take? The reason is simple: you can't predict what the trustee may need to do to manage the trust properly, and if you don't give him or her broad powers, you may hamper the trustee and damage your trust estate. For example, if you don't own any stocks, why give the trustee power to manage them? Because at some point it might be in your best interest for your trustee to purchase securities, and you don't want you trust agreement to prevent him or her from doing so.

Part VI(C) provides for certain payments from your trust upon your death. If the representative of your estate (such as the executor or administrator) decides that the funds left in your estate (not in your trust) are insufficient to pay your estate taxes, expenses of administration, or funeral expenses, he or she can require the trustee to cover those costs. The trustee does not have to get anything in return and your estate representative does not have to repay the money. Once the trustee has paid the representative of your estate, the trustee has no further obligation to monitor the use of these funds.

Part VI(D) is designed to encourage people to deal with the trustee by relieving them of liability in case the trustee takes some action beyond his or her power. For example, if the trustee attempts to sell stock, the buyer can go ahead with the transaction and pay the trustee without worrying about whether the trust really allows the trustee to make that deal.

Part VI(E) gives any successor trustee all of the same powers and duties as the original trustee. It also encourages your chosen successor trustee to accept the job by providing that he or she has no responsibility for anything done by the earlier trustee.

Part VI(F) concerns discretionary distributions by the trustee. Trustees may consider the financial status of any potential beneficiary.

Part VI(G) provides that the trustee will serve without compensation. Since the trustee will be family, that should be no problem.

Part VI(H) provides that if one of the children cannot or will not serve as trustee, the other(s) shall serve alone. For example, if you and your two siblings are serving as trustee and one sibling resigns, you and your one remaining sibling may continue to serve.

Part VI(I) discusses how the trustee may manage the trust. If a time comes when only one trustee is serving, that trustee may act alone. That trustee may not make distributions to anyone except your father or mother but may carry out the other terms of the trust. If two trustees are serving, decisions must be made together. If more than two are serving, decisions may be made by a majority. This does not mean that all trustees must sign every check. The trustees may authorize one person to administer the trust on a day-to-day basis.

Part VI(J) states that the trustee does not have to post a bond. A bond is like an insurance policy; it is designed to protect you trust in case the trustee does something wrong, such as steal assets. Depending on the amount in the trust, a bond could easily cost your trust several hundred dollars.

Article VII: Article VII states that any questions about the trust will be answered by the laws of the state of your primary residence. In the blank space you would fill in the name of your state.

Conclusion: The blanks in the final paragraph are for your city and state. Then each child who is creating the trust would sign where it says "Settlor" and each child who is serving as trustee would sign below that. Each person would print his or her name below the signature line. To the left of each signature, two witnesses to each signature must sign. The witnesses can be the same, but they don't have to be; if they are the same, they must sign twice, once for the settlor and once for the trustee. The witnesses cannot be members of your family.

Then each spouse would also sign, with two witnesses signing below. In many states your spouse has a legal interest in your property and must waive his or her rights in writing to the property covered by the trust.

The final section is for a notary public.

Schedule A: Following the end of the trust is Schedule A, on which you would list any items (cash accounts, real estate, personal property, and the like) to be placed under the control of the trustee. Identify each item as best as you can, using addresses, registration numbers, account numbers, and so forth, wherever possible, to avoid confusion.

On Schedule A you would fill in the names of all of your trustees in the first blank, all of the settlors in the second blank, and all of the trustees again in the third blank, then date the schedule.

At the bottom, each of the settlors, trustees, and spouses would sign before two independent witnesses.

Addition of Property Form: Finally, included is a form that can be used to add property to the trust later. At the top, you would fill in the names of the settlors, the date that the trust was originally made, and name of the trustee. In the first paragraph you would fill in the name of the assignor who is assigning property to the trustee. Then, on the lines that follow, you would list any items to be added to the trust. Again, identify each item as best you can. At the end, each of the settlors, trustees, and spouses would sign before two independent witnesses and a notary.

DECLARATION OF TRUST

THIS DECLARATION OF TRUST (hereinafter referred to as the "Trust Agreement") is made at _____, _____, this _____ day of _____, 199__, by _____, of _____, _____, who, depending on the context, is hereinafter sometimes referred to as the Settlor (hereinafter referred to in the first person), and sometimes as the Trustee (hereinafter referred to sometimes as the "Trustee" and sometimes in the third person impersonal).

ARTICLE I

CREATION OF TRUST

Concurrently herewith I have deposited with the Trustee the property listed in Schedule A of this Trust Agreement. The Trustee agrees to hold said property, the receipt of which is hereby acknowledged, for the purposes and on the terms and provisions hereinafter set forth, and agrees that it will similarly hold all other property (including, without limitation, insurance policies (or proceeds) on my or any other person's life) that may be added hereto (a) by me, during my lifetime (any such property added by me, during my lifetime, to be so added only with the consent of the Trustee, which consent shall not be withheld unreasonably), pursuant to the provisions of my Last Will and Testament or any Codicil thereto, or by any other manner, (b) by my **[husband/wife]**, _____, during **[his/her]** lifetime (any such property added by my said **[husband/wife]**, during **[his/her]** lifetime, to be so added only with the consent of the Trustee, which consent shall not be withheld unreasonably), pursuant to the provisions of **[his/her]** Last Will and Testament or any Codicil thereto, or by any other manner, and (c) by any other person, by inter vivos transfer, by last will and testament or codicil thereto, or by any other manner (any such property added by any such other person to be so added only with the consent of the Trustee, which consent shall not be withheld unreasonably). Any property added by me pursuant to the provisions of my Last Will and Testament or any Codicil thereto or by any other manner at or after my death, shall be held, administered and distributed in accordance with the applicable provisions of this Trust Agreement unless I shall expressly specify that a particular trust or part thereof hereinafter established shall be the recipient of such property, in which event such property so added by me shall be so held, administered and distributed. Any property added by my said **[husband/wife]** or any such other person during my lifetime shall be held, administered and distributed pursuant to the provisions of Article III hereof during my lifetime and thereafter in accordance with the other applicable provisions of this Trust Agreement. Any property added by my said **[husband/wife]** or any such other person after my death shall be held, administered and distributed pursuant to the provisions of the applicable provisions of this Trust Agreement unless my said **[husband/wife]** or such other person shall expressly specify that some other trust or part thereof hereinafter established shall be the recipient of such property, in which event such property so added by my said **[husband/wife]** or such other person shall be so held, administered and distributed.

ARTICLE II

RIGHTS RESERVED BY THE SETTLOR

A. I shall have the right, by written instrument signed by me and delivered to the Trustee during my lifetime, to terminate this Trust as to all or any part of the trust estate, to withdraw any assets at any time held hereunder and to change the Trustee hereunder.

B. This Trust Agreement may be amended or modified by an instrument in writing signed by me and the Trustee.

C. Except as otherwise provided in Paragraph D of Article III hereof, the rights reserved by me in the preceding Paragraphs A and B of this Article II are personal to me and shall not be exercisable by any other person or persons, including, without limitation, any guardians, conservators, or attorneys-in-fact.

ARTICLE III

DISTRIBUTIONS DURING LIFETIME OF SETTLOR

A. During my lifetime and prior to the time any additional property is added to this Trust pursuant to the provisions of Article I hereof, the Trustee shall accumulate and add to the principal the net income, if any, derived from the trust estate.

B. During my lifetime and subsequent to the time additional property is added to this Trust pursuant to the provisions of Article I hereof, the Trustee, except as otherwise provided in the first sentence of Paragraph C of this Article III, shall distribute to or for the benefit of myself and/or such persons, institutions, charitable purposes or otherwise, such amounts, from the income and principal of the trust estate, as I may from time to time direct the Trustee in writing.

C. If, during my lifetime, I shall be unable to make such directions because of incompetency, incapacity or otherwise, the Trustee shall distribute to or for the benefit of me and my **[husband/wife]**, _____, out of the net income or principal or both of the trust estate being held hereunder, such amount or amounts which shall be necessary to provide for our maintenance, support, health and education; provided, however, the Trustee shall not be authorized, in the exercise of the discretionary power conferred upon it under this Paragraph C, to distribute all of the principal of the trust estate and thereby cause the termination of this Trust, it being my intent that at all times at least Ten Dollars ($10.00) shall be held in this Trust. At the end of each taxable year the Trustee shall add any undistributed income to the principal of the trust estate being held hereunder; provided, however, that upon my death the Trustee shall pay to my estate all accrued and undistributed income to the date of my death. As I do not intend that any taxable gift be deemed made by reason of my becoming incompetent, incapacitated or otherwise unable to exercise the rights reserved by me in Article II hereof or to make the directions provided for in the last sentence of Paragraph B of this Article III, then, notwithstanding any other provisions of this Trust Agreement to the contrary, I shall at all times have the power to appoint to or for the benefit of any persons or entities any and all assets contained in the trust estate held under this Trust Agreement at the time of my death; provided, however, that in order for the exercise of said power of appointment to be effective, I must exercise such power by specific reference to this Trust Agreement in the provisions of my Last Will and Testament or any Codicil thereto. In the event that I fail to exercise such power of appointment, or insofar as any such appointment shall be void or shall not take effect, then upon my death all of the trust estate, or any part thereof not effectively appointed by me, shall be distributed in accordance with the applicable provisions of Article IV hereof.

D. In the event there shall be added to or held as a part of the trust estate any interest in any residential real property which is used by me and/or my said **[husband/wife]** from time to time as a residence, whether permanent or seasonal, including all improvements situated thereupon and all adjoining land used as a part thereof (such interest in any such residential property being hereinafter in this Trust Agreement referred to as the "Real Property"), the Trustee shall permit either of us to occupy the Real Property, and shall pay all expenses for the maintenance and ownership of the Real Property (including but not limited to mortgage payments of interest and principal on any loan secured by a mortgage on the Real Property, utilities, real estate taxes and assessments (both general and special), insurance (casualty and liability), repairs, condominium fees, maintenance, replacements and alterations) until (a) my death or (b) the Trustee determines that the Real Property is no longer a residence of either of ours (which determination shall be final and binding upon all interested parties), whichever event shall first occur, whereupon the Trustee shall hold the Real Property free of the conditions imposed hereunder, as a part of the trust estate held pursuant to this Article, with full power and authority to dispose of the same and hold the proceeds as a part of the trust estate; provided, however, that if I request the Trustee to sell the Real Property and to purchase another residence for us, the Trustee shall do so.

ARTICLE IV

ADMINISTRATION AND DISTRIBUTION OF TRUST ESTATE UPON SETTLOR'S DEATH

Upon my death, the Trustee shall hold, administer and distribute the property held hereunder, as the same shall be constituted after being (a) augmented by property received or to be received by the Trustee as a consequence of my death, including, without limitation, any property received or to be received under the terms of my Last Will and Testament or any Codicil thereto and (b) depleted by any funds disbursed by the Trustee pursuant to the provisions of Paragraph C of Article VI hereof (said property as so constituted being hereinafter in this Article IV referred to as the "Remaining Trust Estate") as follows:

A. Upon my death, the Trustee shall distribute the Remaining Trust Estate, in equal shares, to my children who survive me, treating as a surviving child of mine for this purpose the collective issue surviving me of any child of mine who shall have predeceased me, the distribution to such issue to be *per stirpes*, the root of the *per stirpes* distribution to be such predeceased child.

B. If, at the time for distribution of any share or portion of the Remaining Trust Estate being held pursuant to this Article IV, there is no person entitled under the provisions of this Article IV other than this Paragraph B to take such distribution, the Trustee shall divide the entire remaining trust estate into two (2) equal shares. One such share shall be distributed free of the trust to such person or persons as would be entitled to inherit from me and in the proportions they would so inherit under the laws of the State of _____ as though I had died intestate, not survived by a spouse and domiciled in the State of _____ at the time distribution is so to be made. The other such share shall be distributed free of the trust to such person or persons as would be entitled to inherit from my said **[husband/wife]** and in the proportions they would so inherit under the laws of the State of _____ as though **[he/she]** had died intestate, not survived by a spouse and domiciled in the State of _____ at the time distribution is so to be made.

C. If the Trustee is authorized or directed pursuant to the provisions of this Trust Agreement to make distributions or payments of the Remaining Trust Estate to any person (including distributions or payments to be made to a person who is under legal disability or, in the reasonable opinion of the Trustee, is unable properly to administer such distributions or payments), then the Trustee may make such distributions or payments from the Remaining Trust Estate in any one or more of the following ways, as the Trustee may deem advisable: (1) directly to such beneficiary; (2) to the legal guardian of such beneficiary or (3) to a Custodian then serving for such beneficiary or to a person designated by the Trustee to serve as a Custodian for such beneficiary (any such Custodian or person may be the Trustee). The Trustee shall not be required to see to the application of any distribution or payment so made, but the receipt of any of the persons mentioned in Clause (1), (2), or (3) in the immediately preceding sentence shall be a full discharge for the Trustee.

D. No interest whatsoever in the principal and/or income of any trust estate subject to the provisions of this Article IV shall be alienated, disposed of, or in any manner assigned or encumbered by the person for whom held, voluntarily or involuntarily, while such principal and/or income is in the possession or control of the Trustee. For purposes of this Paragraph D, the exercise of any disclaimer by a beneficiary of any rights or benefits under this Trust Agreement shall not cause or result in the provisions of this Paragraph D becoming applicable.

E. Any provisions of this Trust Agreement to the contrary notwithstanding, if not already distributed, all accrued and undistributed income and the entire principal of every trust estate then held hereunder shall be paid over and distributed outright and free of the trust not later than the end of the day immediately preceding the expiration of twenty-one (21) years from and after the death of the last survivor of my children and my children's issue living at the time of my death. Such payment and distribution shall be made to the person or persons for whose benefit the trust estate or estates respectively shall then be held.

ARTICLE V

DEFINITIONS AND MISCELLANEOUS

A. The words "issue," "child," "children," "grandchild" and "grandchildren," as used herein, shall be deemed to include any legally adopted person as if he or she were the natural child of the adopting parent, provided such adopted person was adopted prior to the age of majority.

B. Whenever the context so requires, the use of words herein in the singular shall be construed to include the plural, and words in the plural, the singular, and words whether in the masculine, feminine or neuter gender shall be construed to include all of said genders.

C. For purposes of this Trust Agreement, (1) I shall be deemed to be unable to direct the Trustee with respect to distributions from the principal of the trust estate for purposes of Paragraph B of Article III hereof and (2) any individual shall be deemed to be unable to continue to serve as Trustee hereunder only when:

(1) My or such individual's attending physician and at least one other physician licensed in the United States (or, if I do not have or such individual does not have an attending physician, at least two physicians licensed in the United States) (provided, however, that neither my nor such person's attending physician or any other physician acting hereunder shall be my **[husband/wife]**, a child or issue of mine, or a spouse of such child or issue) shall have signed and delivered to the Trustee then serving hereunder (or, if such Trustee is the person who is deemed to be unable to continue to serve as Trustee hereunder, then to any fiduciary serving hereunder or to the person who is to succeed such individual as Trustee) their written statements indicating that I am not capable in their judgment of directing effectively the Trustee on my own behalf by reason of mental or physical disability or that such individual is incapable in their judgment of attending effectively to such individual's fiduciary duties by reason of mental or physical disability; provided, that the written statements to which reference is made above shall be acknowledged before a notary public and witnessed by two individuals, one of whom may be the notary public; provided, further, that any person relying on any such written statements by such physicians may presume that the identity and qualifications of the physicians signing any such statement are in fact who and what they purport to be, and such person shall not have any duty to make further inquiry or investigation beyond the review of each written statement itself; provided, further, that no person relying on such written statement shall be liable to any other person or persons for action taken in reliance on such written statement; or

(2) I am or such individual is adjudicated incompetent.

ARTICLE VI

POWERS AND DUTIES OF THE TRUSTEE

A. There shall be no duty on the Trustee to pay or see to the payment of any premiums on any policies of life insurance or to take any steps to keep them in force, until such time as the Trustee holds title to any insurance policies hereunder as a part of the corpus of any trust estate. The Trustee furthermore assumes no responsibility with respect to the validity or enforceability of said policies. However, as soon as practicable after receiving notice of the death of the insured under any of such policies, the Trustee shall proceed to collect all amounts payable thereunder. The Trustee shall have full and complete authority to collect and receive any and all such amounts and its receipt therefor shall be a full and complete acquittance to any insurer or payor, who shall be under no obligation to see to the proper application thereof by the Trustee.

B. In the administration of the trusts created hereunder and in addition to the powers exercised by trustees generally, the Trustee shall have the following powers and authorities without any court order or proceeding, exercisable in the discretion of the Trustee:

1. To purchase as an investment for the trust estate or estates any property, real or personal, belonging to my estate and/or the estate of my **[husband/wife]**, _____ ;

2. To retain as suitable investments for the trust estate or estates any properties received by it from me, my said **[husband/wife]**, my estate and/or the estate of my said **[husband/wife]**, and whether received by purchase or in any other manner, without regard to any law, statutory or judicial, or any rule or practice of court now or hereafter in force specifying or limiting the permissible investments of trustees, trust companies or fiduciaries generally or requiring the diversification of investments, and without liability to any person whomsoever for loss or depreciation in value thereof;

3. To sell, exchange, convey, mortgage, pledge, lease, control, and manage, and to make contracts concerning, any of the properties, real or personal, comprised in the trust estate or estates, all either publicly or privately and for such considerations and upon such terms as to credit or otherwise as may be reasonable under the circumstances, which leases and contracts may extend beyond the duration of any of the trusts created hereunder; to give options therefor; and to execute deeds, transfers, mortgages, leases and other instruments of any kind;

4. To invest and reinvest the properties from time to time comprised in the trust estate or estates in stocks, common and/or preferred, bonds, notes, debentures, loans, mortgages, common trust funds, or other securities or property, real or personal, all limitations now or hereafter imposed by law, statutory or judicial, or by any rule or practice of court now or hereafter in force specifying or limiting the permissible investments of trustees, trust companies or fiduciaries generally or requiring the diversification of investments, being hereby expressly waived, it being the intent hereof that the Trustee shall have full power and authority to deal with the trust estate or estates in all respects as though it were the sole owner thereof, without order of court or other authority;

5. To borrow money, from itself or otherwise, with or without security, whenever it deems such action advisable;

6. To exercise voting rights, execute and deliver powers of attorney and proxies and sim-

ilarly act with reference to shares of stock and other securities comprised in the trust estate or estates in such manner as it deems proper, including, without limitation, the power to participate in or oppose reorganizations, recapitalizations, mergers, consolidations, exchanges, liquidations, arrangements and other corporate actions;

7. To collect all money; in accordance with generally accepted trust accounting principles, to determine whether money or other property coming into its possession shall be treated as principal or income and to charge or apportion expenses, taxes, gains and losses to principal or income;

8. To compromise, adjust and settle claims in favor of or against the trust estate or estates upon such terms and conditions as it may deem best; in the case of any litigation in connection with any part of such trust estate or estates, it may, under advice of its counsel, arbitrate, settle, or adjust any such matter in dispute upon such terms as it may consider just and equitable, and its decision shall be binding upon the beneficiaries;

9. To employ investment counsel, custodians of estate property, brokers, accountants, attorneys, clerical or bookkeeping assistants, and other suitable agents and to pay their reasonable compensation and expenses in addition to any compensation payable to the Trustee, and to execute and deliver powers of attorney; to appoint and remove by written instrument, containing such terms and conditions as it may deem appropriate, any natural or legal person or persons as special Trustee to hold all or any part of any real property or other interest in property held in the trust estate or estates and which the Trustee determines, in its sole discretion, it cannot or, because of legal limitations on its powers, it deems inadvisable to hold as Trustee hereunder, and such special Trustee, except as specifically limited by the appointing instrument, shall have the powers, authorities and discretion under this Paragraph B granted to the Trustee with respect to the trust property held by such special Trustee; the Trustee shall not be liable for any neglect, omission or wrongdoing of such investment counsel, custodians, brokers, accountants, attorneys, assistants, agents or special Trustees, provided reasonable care shall have been exercised in their selection;

10. To hold title to stocks, bonds, or other securities or property, real or personal, in its own name or in the name of its nominee and without indication of any fiduciary capacity or to hold any such bonds or securities in bearer form; the Trustee shall assume full responsibility for the acts of any nominee selected by it;

11. To hold as a single fund or unit any part or all of the property comprising any two or more of the separate and distinct shares or portions of the Remaining Trust Estate and to allot undivided interests in such single fund or unit to such separate shares or portions in proportion to the interest of each therein, except that no such holding shall defer the vesting in possession of any estate;

12. To make all repairs, alterations or improvements of any real property which shall constitute a part of the trust estate or estates; adjust boundaries thereof, and to erect or demolish buildings thereon; and, with respect to such property, to convert for different use, grant easements for adequate consideration, partition, and insure for any or all risks;

13. To pay premiums on any policies of life insurance which may form a part of the trust estate or estates; to cancel, sell, assign, hypothecate, pledge or otherwise dispose of any of said policies; to exercise any right, election, option or privilege granted by any of said policies; to borrow any sums in accordance with the provisions of any of said

policies, and to receive all payments, dividends, surrender values, additions, benefits or privileges of any kind which may accrue to any of said policies;

14. To make any allocation, division or distribution required or permitted hereunder in cash or in kind, in real or personal property, or an undivided interest therein, or partly in cash and partly in kind, and to do so without making pro rata allocations, divisions or distributions of specific assets, property allocated, divided or distributed in kind to be taken at its fair market value at the time of such allocation, division or distribution;

15. To receive, in accordance with the provisions of Article I hereof, additional property from me or any other person, the Trustee being authorized and empowered to merge and hold as one any duplicate trusts held for the same beneficiary; and

16. To make such expenditures and do such other acts as are reasonably required to manage, improve, protect, preserve, invest or sell any of the trust estates or otherwise properly to administer this Trust.

C. 1. Subject to the limitations set forth in the last sentence of this Subparagraph 1 and the next following Subparagraph 2 of this Paragraph C, if the representative of my estate, in such representative's sole discretion, shall determine that sufficient or appropriate assets of my estate are not available in sufficient amount (or if there are no assets in my estate) to pay my legal debts, my funeral expenses, the expenses of my last illness, the expenses of administration of my estate, all death taxes chargeable to my estate, including interest and penalties thereon, and all bequests under my Will, other than a residuary bequest, the Trustee shall, upon the request of the representative of my estate, contribute from the principal of the trust estate the amount of such deficiency; and in connection with any such action the Trustee shall rely upon the written statement of the representative of my estate as to the validity and correctness of the amounts of any such legal debts, expenses, taxes and bequests, and shall furnish funds to such representative so as to enable such representative to discharge the same, or to discharge any part or all thereof itself by making payment directly to the governmental official or agency or to the person entitled or claiming to be entitled to receive payment thereof. If the Trustee hereunder holds any property that is bequeathed under my Will (other than a residuary bequest), then the Trustee to the extent that such property is held under this Trust Agreement shall distribute such property to the persons entitled to receive such bequest under my Will (other than a residuary bequest) after the deduction, if any, of expenses and taxes to be charged to such bequest pursuant to the provisions of my Will. No consideration need be required by the Trustee from the representative of my estate for any disbursement made by the Trustee pursuant hereto, nor shall there be any obligation upon such representative to repay to the Trustee any of the funds disbursed by it hereunder, and all amounts disbursed by the Trustee pursuant to the authority hereby conferred upon it shall be disbursed without any right in or duty upon the Trustee to seek or obtain contribution or reimbursement from any person or property on account of such payment. The Trustee shall not be responsible for the application of any funds delivered by it to the representative of my estate pursuant to the authority herein granted, nor shall the Trustee be subject to liability to any beneficiary hereunder on account of any payment made by it pursuant to the provisions hereof.

2. Any provisions of this Article VI to the contrary notwithstanding, under no circumstances shall the Trustee make any disbursements pursuant to this Paragraph C from (a) assets which are excluded from my gross estate for purposes of the Federal estate tax payable by reason of my death or (b) assets which are not subject to a state inheritance, state estate or other state death tax imposed by reason of my death; provided, however, that assets described in Clause (b) of this sentence (so long as they do not constitute assets described in Clause (a) of this sentence) may be used to the extent that other assets which are included in my gross estate for purposes of the Federal estate tax payable by reason of my death and subject to a state inheritance, state estate or other state death tax imposed by reason of my death shall be insufficient to satisfy the Trustee's obligation hereunder.

D. The Trustee shall keep accurate records showing all receipts and disbursements and other transactions involving the trust estate or estates and shall furnish annually to each income beneficiary of the trust estate (1) a statement of the receipts and disbursements affecting such beneficiary's interest in the trust estate and (2) a complete inventory of the trust estate then held for the benefit of such beneficiary.

E. No person, firm or corporation dealing with the Trustee or a nominee of the Trustee or performing any act pursuant to action taken or order given by the Trustee or such nominee shall be obliged to inquire as to the propriety, validity or legality thereof hereunder, nor shall any such person be liable for the application of any money or other consideration paid to the Trustee or such nominee, but, instead, may rely upon any action taken by the Trustee or such nominee pursuant to the powers and authorities conferred upon it under the provisions of this Article VI in all respects as if the same were completely unlimited. No transfer agent or registrar of any security held hereunder shall be required to inquire as to the propriety, validity or legality of any transfer made by the Trustee or such nominee.

F. Any successor Trustee shall have and enjoy all the powers, authorities, duties and immunities hereby vested in and imposed upon the original Trustee and no successor Trustee shall be obliged to inquire into or be in any way accountable for the previous administration of the trust property.

G. My Trustee is authorized, in its sole discretion, to sell to, purchase from, borrow funds from, lend funds to, or otherwise deal with, upon such terms and conditions as my Trustee shall deem just and equitable and for full and adequate consideration, the Executor of the Last Will and Testament of myself or my said [husband/wife] or the Trustee of any Trust established by me or my said [husband/wife] (whether such Trust is a testamentary or inter vivos trust), even though my Trustee may also be serving as Executor under my Will or my said [husband's/wife's] Will or as Trustee under any such Trust established by me or by my said [husband/wife].

H. In determining the amount of any discretionary distributions of income or principal to a beneficiary of a trust created hereunder, the Trustee shall take into account all other means and resources known to or reasonably ascertainable by the Trustee which are available to such beneficiary for the purposes for which the Trustee is authorized to make said distributions.

I. The Trustee shall not receive any compensation for its services hereunder, however, the Trustee shall be entitled to be reimbursed for any reasonable expenses it incurs which are necessary to carry out its duties as Trustee hereunder.

J. 1. At such time as I shall become unwilling or unable to continue to serve as Trustee hereunder, then my _____, _____, of _____, _____, upon [his/her] formal written acceptance, shall serve as Trustee hereunder. In the event that my said _____ shall not survive me or shall be unwilling or unable to serve or to continue to serve as Trustee hereunder, then my _____, _____, of _____, _____, upon [his/her] formal written acceptance, shall serve as Trustee hereunder. In the event that both my said _____ and my said _____ shall not survive me or shall be unwilling or unable to serve or to continue to serve as Trustee hereunder, then my _____, _____, of _____, _____, upon [his/her] formal written acceptance, shall serve as Trustee hereunder. In the event that my said _____, my said _____ and my said _____ shall not survive me or shall be unwilling or unable to serve or to continue to serve as Trustee hereunder, then my _____, _____, of _____, _____, upon [his/her] formal written acceptance, shall serve as Trustee hereunder.

2. Any Trustee shall be entitled to resign as Trustee for any reason whatsoever by giving written notice to the Trustee designated to succeed it, provided that such successor Trustee shall first execute a formal written acceptance of the duties and obligations of the Trustee hereunder and file an executed copy of such acceptance with the preceding Trustee. After this is done, and when all sums then due from the trust estate to such predecessor Trustee have been paid, such predecessor Trustee shall transfer the Trust property then in its hands to such successor Trustee and such predecessor Trustee shall thereupon and thereby be discharged of all subsequent duties and obligations under or arising out of its trusteeship.

K. No bond shall be required of the Trustee hereunder or any successor Trustee.

L. Any provisions of this Trust Agreement or otherwise to the contrary notwithstanding, the Trustee shall make no discretionary distribution pursuant to the provisions of this Trust Agreement from the trust estate being held hereunder for the benefit of any beneficiary, the effect of which would be to discharge or satisfy a legal support obligation or other legal obligation of the Trustee in the Trustee's individual capacity. For purposes of this Paragraph L, no Trustee shall be deemed to have any legal obligation to support himself or herself.

ARTICLE VII

GOVERNING LAW

This Trust Agreement shall be construed under and in accordance with the laws of the State of _____.

IN WITNESS WHEREOF, I have hereunto set my hand, as Settlor and as Trustee, at _____, _____, **on the day and year first above written.**

Signed in the presence of:

_____   _____

_____   _____
                                                                    "Settlor"

_____   _____

_____   _____
                                                                    "Trustee"

I, the undersigned legal spouse of the Settlor, hereby waive all community property, dower or courtesy rights which I may have in the hereinabove-described property and give my assent to the provisions of the trust and to the inclusion in it of the said property.

                                   _____

                                   _____

Witness: _____   Witness: _____

STATE OF _____   City
                                    or
COUNTY OF _____   Town _____

On the _____ day of _____, 19___, personally appeared _____, known to me to be the individual(s) who executed the foregoing instrument, and acknowledged the same to be **[his/her]** free act and deed, before me.

My commission expires: _____   _____
                                                   Notary Public

SCHEDULE A

The following is a true and correct Schedule A of the property assigned, delivered and conveyed to _____, Trustee, to be held, treated and disposed of in accordance with the terms of a certain Declaration of Trust by _____, as Settlor and Trustee, dated _____, 19____, to which Agreement this Schedule A is attached and made a part hereof.

_____
_____
_____
_____
_____
_____
_____
_____
_____
_____
_____
_____
_____
_____
_____
_____
_____
_____
_____

Signed in the presence of:

_____   _____

_____   _____
                                                                          "Settlor"

_____   _____

_____   _____
                                                                          "Trustee"

    I, the undersigned legal spouse of the Settlor, hereby waive all community property, dower or courtesy rights with I may have in the hereinabove-described property and give my assent to the provisions of the trust and to the inclusion in it of the said property.

                                      _____

                                      _____

Witness: _____   Witness: _____

_____   _____

ADDITION OF PROPERTY TO DECLARATION OF TRUST

BY _____

DATED _____ _____, 19____

WITH_____, TRUSTEE

_____ (the "Assignor"), pursuant to the terms of the above-described Declaration of Trust, does hereby assign, transfer and convey to _____, Trustee, and _____, Trustee, does hereby acknowledge receipt of, the following assets from the Assignor:

_____
_____
_____
_____
_____
_____
_____
_____
_____
_____
_____
_____
_____
_____
_____
_____
_____
_____
_____

The Trustee agrees to hold, manage and administer the above assets as a part of the trust estate created under such Declaration of Trust.

At the request of the Trustee, the Assignor shall fully cooperate and execute any and all documents deemed necessary or desirable by it in order to cause the assignment made hereby to be properly recorded.

IN WITNESS WHEREOF, the Assignor and the Trustee have signed their names at _____, _____, on this _____ day of _____, 19____,

Signed in the presence of:

_____   _____

_____   _____, Assignor

_____   _____

_____   _____, Trustee

I, the undersigned legal spouse of the Assignor, hereby waive all community property,. dower or courtesy rights which I may have in the hereinabove-described property and give my assent to the inclusion in the trust of the said property.

_____

_____

Witness: _____   Witness: _____

STATE OF _____   City
                                      or
COUNTY OF _____   Town _____

On the _____ day of _____, 19___, personally appeared _____, known to me to be the individual(s) who executed the foregoing instrument, and acknowledged the same to be **[his/her]** free act and deed, before me.

_____
Notary Public

My commission expires:

_____

Declaration of Trust

Explanation

As you can see, this revocable living declaration of trust agreement is filled with legalese. Don't be scared off by the confusing language. The explanations that follow should provide you with a clear understanding of the terms.

Introduction: In the first blanks you would fill in your city and state and the day, month, and year in which the trust is to be executed, then your name and the city and state of your residence. This trust, unlike the others in the appendixes, is set up for you to serve as your own trustee, so you can stay in control for as long as possible.

Article I: This paragraph transfers into the trust all of the items listed on Schedule A at the end of the trust. You can include on Schedule A just about any item imaginable, including real estate, personal property, savings and checking accounts, boats, cars, and even clothing.

If the property you put into the trust increases in value, the increased value is part of the trust. And if an asset changes form, the new asset remains in the trust. For example, if the trustee takes $5,000 from a bank account and buys $5,000 worth of stock, the stock remains in the trust. You and your spouse can always add to the trust by using the Addition to Trust form following Schedule A.

Article II: This section is very important. It provides that you may revoke or change the trust or withdraw assets at any time.

Article III: This section requires the trustee to distribute income and principal from the trust to anyone you designate. There may come a time when you step down as trustee, but this provision still allows you to dictate distributions. If at some time you become unable to serve as trustee and to direct the distributions, then Part C requires the trustee to distribute any assets needed by you and/or your spouse. Part D gives you and your spouse the right to live in your home (if in the trust) until your death or until neither of you is living in the home any longer. House-related expenses should be paid by the trustee from the trust.

Article IV: This section describes how your trust principal, less any of your estate taxes, estate administration costs, or funeral expenses, as provided in Article VI(C), will be distributed after you die.

Paragraph IV(A) provides that after you die, the balance of your trust principal will be distributed equally to your children. If any of your children has died before you, that child's portion goes to that child's children.

Paragraph IV(B) provides for the distribution of the trust if there's no one to receive the principal from your trust under Paragraph IV(A). If you die leaving no living children or grandchildren, Paragraph IV(B) takes over.

Under IV(B), the remaining principal of the trust would be divided into two parts. One part would go to those persons who would inherit from you under the laws of your state as if you had died without a will or a trust. Every state has a law that dictates to whom an estate of someone who dies without a will is to be distributed—usually it is the closest living relative(s) of the deceased. For example, if you die without children or grandchildren, Paragraph IV(B) may mean that your parent or brother collects part of the trust estate. The other half of the trust estate will be distributed to those persons who would inherit from your deceased spouse under the laws of your state as if he or she had died without a will.

The estate is split into two parts so that relatives on both sides of your family are treated equally. For example, rather than having everything go to your cousin, half may go to your cousin and half to your deceased spouse's sister.

The blanks in Paragraph IV(B) are for the names of your state and your spouse (if any).

Part IV(C) discusses distributions, after you die, to beneficiaries named in your trust who are under some legal disability or are unable to administer their distributions. For example, if your child is senile or suffering from Alzheimer's disease, he or she may be under a legal disability or unable to manage his or her money. Or if a distribution under your trust is to go to a young child (perhaps the children of a deceased child of yours), Part IV(C) may come into play.

If a distribution from your trust is to go to someone who is under a legal disability or unable to manage their money, the trustee has three options:

1. Pay the money to the beneficiary.
2. Make the distribution to a legal guardian of the beneficiary.
3. Distribute the beneficiary's portion to a custodian for the beneficiary.

If, when you make up your trust, you could predict the ages and physical and mental conditions of all of your beneficiaries at the time of your death, you could spell out which of these three options you would want the trustee to pursue. But since you can't, this trust allows the trustee to choose which option he or she believes is best.

The last sentence of Part IV(C) says that once the trustee has made his or her choice and distributed a beneficiary's portion to the beneficiary or to the beneficiary's guardian or custodian, the trustee is off the hook; he or she doesn't have to monitor the use of the distribution after that.

Part IV(D), often called a spendthrift clause, provides that nobody but your intended beneficiary can obtain an interest in a distribution under your trust. For example, your child, who will receive a portion of your trust after you're gone, can't sell his or her expected distribution in the future to someone for cash now. And a beneficiary can't put up his or her interest in a distribution as collateral for a loan. After all, you want the person you name in the trust to receive a distribution, not some stranger.

Spendthrift clauses like this are enforced in most, but not all, states. If you have a serious concern that a beneficiary has or may have creditor problems, consult with a local attorney to determine whether this clause will be effective in your state.

Trusts cannot legally tie up assets forever, so Part IV(E) is designed to avoid potential problems by limiting the life of the trust.

Article V: This is the definition section. The most important point here is to recognize that a legally adopted child will be considered a child for purposes of the trust agreement. So by leaving everything to your children equally after you die, any adopted child would be treated the same as a natural child.

Article VI: This section deals with the powers and duties you are giving to the trustee, who will be you initially but someone else eventually.

Part VI(A) says that after your death, the trustee

must collect the money due under any insurance policy on your life. The trustee does not have a duty to pay your life insurance premiums during your lifetime until and unless the trustee takes title to any insurance policy.

Part VI(B) is very important, setting forth the powers of the trustee. As you can see, this trust agreement gives the trustee very broad powers to administer the funds and property in the estate, including the power to:

1. Buy real estate or personal property from your or your spouse's estate. Without this power, purchases by your trustee from your estate or your spouse's estate at death might not be allowed.
2. Keep in your trust anything received from you or your estate or your spouse or your spouse's estate.
3. Sell, exchange, mortgage, and do just about anything else with property in the trust.
4. Invest the assets in the trust in just about anything.
5. Borrow money for the trust.
6. Manage stock and other securities.
7. Collect money for the trust.
8. Handle claims and lawsuits for or against the trust.
9. Hire and pay counselors and assistants, like lawyers and accountants, for the trust.
10. Hold property in his or her own name, in the name of a nominee, or in bearer form.
11. Maintain one fund for different trust shares.
12. Manage real estate in the trust, including repairing, improving, or converting property.
13. Handle life insurance policies in the trust, including paying premiums, canceling or selling policies, cashing in policies, or borrowing against them.
14. Make distributions under the trust in cash or in property.
15. Receive additional property for the trust.
16. Do anything else reasonably required to manage, protect, or preserve the trust assets.

Why put in many specific powers instead of just having item 16, which generally allows the trustee to do anything reasonably necessary? Because with only a general statement, someone with whom the trustee must deal may question his or her power and may refuse to do business with him or her. For example, without specifically giving the trustee the power to sell real estate, buyers, lenders, and escrow agents may be hesitant to deal with the trustee, even if your trust agreement generally gives him or her broad powers. By listing specific powers, you can ensure the trustee's ability to manage the trust properly.

Why give the trustee such broad powers anyway? Why not just specify a few actions he or she may take? The reason is simple: you can't predict what the trustee may need to do to manage your estate properly, and if you don't give him or her broad powers, you may hamper him or her and damage your trust estate. For example, if you don't own any stocks, why give the trustee power to manage them? Because at some point it might be in your best interest for your trustee to purchase securities, and you don't want your trust agreement to prevent him or her from doing so.

Part VI(C) provides for certain payments from your trust upon your death. If the representative of your estate (such as the executor or administrator) decides that the funds left in your estate (not in your trust) are insufficient to pay your estate taxes, expenses of administration, or funeral expenses, he or she can require the trustee to cover those costs. The trustee does not have to get anything in return and your estate representative does not have to repay the money. Once the trustee has paid the representative of your estate, the trustee has no further obligation to monitor the use of these funds.

Part VI(D) requires the trustee to keep accurate records showing all transactions in the trust. Every year the trustee must give to certain beneficiaries a statement listing the trust transactions for the year and a current inventory of assets in the trust. Not every possible future beneficiary of the trust gets this report. For example, if the trust agreement provides income to you for your lifetime, and then on your death the assets will be distributed to your children or their children, only you are entitled to the trustee's report.

Part VI(E) is designed to encourage people to deal with the trustee by relieving them of liability in case the trustee takes some action beyond his or her power. For example, if the trustee attempts to sell a house, the buyer can go ahead with the transaction and pay the trustee without worrying about whether the trust really allows the trustee to make that deal.

Part VI(F) gives any successor trustee all of the same powers and duties as the original trustee. It also encourages your chosen successor trustee to accept the job by providing that he or she has no responsibility for anything done by the earlier trustee.

Part VI(G) authorizes the trustee to engage in transactions with the executor of your or your spouse's estate or any trustee of any other trust established by you or your spouse. Without this language, a conflict-of-interest issue could arise over these types of dealings.

Part VI(H) concerns discretionary distributions by the trustee. The trustee shall consider the financial status of any potential beneficiary before making discretionary distributions.

In Part VI(I) you are providing that the trustee will serve without compensation. Since the trustee (after you) will probably be your child or someone else close to you, that should be agreeable. Other possible trustees, such as a bank, will want to be paid.

Part VI(J) allows you to name alternative trustees. In the first blank, you would fill in the relationship, name, and address of your first choice. In the next blanks, you would do the same for your next choices.

Part VI(K) states that the trustee does not have to post a bond. A bond is like an insurance policy; it is designed to protect your trust in case the trustee does something wrong, such as steal assets. Depending on the amount in the trust, the bond could easily cost your trust several hundred dollars. If you've followed the tips in this book and selected the right trustee, you shouldn't need a bond.

Part VI(L) is a protection for the trustee to avoid the remote possibility of having the trust property included in the trustee's estate, causing adverse tax consequences.

Article VII: Article VII states that any questions about the trust will be answered by the laws of the state of your primary residence. In the blank space you would fill in the name of your state.

Conclusion: The blanks in the final paragraph are for your city and state. Then you would sign where it says "Settlor" and again where it says "Trustee," then print your name below the signature lines. To the left of your signatures, two witnesses to each signature would sign. The witnesses can be the same, but they don't have to be; if they are the same, they must sign twice, once for the settlor and once for the trustee. The witnesses cannot be members of your family.

Your spouse would also have to sign with two witnesses signing below. In many states your spouse has a legal interest in your property and must waive his or her rights in writing to the property covered by the trust.

The final section is for a notary public.

Schedule A: Following the end of the trust is Schedule A, on which you would list any items (cash accounts, real estate, personal property, and the like) to be placed under the control of the trustee. Identify each item as best as you can, using addresses, registration numbers, account numbers, and other information wherever possible, to avoid confusion.

On Schedule A you would fill in your name as trustee in the first blank and your name as settlor and trustee again in the second blank, then date the schedule.

At the bottom, you and your spouse would sign before two independent witnesses.

Addition of Property Form: Finally, included is a form that you can use to add property to the trust later. At the top, you would fill in your name, the date that the trust was originally made, and the name of the trustee. Then you would fill in your name as the assignor, the one assigning property to the trustee. On the lines that follow, you would list any items to be added to the trust. Again, identify each item as best you can. At the end, you would sign both as assignor and trustee, and then your spouse would sign, before two independent witnesses and a notary.

Notes

PROLOGUE

1. Walter and Ruth Griffith, of Noorhfield, Ohio, letter to Ohio governor George Voinovich, copy to Armond Budish, dated February 16, 1993.

2. John and Jane Surdock, of Grafton, Ohio, letter to Ohio governor George Voinovich, copy to Armond Budish, dated February 10, 1993.

3. Jim Baechle, of Brook Park, Ohio, letter to Ohio governor George Voinovich, copy to Armond Budish, dated February 13, 1993.

4. Mrs. R. J. McCarthy, of Sagamore Hills, Ohio, letter to Ohio governor George Voinovich, copy to Armond Budish, dated February 22, 1993.

5. Isabel Kennedy, of Cleveland, Ohio, letter to Ohio governor George Voinovich, copy to Armond Budish, dated April 27, 1992.

INTRODUCTION

1. Statement of Congressman Claude M. Pepper, "Catastrophic Health Insurance: Filling the Long-Term Care Gap," Hearing before the Subcommittee on Health and Long-Term Care, Select Committee on Aging, July 2, 1987 (hereafter "July 2 Hearing"), p. 5.

2. Eleanore Csontos, of Macedonia, Ohio, letter to Ohio governor George Voinovich, copy to Armond Budish, dated February 11, 1993.

3. Statement of Jack Ossofsky, "Paying the Price of Catastrophic Illness: From Accidents to Alzheimer's," Hearing before the Subcommittee on Health and Long-Term Care, House Select Committee on Aging, January 28, 1987, p. 29.

4. Alfred Pflaum, letter to Armond Budish, dated February 9, 1993.

5. Statement of Grace Still, "Catastrophic Health Insurance: The Pennsylvania Perspective," Hearing before the Subcommittee on Health and Long-Term Care, Select Committee on Aging, April 10, 1987 (hereafter "April 10 Hearing"), pp. 13–14.

6. Statement of Nathan Mendelsohn, April 10 Hearing, pp. 12–13.

7. Linda O'Donnell, R. N., letter to Armond Budish, undated.

8. Eleanor Melzak, letter to Ohio governor George Voinovich, copy to Armond Budish, dated February 9, 1993.

9. Linda Ellis, letter to Ohio governor George Voinovich, copy to Armond Budish, dated February 7, 1993.

10. H. E. Gallagher, letter to Armond Budish, dated February 10, 1993.

11. Statement of Congressman Robert A. Borski, April 10 Hearing, p. 3.

12. Raymond J. Hanley and Joshua M. Weiner, "A Non-problem: Scheming Oldsters Bilking Medicaid," *The Philadelphia Inquirer,* May 11, 1992, p. A11.

13. Walter and Ruth Griffith, of Noorhfield, Ohio, letter to Ohio governor George Voinovich, copy to Armond Budish, dated February 16, 1993.

14. Charles Morelli, letter to Armond Budish, dated February 9, 1993.

15. Sue Hildebrand, letter to Ohio governor George Voinovich, copy to Armond Budish, dated May 5, 1992.

16. Mrs. Mildred Stith, letter to Ohio governor George Voinovich, copy to Armond Budish, dated February 12, 1993.

17. Shirley Hazle, letter to Ohio governor George Voinovich, copy to Armond Budish, dated March 15, 1993.

18. Michael Gilfix and Peter J. Strauss, "New Age Estate Planning: The Emergence of Elder Law," *Trusts and Estates,* April 1988.

19. Ibid.

20. Statement of Congressman Claude M. Pepper, July 2 Hearing, p. 4.

21. Federal Affairs Health Team, AARP, "The Omnibus Budget Reconciliation Act of 1993 (OBRA 1993), Analysis of Medicare and Medicaid Cuts," August 11, 1993.

22. Statement of Esther Peterson in article by Ken Franckling, United Press International, December 7, 1987.

23. Statement of Senator John Heinz in article by Margaret Scherf, Associated Press, September 21, 1984.

CHAPTER 1

1. Figures are from the U.S. Department of Health and Human Services, set forth in "Long Term Care and Personal Impoverishment: Seven in Ten Elderly Living Alone Are at Risk," reported presented by the chairman of the House Select Committee on Aging, One Hundredth Congress, First Session, October 1987, p. 5.

2. Christopher Murtaugh, Peter Kemper, and Brenda Spillman, "The Risk of Nursing-Home Use," report presented at the American Public Health Association, November 1988; see also P. Kemper and C. Murtaugh, "Lifetime Use of Nursing-Home Care," *New England Journal of Medicine* 324, no. 9, February 28, 1991, p. 595.

3. Esther Peterson, *Choice Time: Thinking Ahead on Long Term Care,* prepared by Aetna Life Insurance and Annuity Company, n.d., p. 3.

4. Cynthia M. Taeuber, *Sixty-five Plus in America,* U.S. Department of Commerce, Economics and Statistics Administration, Bureau of the Census, August 1992, p. v, 2-1–2-18, 3-11–3-15, 3-17–3-19, 6-8–6-13.

5. Statement of Congresswoman Mary Rose Oakar, Hearing before the Subcommittee on Health and Long-Term Care, House Select Committee on Aging, July 2, 1987 (hereafter "July 2 Hearing"), p. 16.

6. Statement of Congressman Edward R. Roybal, news release of the House Select Committee on Aging, November 9, 1987.

7. Mrs. Bellamy, of Knoxville, Tennessee, letter presented in Statement of William A. Lessard, July 2 Hearing, p. 84.

8. Testimony of Dr. Samuel L. Baily, Hearing before the Sub-

committee on Health and Long-Term Care, House Select Committee on Aging, January 28, 1987, p. 136.

9. "Long Term Care and Personal Impoverishment," pp. 9, 15.

CHAPTER 2

1. Statement of Congressman Borski, Hearing before the Subcommittee on Health and Long-Term Care, House Select Committee on Aging, April 10, 1987, p. 15 (hereafter "April 10 Hearing").

2. Anne McGrath, "The Financial Agony of Long-Term Illness," *U.S. News and World Report,* February 9, 1987; Esther Peterson, *Choice Time: Thinking Ahead on Long Term Care,* prepared by Aetna Life Insurance and Annuity Company, n.d., p. 3.

3. Statement of Jack J. Lomas, April 10 Hearing, p. 10.

4. Statement of Congressman Borski, April 10 Hearing, p. 3.

5. Statement of Congressman Pepper, April 10 Hearing, p. 8.

6. Statement of Gail Shearer, Hearing before the Subcommittee on Health and Long-Term Care, House Select Committee on Aging, January 28, 1987, pp. 53, 57.

7. From Statement of William A. Lessard, Hearing before the Subcommittee on Health and Long-Term Care, House Select Committee on Aging, July 2, 1987, p. 84.

8. "Long Term Care and Personal Impoverishment: Seven in Ten Elderly Living Alone Are at Risk," report presented by the chairman of the House Select Committee on Aging, One Hundredth Congress, First Session, October 1987, p. 3.

CHAPTER 6

1. Statement of Congressman Claude M. Pepper, "Paying the Price of Catastrophic Illness: From Accidents to Alzheimer's," Hearing before the Subcommittee on Health and Long-Term Care, House Select Committee on Aging, January 28, 1987, pp. 1–2.

CHAPTER 7

1. Beverly Newton, "What, Me Pay for Nursing Home Costs?" videotape produced by Thomas & Partners Company, Westport, Conn., 1992.

2. Ludvik Roch, "What Me Pay?"

CHAPTER 11

1. Pauline Thoma, "What, Me Pay for Nursing Home Costs?" videotape produced by Thomas & Partners Company, Westport, Conn., 1992.

2. Norman Dacey, *How to Avoid Probate!* (New York: Crown, 1983), p. 15.

3. AARP, *A Report on Probate: Consumer Perspectives and Concerns* (Washington, D.C.: AARP, 1990).

CHAPTER 15

1. Judge Jeffrey H. Gallet, *In re Rose Septuagenarian*, 126 Misc. 2d 699, Family Court, Queens County.

CHAPTER 16

1. Families USA Foundation, "Nursing Home Insurance: Who Can Afford It?" (Washington, D.C.: Families USA Foundation, 1993), p. 10.

2. D. Spence and J. Wiener, "Nursing Home Length of Stay Patterns: Results from the 1985 National Nursing Home Survey," *Gerontologist* 30 (February 1990).

3. Families USA Foundation, "Nursing Home Insurance," p. 10.

CHAPTER 18

1. Federal Affairs Health Team, AARP, "The Omnibus Budget Reconciliation Act of 1993 (OBRA 1993), Analysis of Medicare and Medicaid Cuts," August 11, 1993, pp. 12–13.

Index